Office Procedures in Urology

Editor

J. STEPHEN JONES

UROLOGIC CLINICS OF NORTH AMERICA

www.urologic.theclinics.com

Consulting Editor

SAMIR S. TANEJA

November 2013 • Volume 40 • Number 4

ELSEVIER

1600 John F. Kennedy Boulevard • Suite 1800 • Philadelphia, Pennsylvania, 19103-2899

http://www.theclinics.com

UROLOGIC CLINICS OF NORTH AMERICA Volume 40, Number 4
November 2013 ISSN 0094-0143, ISBN-13: 978-0-323-24239-4

Editor: Kerry Holland
Developmental Editor: Susan Showalter

Urologic Clinics of North America (ISSN 0094-0143) is published quarterly by Elsevier Inc., 360 Park Avenue South, New York, NY 10010-1710. Months of issue are February, May, August, and November. Business and Editorial Offices: 1600 John F. Kennedy Blvd., Suite 1800, Philadelphia, PA 19103-2899. Periodicals postage paid at New York, NY and additional mailing offices. Subscription prices are $339.00 per year (US individuals), $583.00 per year (US institutions), $396.00 per year (Canadian individuals), $713.00 per year (Canadian institutions), $492.00 per year (foreign individuals), and $713.00 per year (foreign institutions). Foreign air speed delivery is included in all *Clinics* subscription prices. All prices are subject to change without notice. **POSTMASTER:** Send address changes to *Urologic Clinics of North America*, Elsevier Health Sciences Division, Subscription Customer Service, 3251 Riverport Lane, Maryland Heights, MO 63043. Customer Service: 1-800-654-2452 (US). From outside the United States, call 1-314-447-8871. Fax: 1-314-447-8029. E-mail: JournalsCustomerServiceusa@elsevier.com (for print support) and JournalsOnlineSupport-usa@elsevier.com (for online support).

Reprints. For copies of 100 or more, of articles in this publication, please contact the Commercial Reprints Department, Elsevier Inc., 360 Park Avenue South, New York, New York 10010-1710. Tel.: 212-633-3874; Fax: 212-633-3820; E-mail: reprints@elsevier.com.

Urologic Clinics of North America is covered in MEDLINE/PubMed (*Index Medicus*), *Excerpta Medica, Current Contents/Clinical Medicine, Science Citation Index,* and *ISI/BIOMED*.

Printed and bound by CPI Group (UK) Ltd, Croydon, CR0 4YY

Transferred to digital print 2012

PROGRAM OBJECTIVE
The goal of Urologic Clinics of North America is to keep practicing urologists and urology residents up to date with current clinical practice in urology by providing timely articles reviewing the state of the art in patient care.

TARGET AUDIENCE
Practicing urologists, urology residents and other health care professionals practicing in the discipline of urology.

LEARNING OBJECTIVES
Upon completion of this activity, participants will be able to:
- Review office-based management of impotence and Peyronie's disease and non-muscle invasive bladder cancer.
- Discuss infusion therapy and implantables for the Urologist.
- List coding for office procedures.

ACCREDITATION
The Elsevier Office of Continuing Medical Education (EOCME) is accredited by the Accreditation Council for Continuing Medical Education (ACCME) to provide continuing medical education for physicians.

The EOCME designates this enduringmaterial for a maximum of 15 *AMA PRA Category 1 Credit*(s)™. Physicians should claim only the credit commensurate with the extent of their participation in the activity.

All other health care professionals requesting continuing education credit for this enduring material will be issued a certificate of participation.

DISCLOSURE OF CONFLICTS OF INTEREST
The EOCME assesses conflict of interest with its instructors, faculty, planners, and other individuals who are in a position to control the content of CME activities. All relevant conflicts of interest that are identified are thoroughly vetted by EOCME for fair balance, scientific objectivity, and patient care recommendations. EOCME is committed to providing its learners with CME activities that promote improvements or quality in healthcare and not a specific proprietary business or a commercial interest.

The planning committee, staff, authors and editors listed below have identified no financial relationships or relationships to products or devices they or their spouse/life partner have with commercial interest related to the content of this CME activity:
Raymond Borkowski, MD; Quentin Clemens, MD, FACS, MSCI; Raoul S. Concepcion, MD, FACS; Nicole Congleton; Shubha De, MD; Ursula Galway, MD; Larry Hakim, MD; Harry Herr, MD; Kerry Holland; Brynne Hunter; Mohamed Ismail, MD; Ravi Kacker, MD; Kiranpreet K. Khurana; Zachary Klaassen, MD; Peter N. Kolettis, MD; Indu Kumari; Sandy Lavery; Aaron Lay, MD; Sara M. Lenherr, MD; Joshua J. Meeks, MD, PhD; Jill McNair; Diane K. Newman, DNP, FAAN, BCB-PMD; Jennifer Rothschild, MD; Matthew Rogers; Edmund Sabanegh Jr, MD; Ashley H. Tapscott, DO; Martha K. Terris; Yvette Williams.

The planning committee, staff, authors and editors listed below have identified financial relationships or relationships to products or devices they or their spouse/life partner have with commercial interest related to the content of this CME activity:
Anurag Das, MD, FACS has stock ownership in Amgen, Astellas, Johnson and Johnson, Novartis, Novo Nordisk, and Sanofi-Aventis.
Robert Dowling, MD is a consultant for Healthtronics IT Solutions and is employed by Dowling Medical Director Services LLC.
Leonard Gomella, MD is a consultant/advisor for Astellas, Bayer, Dendreon, Ferring and Photocure; has research grants from Astellas and Dendreon.
J. Stephen Jones, MD is a consultant for Healthronics and Cook; has a research grant from Photocure.
Bodo Knudsenis a consultant/advisor for Boston Scientifc and Olympus Surgical.
Manoj Monga, MD, FACS is a consultant/advisor for Bard, Olympus, Cook, Fortec, Coloplast, and Histosonics.
Mark Painter has stock ownership and an employment affiliation in Physician Reimbursement System.
Neal D. Shore, MD, FACS is a consultant/advisor for and has research grants with Amgen, Bayer, Janssen, Dendreon, Astellas, Sanofi, and Ferring.
Samir S. Taneja, MD is on Speakers Bureau for Janssen, and is a consultant/advisor for Elgen, GTX, Bayer and Healthtronics.
Ian M. Thompson III, MD is the owner of Urology Job Search, LLC.
Alan J. Wein, MD, PhD is a consultant/advisor for Merck, Allergan, Medtronic, FerringPharmaceuticals, Pfizer, and Astellas.

UNAPPROVED/OFF-LABEL USE DISCLOSURE
The EOCME requires CME faculty to disclose to the participants:
1. When products or procedures being discussed are off-label, unlabelled, experimental, and/or investigational (not US Food and Drug Administration (FDA) approved); and
2. Any limitations on the information presented, such as data that are preliminary or that represent ongoing research, interim analyses, and/or unsupported opinions. Faculty may discuss information about pharmaceutical agents that is outside of FDA-approved labelling. This information is intended solely for CME and is not intended to promote off-label use of these medications. If you have any questions, contact the medical affairs department of the manufacturer for the most recent prescribing information.

TO ENROLL

To enroll in the *Urologic Clinics of North America* Continuing Medical Education program, call customer service at 1-800-654-2452 or sign up online at http://www.theclinics.com/home/cme. The CME program is available to subscribers for an additional annual fee of $243 USD.

METHOD OF PARTICIPATION

In order to claim credit, participants must complete the following:
1. Complete enrolment as indicated above.
2. Read the activity.
3. Complete the CME Test and Evaluation. Participants must achieve a score of 70% on the test. All CME Tests and Evaluations must be completed online.

CME INQUIRIES/SPECIAL NEEDS

For all CME inquiries or special needs, please contact elsevierCME@elsevier.com.

Contributors

CONSULTING EDITOR

SAMIR S. TANEJA, MD
The James M. Neissa and Janet Riha Neissa
Professor of Urologic Oncology, Professor of
Urology and Radiology, Director, Division of
Urologic Oncology, Department of Urology,
Co-Director, Smilow Comprehensive Prostate
Cancer Center, NYU Langone Medical Center,
New York, New York

EDITOR

J. STEPHEN JONES, MD, FACS, MBA
Chief of Surgical Operations, Professor and
Miller/Horvitz Chair in Urological Oncology,
Cleveland Clinic Regional Hospitals,
Cleveland, Ohio

AUTHORS

RAYMOND BORKOWSKI, MD
Staff Anesthesiologist, Department of
Anesthesiology, Cleveland Clinic, Cleveland,
Ohio

J. QUENTIN CLEMENS, MD, MSCI
Department of Urology, University of Michigan,
Ann Arbor, Michigan

RAOUL S. CONCEPCION, MD, FACS
Director of Clinical Research, Urology
Associates, Nashville, Tennessee

ANURAG DAS, MD, FACS
Division of Urology, Beth Israel Deaconess
Medical Center, Harvard Medical School,
Boston, Massachusetts

SHUBHA DE, MD
Endourology Fellow, Cleveland Clinic,
Cleveland, Ohio

ROBERT A. DOWLING, MD
Dowling Medical Director Services LLC,
Fort Worth, Texas

URSULA GALWAY, MD
Staff Anesthesiologist, Department of
Anesthesiology, Associate Professor,
Cleveland Clinic Lerner College of Medicine
of Case Western Reserve, Cleveland Clinic,
Cleveland, Ohio

LEONARD G. GOMELLA, MD, FACS
The Bernard W. Godwin Professor of Prostate
Cancer, Chairman, Department of Urology,
Associate Director, Jefferson Kimmel Cancer
Center, Thomas Jefferson University,
Philadelphia, Pennsylvania

LAWRENCE S. HAKIM, MD
Chairman, Department of Urology, Cleveland
Clinic Florida, Weston, Florida

HARRY W. HERR, MD
Attending Physician, Department of Surgery,
Urology Service, Sidney Kimmel Center for
Prostate and Urologic Cancers, Memorial
Sloan-Kettering, New York, New York

MOHAMED T. ISMAIL, MD
Chief, Department of Urology, VA Medical
Center, Wilmington, Delaware; Assistant
Professor, Department of Urology, Thomas
Jefferson University, Philadelphia, Pennsylvania

RAVI KACKER, MD
Division of Urology, Beth Israel Deaconess
Medical Center, Harvard Medical School,
Boston, Massachusetts

KIRANPREET K. KHURANA, MD
Urology Resident, Department of Urology,
Glickman Urologic & Kidney Institute,
Cleveland Clinic, Cleveland, Ohio

ZACHARY KLAASSEN, MD
Department of Surgery, Section of Urology,
Medical College of Georgia-Georgia Regents
University; Resident, Department of Surgery,
Section of Urology, Charlie Norwood Veterans
Affairs Medical Center, Augusta, Georgia

BODO KNUDSEN, MD, FRCS(C)
Assistant Professor and Vice-Chair,
Department of Urology, Ohio State University,
Columbus, Ohio

PETER N. KOLETTIS, MD
Professor, Department of Urology, University
of Alabama at Birmingham, Birmingham,
Alabama

AARON LAY, MD
Division of Urology, Beth Israel Deaconess
Medical Center, Harvard Medical School,
Boston, Massachusetts

SARA M. LENHERR, MD
Department of Urology, University of Michigan,
Ann Arbor, Michigan

JOSHUA J. MEEKS, MD, PhD
Assistant Professor, Department of Urology,
Northwestern University, Feinberg School of
Medicine, Chicago, Illinois

MANOJ MONGA, MD, FACS
Director, Stevan Streem Center for
Endourology & Stone Disease, Cleveland
Clinic, Cleveland, Ohio

DIANE K. NEWMAN, DNP, ANP-BC, FAAN
Adjunct Associate Professor of Urology in
Surgery, Research Investigator Senior,

Perelman School of Medicine, University of
Pennsylvania; Co-Director, Penn Center for
Continence and Pelvic Health; Division of
Urology, Penn Medicine, Philadelphia,
Pennsylvania

MARK PAINTER
PRS Network, Thornton, Colorado

MATTHEW D. ROGERS, MD
Resident, Department of Urology, University of
Alabama at Birmingham, Birmingham,
Alabama

JENNIFER ROTHSCHILD, MD, MPH
Assistant Professor, Department of Urology,
University of California at Davis Medical
Center, Sacramento, California

EDMUND S. SABANEGH Jr, MD
Chair, Department of Urology, Glickman
Urologic & Kidney Institute, Cleveland Clinic,
Cleveland, Ohio

NEAL D. SHORE, MD, FACS
Director, CPI, Carolina Urologic Research
Center, Myrtle Beach, South Carolina

ASHLEY H. TAPSCOTT, DO
Fellow, Department of Urology, Cleveland
Clinic Florida, Weston, Florida

MARTHA K. TERRIS, MD
Department of Surgery, Section of Urology,
Medical College of Georgia-Georgia Regents
University, Witherington Chair of Urology,
Residency Program Director; Department of
Surgery, Section of Urology, Charlie Norwood
Veterans Affairs Medical Center; Co-Director,
Multidisciplinary Genitourinary/Prostate Team,
Georgia Regents University Cancer Center,
Augusta, Georgia

IAN M. THOMPSON III, MD
Assistant Professor, Department of Urology,
University of Texas Health Science Center at
San Antonio, San Antonio, Texas

ALAN J. WEIN, MD, PhD (Hon), FACS
Founders Professor & Chief of Urology,
Director, Urology Residency Program, Penn
Medicine, Perelman School of Medicine,
University of Pennsylvania Health System,
Philadelphia, Pennsylvania

Contents

Mohamed T. Ismail and Leonard G. Gomella

Grayscale transrectal ultrasonographic prostate biopsy using local anesthesia remains the standard approach to the definitive diagnosis of prostate cancer. Careful patient evaluation and preparation are essential to maximize the results and minimize the complications of the biopsy procedure.

Joshua J. Meeks and Harry W. Herr

Bladder cancer is extremely common in the United States and extremely costly because of the high cost of surveillance. In some patients, office-based surveillance may be a safe, cost-reducing alternative. This article attempts to identify ideal candidates and highlights surveillance strategies that can be employed in an office-based setting.

Shubha De, Manoj Monga, and Bodo Knudsen

As hospital resources are becoming strained, ambulatory surgical centers and day hospitals are being increasingly utilized. For the urologist, a working knowledge of local anesthetics and conscious sedation protocols are important, as many surgical kidney-stone procedures can be performed without general anesthetic. With any anesthesia, the key goal is to maximize patient comfort while minimizing respiratory depression and avoiding prolonged sedation. When using these medications, a working knowledge of emergency reversal, ventilation (bag mask/laryngeal mask airway/intubation), and cardiopulmonary resuscitation is recommended.

Ursula Galway and Raymond Borkowski

This article describes office-based surgery and office-based anesthesia (OBA), including the safe setup of OBA and safety concerns regarding OBA. Also discussed are the preoperative selection and workup of a patient undergoing OBA, anesthetic options, the prevention and treatment of postoperative nausea, vomiting, and pain, and planning for safe discharge.

Erectile dysfunction (ED) impacts more than 50% of men older than 40 years; Peyronie disease (PD) affects up to 10% of men, with an adverse impact on normal sexual function and overall well-being. ED can also be the first sign of other underlying disease. The office-based evaluation of ED and PD is the first step in the management of these devastating conditions of men's health. New and exciting nonsurgical therapies are now available to help treat these conditions and restore sexual function and quality of life.

The purpose of this article is to update urologists on contemporary indications and techniques for adult urodynamic testing. The discussion includes examples of specific clinical questions and appropriate urodynamic testing techniques to address these questions. It includes quality control measures and examples of testing pitfalls with troubleshooting methods.

This article is intended to familiarize the surgeon with all aspects of vasectomy including preoperative counseling, anesthetic techniques, surgical techniques, postoperative follow-up, and postvasectomy semen analysis. The latest literature regarding the complication rates and failure rates of various vas occlusion techniques is also discussed.

This article describes sperm retrieval procedures that may be performed in an office setting. Indications for sperm retrieval, preprocedural preparation, and anesthetic considerations are discussed. Vasal sperm aspiration, percutaneous epididymal sperm aspiration, microsurgical epididymal sperm aspiration, testicular sperm aspiration, conventional, and microdissection testicular sperm extraction are reviewed. Success and complication rates as well as factors that may influence success (histopathology, cancerous cause, Klinefelter syndrome, Y microdeletions, varicocele, and hormone administration) are reviewed.

Overactive bladder (OAB) is commonly encountered in urologic practice. Treatment algorithms begin with conservative therapy and pharmacotherapy with antimuscarinics. Some patients do not receive adequate relief from these methods or they do not tolerate side effects from pharmacotherapy. A test stimulation for sacral neuromodulation and percutaneous tibial nerve stimulation are office-based techniques that are commonly used as the next step in the algorithm of care in patients with OAB. These techniques are efficacious and approved by the Food and Drug Administration for treatment of overactive bladder and its associated symptoms.

UROLOGIC CLINICS OF NORTH AMERICA

NOW AVAILABLE FOR YOUR iPhone and iPad

Foreword
The Contemporary Ambulatory Urologic Practice

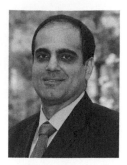

Samir S. Taneja, MD
Consulting Editor

The vast majority of contemporary urologic practice is carried out in the ambulatory setting, including urologic surgery. From a financial perspective, much of the income of the average urologist arises from his/her office practice, and, indeed, the need for urologists, now and in the future, may be largely in the office setting. While the implications of this observation on future urologic training continue to be debated, there is no doubt that for current urologic trainees, more time should be invested in learning the management of urologic disease in the outpatient setting. At present, most urologic residencies are focused on the operating room, and most trainees primarily seek operative training.

Because time in the operating room is not well-reimbursed, and because it takes away time from the office, urologists have found ways to bring many of the simpler urologic surgical services back to the office or ambulatory setting, thereby improving efficiency and time management and providing more convenient care for the patient.

In this issue of the *Urologic Clinics* I have asked Dr Stephen Jones of the Cleveland Clinic Foundation to assemble up-to-date articles on the spectrum of contemporary ambulatory urologic practice. Not only is Dr Jones renowned as a urologic surgeon, but he has a wealth of experience in oversight of clinical practice, ambulatory care, and office efficiency. I have asked him to provide perspective, not only on the urologic issues surrounding disease management in the ambulatory setting but also on the practical issues of office efficiency, billing and coding, quality control, and safety. As urologists push the envelope of what can be done in the ambulatory setting, these aspects will be critical.

I am deeply indebted to Dr Jones and the outstanding authors he has invited to contribute to this issue. Each of the articles provides a very unique perspective that I feel will be incredibly informative to the reader. For those starting in practice, much of the content will not likely have been provided in training, and for those already experienced in ambulatory care, I am confident the pearls included will enhance their clinical practice in many ways.

Samir S. Taneja, MD
Division of Urologic Oncology
Smilow Comprehensive Prostate Cancer Center
Department of Urology
NYU Langone Medical Center
150 East 32nd Street, Suite 200
New York, NY 10016, USA

E-mail address:
samir.taneja@nyumc.org

Urol Clin N Am 40 (2013) xi
http://dx.doi.org/10.1016/j.ucl.2013.09.002
0094-0143/13/$ – see front matter © 2013 Elsevier Inc. All rights reserved.

Preface
Urologic Office Procedures

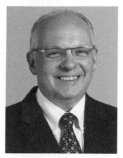

J. Stephen Jones, MD, FACS, MBA
Editor

Throughout the quarter century of my career, change has been in the fabric of medical life. Nevertheless, the monumental transformation we now face could not have been envisioned even a decade ago. We have seen an inexorable shift from inpatient to outpatient care, and nowhere is that more intense than in surgery.

As a resident, we automatically hospitalized prostatectomy patients for 5 days regardless of their clinical status. In my early practice one patient objected to staying for a second postoperative night because he "felt fine" during afternoon rounds. The charge nurse and I looked at each other, each trying to get the other to come up with a good reason for him to remain hospitalized. Neither of us could, so I discharged him and was immediately scorned by older colleagues for the seemingly haphazard decision. Twenty years later, half of my radical retropubic prostatectomy patients as well as many of our robotic prostatectomy patients go home on that timetable, and rarely, even on the evening of surgery. Innumerable patients have been put at lower risk of hospital acquired conditions and unnecessary costs as a result of this trend across all surgical specialties.

With the shift to outpatient surgery comes its natural partner—a shift of more and more procedures into the office setting—the subject of this edition of *Urologic Clinics*. Beyond the obvious financial benefits are a multitude of other advantages. Care is more likely to be delivered closer to the patient's home, and in a more comfortable and usually less intimidating setting than a traditional operating room. Safety and quality should never be sacrificed, but the office setting incurs less excessive regulatory oversight and complexity. If systemic medications or anesthetics are foregone, patients avoid potential side effects and additional costs. They can also drive themselves to and from the procedure appointment, so neither they nor a driver must take off a full day of work. This trend is a big satisfier for most patients and certainly is to the urologist who is far more efficient and has to do much less redundant paperwork.

The authors have been carefully selected based on leadership and expertise in this trend. These nationally known experts have played key roles in defining their respective fields and are regarded as critical thought leaders in both academic and private practice, where many of the innovations occur. Importantly, they present the topics in a practical manner. I learned from each of them and know much of their advice will be integrated into the practices of the readership.

J. Stephen Jones, MD, FACS, MBA
Cleveland Clinic Regional Hospitals
Urological Oncology
9500 Euclid Avenue, Q10-1
Cleveland, OH 44195, USA

E-mail address:
Joness7@ccf.org

http://dx.doi.org/10.1016/j.ucl.2013.08.015
0094-0143/13/$ – see front matter © 2013 Published by Elsevier Inc.

Dedication

This issue is dedicated to Sam and Maria Miller. Their leadership, wisdom, and generosity make our community and world a better and more beautiful place. Their friendship to me and my wife Kathy continues to teach us ways to value the goodness in mankind.

J. Stephen Jones, MD, FACS, MBA
Cleveland Clinic Regional Hospitals
Urological Oncology
9500 Euclid Avenue, Q10-1
Cleveland, OH 44195, USA

E-mail address:
Joness7@ccf.org

Urol Clin N Am 40 (2013) xv
http://dx.doi.org/10.1016/j.ucl.2013.08.016
0094-0143/13/$ – see front matter

urologic.theclinics.com

Transrectal Prostate Biopsy

Mohamed T. Ismail, MD[a,b], Leonard G. Gomella, MD[b,*]

KEYWORDS

- Prostate cancer • Prostate biopsy • Detection • Diagnosis • Transrectal ultrasonography
- Technique

KEY POINTS

- Grayscale transrectal ultrasound (TRUS)-guided prostate biopsy using local anesthesia remains the standard approach to the definitive diagnosis of prostate cancer.
- Careful patient evaluation and preparation are essential to maximize the results and minimize the complications of the biopsy procedure.
- Image guided enhancement for prostate biopsy allows for better visualization and their role in the diagnosis is evolving.

INTRODUCTION

Prostate cancer (PCa) is the most common neoplasm in the Western hemisphere, and the incidence is still increasing.[1] Screening, detection, and diagnosis of PCa are currently based on serum prostate-specific antigen (PSA) level; digital rectal examination (DRE) and transrectal ultrasound (TRUS)-guided systemic biopsies. Although there is intense controversy concerning PCa screening, when a decision is made to perform a diagnostic prostate biopsy (PB), TRUS is the preferred and standard-of-care technique.[2]

TRUS has many advantages over other medical imaging modalities. The lack of ionizing radiation, low cost, and the proximity of the prostate to the rectal wall resulted in TRUS being the most commonly used prostate imaging modality. After the initial introduction of the sextant PB technique proposed by Hodge, little refinement of the technique was carried out until Stamey[3] suggested directing the biopsies more laterally. It was then recognized that even lateral sextant biopsies could miss up to 30% of cancers, because more extended biopsy schemes result in higher cancer detection rates.[4,5] As defined by the National Comprehensive Cancer Network (NCCN), an extended PB (EPB) is essentially a sextant template with at least 4 additional cores from the lateral peripheral zones as well as biopsies directed to lesions found on palpation or imaging.[6] Little controversy exists in the urologic community regarding the usefulness of EPB compared with sextant biopsy in increasing the detection rate of PCa.

INDICATIONS

PB is indicated when there is suspicion of advanced or metastatic PCa based on factors such as bony metastasis or pelvic/retroperitoneal adenopathy or suggestive symptoms. More commonly, the decision to perform PB has been traditionally based on abnormal DRE or increased PSA level. Abnormal DRE usually indicates an initial PB irrespective of PSA level. In the Washington PCa screening study,[7] 14% of the cancers were diagnosed by DRE alone. Among those patients who underwent radical prostatectomy (RP) based on abnormal DRE, 20% were non–organ confined and 20% had a Gleason score of 7 or greater.

Disclosures: The authors have nothing to disclose.
[a] Department of Urology, VA Medical Center, 1601 Kirkwood Highway, Wilmington, DE 19805, USA;
[b] Department of Urology, Thomas Jefferson University, 1025 Walnut Street, 1102, Philadelphia, PA 19107, USA
* Corresponding author.
E-mail address: leonard.gomella@jefferson.edu

Urol Clin N Am 40 (2013) 457–472
http://dx.doi.org/10.1016/j.ucl.2013.07.012

The debate regarding the pros and cons of PSA-based screening continues and is beyond the scope of this review.[8,9] If a patient opts for PSA-based screening, there is no absolute cutoff for PB (**Table 1**). Most sources recommend repeating an abnormal PSA value before making the decision to perform PB with a normal DRE, and there is general agreement that PSA higher than 4 is suggestive of the presence of PCa for a biopsy. A PSA threshold of 2.6 ng/mL doubles cancer detection rates in men younger than 60 years with little loss in specificity.[10] There are several other factors to consider in proceeding to biopsy, potentially including PSA velocity, % free PSA, PSA density (PSAD), age, family history, ethnicity, and comorbidities. The NCCN recommends the use of a PSA velocity of 0.35 ng/mL/y or greater as indication for biopsy in men with PSA 2.5 ng/mL or less.[6] In addition, the group recommends the use of % free PSA as alternative indication of initial biopsy, with the intention of avoiding unnecessary biopsies. The % free/total PSA ratio can be used to indicate biopsy if less than 10%, consider PB intermediate if between 10% and 25%, and no PB if greater than 25%. PSAD and age-referenced PSA have been investigated but are controversial.[6] Recent data from the dutasteride REDUCE (reduction by dutasteride of prostate cancer events) chemoprevention trial again confirmed that family history is a significant risk factor for cancer.[11] Several researchers found that African American race remains an independent predictor of PCa detection in men undergoing initial PB.[12,13]

Newer tests such as kallikrein markers in blood, genomics, proteomics, and a variety of urinary markers such as PCA3 and TMPRSS2-ERG remain under investigation to aid in the decision making for PB.[14] **Box 1** lists the factors to be considered as an indication for PB.

Predictive models have been developed to reduce unnecessary biopsies and still detect most clinically important cancers and are available on the Internet. The finasteride-based PCa Prevention Trial model (http://deb.uthscsa.edu/URORiskCalc/Pages/uroriskcalc.jsp) uses variables such as PSA, age, family history, race, DRE, and previous negative biopsy.[15] The European Randomized Study of Screening for PCa (ERSPC)-based model has several calculators (http://www.prostatecancer-riskcalculator.com/) that rely on additional items such as TRUS-estimated prostate volume and the presence of hypoechoic lesions.[16] Other indications for PB include as a part of an active surveillance (AS) protocol[14] and in the evaluation of recurrence after local radiation therapy.[17]

PATIENT PREPARATION

A complete history and physical examination, urinalysis and culture, and PSA determination are mandatory before a PB. Attention to any anorectal

Table 1
Summary of some major organizations recommendations for PSA cutoff for initial biopsy

Organization	PSA Cutoff	Reference
American Urological Association PSA best practice statement: 2009 update	No longer recommending a single cutoff	http://AUAnet.org
NCCN guideline version 2012	PSA ≤2.5 ng/mL and PSA velocity ≥0.35 ng/mL/y PSA 2.6–4.0 ng/mL PSA ≥4.0 ng/mL especially if free PSA ≤10%	http://www.nccn.org
European Association of Urology guidelines on prostate cancer, 2012 update	No longer recommending a single cutoff For young men, PSA values <2–3 ng/mL are often used	http://www.uroweb.org
National Institute for Health and Clinical Excellence, UK clinical guideline 58, prostate cancer 2008	No longer recommending a single cutoff	http://www.nice.org
Australian Cancer Network Localized prostate cancer: a guide for men and their families in 2010	No longer recommending a single cutoff	http://www.cancer.org.au
Canadian Urological Association PSA screening: The Canadian perspective	No longer recommending a single cutoff	http://www.cua.org

---

Box 1
Factors to be considered as an indication for PB

DRE

PSA value

PSA velocity

% Free PSA

Family history

Race

PSAD

Comorbidities

Kallikrein markers, genomics, and proteomics

PCA3 and TMPRSS2-ERG

Box 2
Factors to consider before a PB

History and physical examination including DRE

PSA

Urinalysis and culture

Use of oral anticoagulants

Use of antiplatelet medications

Use of a rectal enema

---

disease that may interfere with the probe or needle insertion should be noted. The use of low-dose aspirin does not seem to increase bleeding and should be continued if deemed medically necessary. Oral anticoagulants should be stopped 5 days before the biopsy and low-molecular-weight heparin bridging used if medically indicated.

The use of rectal enema to reduce infectious complications is contentious, with 81% of urologists in the United States using an enema in preparation for a TRUS biopsy.[18] Several studies showed that the risk of infectious complications is lower if a rectal enema is used.[19,20] In a large study from Korea, infectious complications developed in 1.3% of patients who had rectal preparation, but in 9.5% of those who did not.[21] In another nonrandomized Korean study,[22] the use of a povidone-iodine suppository before biopsy markedly reduced infectious complications.

However, a study by Carey and Korman[23] reported that enema before biopsy provides no significant advantage in clinical outcome. Moreover, in a recent study from Canada,[24] rectal cleansing with povidone-iodine before TRUS biopsy did not significantly reduce the risk of infectious complications. **Box 2** lists the factors to consider before a PB.

ANTIBIOTIC PROPHYLAXIS

Infectious complications associated with TRUS biopsies are a growing concern. More frequent complications are being observed,[25,26] and the rate of resistance to commonly used antibiotics is increasing.[27,28] Infectious complications related to TRUS biopsy range from transient fever to urinary tract infection (UTI), sepsis, and possible death. The rate of sepsis after TRUS biopsy is estimated to be between 0.1% and 5%, with UTIs occurring in 3% to 11% of patients.[25,26,28,29] The standard of care is to use antibiotics at the time of TRUS biopsy. Traditionally, fluoroquinolones have been used.[30] In a survey of more than 900 US urologists,[18] more than 85% reported using fluoroquinolones. There is no evidence whether a single or a more extended protocol is needed. Recent studies suggest that the escalating rates of infectious complications and need for hospitalization are often caused by fluoroquinolone-resistant bacteria.[25,27,31] Two antibiotic prophylactic strategies are being used (**Box 3**). Studies have shown reduced risk of infection in patients by adding a single dose of aminoglycoside just before biopsy.[32,33] Another proposed strategy is the use of rectal swabs before TRUS biopsy to screen patients for colonization with fluoroquinolone-resistant bacteria and then to use targeted antimicrobial prophylaxis.[34,35] The antibiotics for PB recommended by the American Urological Association (AUA) include fluoroquinolones or first-generation/second-generation/third-generation cephalosporins.

Alternatively, aminoglycoside or aztreonam + metronidazole or clindamycin may be used. The only agents for which oral administration is acceptable for PB are the quinolones.

ULTRASOUND PROBE CONFIGURATION

Two different types of probes are available: end-fire and side-fire probe configurations and transmit frequencies of 6 to 10 MHz (**Figs. 1** and **2**). End-fire probes execute the biopsy in a more

---

Box 3
Strategies to reduce infectious complications associated with PB

Addition of single-dose aminoglycoside

Rectal swab and targeted antibiotic coverage

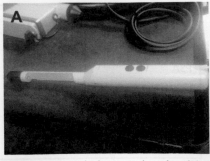
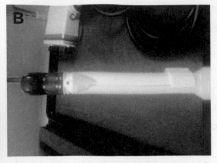

Fig. 1. (A) Side-fire transrectal ultrasound probe. (B) Side-fire transrectal ultrasound probe with needle guide attached.

anteroposterior plane and might therefore allow better access to the most lateral part of the peripheral zone. In addition, targeting the anterior horn of the prostate might be simplified. Evidence form retrospective studies suggests that an end-fire configuration results in greater detection of PCa.[36,37] However, in a recent prospective randomized multicenter trial,[38] no difference was seen in PCa detection rates when a systematic biopsy scheme was adopted. In another study, the side-fire probe was associated with a better patient tolerance profile, which may be related to the size of the tip and the fact that the insertion procedure for the side-fire probe seems to be gentler and better tolerated.[39] With these considerations, the choice of probe remains operator dependent. The acoustic properties of soft tissue are similar to those of water, but clinically useful ultrasound energy does not propagate through air. For this reason, a water-density substance, termed a coupling medium, is used. The coupling medium, usually sonographic jelly or lubricant, is placed between the probe and the rectal surface. If the probe is covered with a protective condom, the coupling medium is placed between the probe and the condom, as well as between the condom and the rectal surface. TRUS should be performed in both transverse and sagittal planes.

ANESTHESIA AND PATIENT POSITIONING

Patients are usually placed in the left-lateral decubitus position, with the hips flexed up to 90°. A pillow placed between the knees helps maintain positioning. Make certain that the buttocks are flush with the end of the table to allow manipulation of the probe and biopsy gun without obstruction. Alternatively, some use the dorsal lithotomy position. A repeat DRE should be performed before insertion of the TRUS probe and abnormalities documented.

An important topic is pain control during and after biopsy. The overall sensitivity of the PB is probably only 70%. Many patients have to undergo a repeat biopsy, and this is an important part of AS protocols. If the patient experiences significant pain, it is difficult to convince them about the necessity of repeat biopsy. Periprostatic nerve block (PPNB) with 1% lidocaine is considered the standard anesthetic technique.[40] The most common site of injection is bilaterally at the junction of the base of the prostate and seminal vesicles, because of the results of anatomic studies showing that the neuroatonomic pathway originates from the inferior hypogastric plexus located at the tip of seminal vesicles and passes between the prostate and rectum.[41] Various infiltration sites

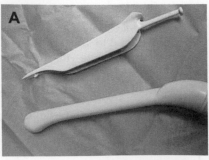
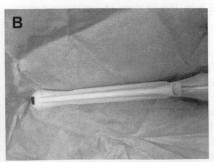

Fig. 2. (A) End-fire transrectal ultrasound probe with needle guide. (B) End-fire transrectal ultrasound probe with needle guide attached.

have been studied (**Box 4**), including the apex only,[42,43] bilateral neurovascular bundles,[44,45] apex and neurovascular regions,[42,46] 3 locations (base, mid, and apex) posterolateral,[47] and lateral to the tip of seminal vesicles.[48] Ismail and colleagues[49] reported that combined bilateral neurovascular bundles with apical infiltration resulted in more effective reduction in pain associated with TRUS biopsy than bilateral neurovascular infiltration alone, especially in younger patients. However, PPNB does not address somatic pain related to probe insertion and movement, which can be more painful than the biopsy, or pain caused by the infiltration itself. Cormio and colleagues[46] recently reported their results on using 3 noninfiltrative anesthesia (NIA) protocols for TRUS biopsy. These investigators found that lidocaine-prilocaine cream was most effective in probe-related pain, whereas lidocaine-ketorolac gel was most effective in sampling-related pain. Some investigators have discussed the issue of whether PPNB should be associated with NIA or oral medications.[50,51] Obek and colleagues[50] have shown that the combination of PPNB with NIA was superior to PPNB alone. Pendleton and colleagues[51] reported that oral administration of 75 mg tramadol/650 mg acetaminophen 3 hours before PNB seems to provide more effective pain control that PNB alone, without causing any additional side effects.

GRAYSCALE EXAMINATION

Grayscale TRUS is the classic technique for prostate imaging and enables a detailed visualization of the prostate (**Fig. 3**). Prostate volume should be calculated and PSAD obtained in all patients undergoing TRUS. Volume is determined using the prolate ellipse formula (height × length × width × 1.83), which is intrinsic to most modern ultrasonography units. As a general reference, the average prostate volume in a 60-year-old to 70-year-old is approximately 48 mL.

The debate over targeting hypoechoic lesions in the prostate is still unsettled. A biopsy study of

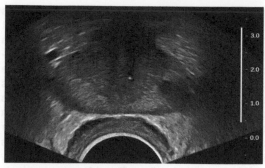

Fig. 3. Grayscale examination of prostate with classically described hypoechoic lesion at left base. Lesion was biopsy proven Gleason 8 (4 + 4) adenocarcinoma of the prostate.

3912 patients published in 2004[52] revealed that PCa was detected in 25.5% with a hypoechoic lesion and in 25.4% without such a lesion. Even more interesting is the per core distinction, which was 9.3% for hypoechoic and 10.4% for isoechoic areas. On the other hand, Toi and colleagues[53] found that biopsies taken when a prostate lesion is identified by TRUS are almost twice as likely to show cancer than when no lesion is visible. The cancers were found to be of higher volume and grade. The investigators concluded that the search for and targeting hypoechoic lesion on TRUS remains important for PCa diagnosis.

BIOPSY TECHNIQUE

The standard device used is a spring-driven 18-gauge needle core biopsy device or biopsy gun, which is passed through the needle guide attached to the ultrasound probe (**Fig. 4**). The best visualization of the biopsy needle path is often in the sagittal plane. Grayscale images are superimposed with a ruled puncture path that corresponds to the needle guide of the TRUS unit. By

---

Box 4
Sites of injection of PPNB

Bilateral neurovascular bundles

Apex only

Apex and neurovascular bundles

Three locations: base, mid, and apex posterolateral

Lateral to tip of seminal vesicles

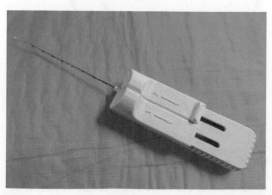

Fig. 4. Example of a spring-loaded automatic 18-gauge PB needle.

design, the spring-loaded biopsy gun advances the needle 0.5 cm and samples the subsequent 1.5 cm of tissue, with the tip extending 0.5 cm beyond the area sampled. Place the tip of the needle approximately 0.5 cm posterior to the prostate capsule before activation. If the needle is advanced through the capsule before firing, this may result in sampling more anterior tissue. As a consequence, the most common site of cancer may be missed. Using the probe to compress the rectal mucosa before firing the needle may reduce rectal bleeding. The biopsy sample is placed in formalin solution provided by the reference laboratory. Sample submission can vary and is discussed later.

NUMBER AND SITE OF BIOPSY CORES

A laterally directed systematic TRUS-guided PB with 12 cores is considered the standard procedure for PCa detection, resulting in a positive biopsy rate of 25% to 50%.[6,54,55] **Fig. 5** shows the recommended biopsy location and direction of a typical TRUS 12-core biopsy template.

Several studies have reported the higher yield of an EPB versus the old standard sextant biopsy, without an increase in the detection of insignificant cancer.[55,56] The debate continues as to whether there is a value in adjusting the number of cores based on age or prostate volume.[57–59] Sampling

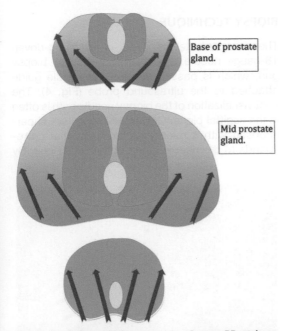

Fig. 5. Recommended systematic 12-core PB at base, mid, and apical prostate gland. Blue represents peripheral zone, the focus of the biopsy needle. Green represents the transition zone and tan represents the urethra.

accuracy tends to decrease progressively with an increasing prostate volume. Ploussard and colleagues[60] proposed that an extended biopsy scheme, with 21 cores obtained, increases cancer detection rates, especially if PSAD is less than 0.20 ng/mL.

On the other hand, it has been shown that the saturation technique as an initial PB strategy does not improve cancer detection. Jones[61] has suggested that further efforts at extended biopsy strategies beyond 10 to 12 cores are not appropriate as initial biopsy strategy. In a systemic review, Eichler and colleagues[62] showed that there is no significant benefit in taking more than 12 cores and methods requiring more than 18 cores have a poor side-effect profile. The AUA consensus has suggested that a 12-core biopsy is the recommended initial biopsy scheme; other investigators have advocated for additional biopsies, such as the 14-core biopsy by Mousa and colleagues.[63]

In addition to the number of cores and prostate volume, the concept of biopsy core direction is equally important. The apex and the base of the peripheral gland are the most common cancer sites, which is where biopsies should be directed, whereas the parasagittal biopsies have been shown to have the lowest possibility of PCa at the initial biopsy.[57,64–66] Based on landmark anatomic PCa location studies[67] and furthered by knowledge of tumor location by Stamey,[3] the addition of laterally directed biopsies has been shown to yield an approximately 5% to 35% increase in cancer detection rates.[56,64] Most of the extradetected cancers were in anterior apical and far lateral midlobar regions, 2 areas well sampled by EPB. Contrary to earlier findings regarding the importance of parasagittally directed cores to detect transitional zone (TZ) cancer,[67] it now seems established that because of their low prevalence at initial biopsy, cores of this area should be abandoned.[54] Researchers form the University of Washington reported their experience with obtaining biopsies from the anterior apical region.[66] These biopsies were directed under the capsule with the goal of sampling the peripheral zone anterior and distal to the TZ at apex. These investigators reported that the most common unique site of cancer was the anterior apex, where 17% of cancers would have been missed if not sampled. The use of EPB has resulted in more Gleason score concordance. San Francisco and colleagues[68] reported an improvement on concordance rate from 63% to 72%. Milan and colleagues[69] reported that rate of upgrading to worsening cancer was significantly reduced with EPB. With EPB, the risk of significant upgrading decreases because of higher sampling density and more accurate pathologic biopsy evaluation. The AUA has recently completed a white paper confirming that a 12-core systematic biopsy is optimal and that there was not compelling evidence that individual site-specific labeling of cores benefits clinical decision making regarding the initial management of PCa. The investigators recommend packaging no more than 2 cores in each jar to avoid reduction of cancer detection rates through inadequate tissue sampling.[70]

QUALITY ASSURANCE

Benign or malignant conditions of the prostate are diagnosed by nuclear and architectural examination of prostate tissue. Therefore, 2 important factors are important in assessing the adequacy of a biopsy, namely, core length and the presence of glandular elements (**Box 5**). Boccon-Gibod and colleagues[71] suggested that the average needle biopsy length should serve as a measure of quality control, with 10 mm of tissue as the shortest acceptable length. Iczkowski and colleagues[72] noted that the length of a single core sampled by sextant biopsy varied more than 3.6-fold. These investigators reported that a longer total tissue length increased the cancer detection rate, but this finding attained statistical significance only for cores obtained at apex. Obek and colleagues[73] showed that a significant correlation with needle core length and cancer detection rates exists for all biopsy cores and is not limited to a specific prostate site. These investigators established a cutoff to predict a higher cancer detection rate and, thus, a potential core quality assessment tool. Obtaining cores longer than 11.9 mm was associated with 2.5 times higher likelihood of detection of PCa. Core length may vary according to different factors, including but not limited to the urologist who performs the biopsy, the needle, the biopsy retrieval and tissue handling methods, and the pathologic analysis.[71,72] To investigate the adequacy of the samples obtained by PBs, Dogan and colleagues[74] evaluated cores obtained form 378 patients. These investigators found that the highest incidence of absence of glandular elements was detected at apical and far lateral biopsy samples. Absence of glandular elements in 1, 2,

and 5 biopsy samples were 50%, 27.8%, and 16.1%, respectively. The results have been found to be operator dependent. For patients with PSA between 4 and 10 ng/mL, cancer detection rates was lower in patients with absence of glandular elements. Collectively, these data suggest that clinicians must evaluate the pathology report in detail regarding core length and the presence of glandular elements. Pathologists must inform clinicians if they notice inadequacy of samples, and clinicians should even repeat the biopsy in necessary cases.

REPEAT PB AFTER INITIAL NEGATIVE BIOPSY

Studies of repeat PB after negative EPB indicate that up to 30% of patients have cancers that were not previously identified.[75,76] Repeat PB seems to be justified in men with an initial negative biopsy but persistent suspicion of PCa based on age, comorbidities, DRE findings, repeated PSA measurements, other PSA derivatives (% free PSA, complexed PSA, PSAD, PSA velocity), or urinary PCA3 score.[6] The use of the Progensa PCA3 assay (Hologic Gen-Probe, San Diego, CA, USA), which uses a PCA3 score with a cutoff value of 25 in post-DRE first-catch urine, has been approved by the US Food and Drug Administration to aid in the decision for repeat PB in men with 1 or more previous negative biopsies.[77] The cutoff value remains debatable, because some studies have used 35 as the cutoff of abnormal.[78,79] The superiority of PCA3 score compared with % free PSA was shown, indicating that a lower PCA3 score may prevent unnecessary repeat PB.[80,81] PCA3 seems to have a role in reducing unnecessary PB at first repeat PB but not at second or more repeat PB sessions.[82]

The number of biopsies needed in the repeat settings is still debatable. The NCCN guidelines suggest performing a second extended protocol and considering saturation biopsies only in patients with high risk of cancer after multiple negative biopsies.[6] Several studies support the hypothesis that saturation biopsy (>20 cores) seems appropriate in the repeat biopsy setting.[76,83,84] In a study from Italy,[84] the best re-biopsy scheme varied according to the clinical characteristics of the patients. For patients with no atypical small acinar proliferation (ASAP), the ideal number of cores varied according to % free PSA. If % free PSA was less than 10%, the best scheme was a 14-core biopsy (including 4 TZ biopsies), whereas if % free PSA was greater than 10%, then the ideal scheme would include 20 core biopsy (including 4 TZ biopsies). In addition to the number of biopsies, location is an important issue in repeat biopsy. According to

---

Box 5
Factors important in assessing adequacy of PB

Core length

Presence of glandular elements

the European Association of Urology (EAU) 2013 guidelines, TZ biopsies should be considered in the repeat setting.[85] In addition, the anterior apex seems to be the most common site of single-focus PCa, and repeat biopsies should include this distinct location.[76,86,87] Djavan and colleagues[88] reported in 2001 an original work on the risk of PCa on repeat biopsies performed 6 weeks after an initial negative set. These investigators found that cancer detection rates on biopsies 1, 2, 3, and 4 were 22%, 10%, 5%, and 4%, respectively, and that 58%, 60.9%, 86.3%, and 100% of patients who had RP had organ-confined disease on biopsies 1, 2, 3, and 4. The investigators concluded that biopsy 2 in all cases of a negative finding on biopsy 1 seems justified; however, further biopsies should be obtained only in select patients. Two important points need to be stressed: there was minimal delay between biopsies and these biopsies were all sextant. Thus, these findings may not apply in the modern extended biopsy era. Campos-Fernandes and colleagues[75] in a more recent cohort with extended biopsies found that 18%, 17%, and 14% of patients had PCa in second, third, and fourth biopsies, respectively. Cancer detected at these sets of biopsies was significant in 85% of cases. Similarly, Tan and colleagues[89] found significant PCa detected on third or greater PB, underscoring the importance of repeat biopsy in the setting of increased or increasing PSA despite negative previous PB. Pelvic magnetic resonance imaging (MRI) may be used to further investigate the possibility of an anterior located PCa in selected patients. Thus, no definitive recommendation can be made on when to stop biopsies when there is concern, and the decision should be individualized.

Another issue in the repeat biopsy setting is the role of transurethral resection of the prostate (TURP). Several investigators have reported the PCa detection rate offered by TURP.[90,91] However, the 2013 EAU guidelines[92] state "the use of diagnostic TURP instead of repeat biopsies is a poor tool for cancer detection." The NCCN 2012 guidelines[6] recommend TZ biopsies as part of repeat biopsy strategy, but they do not specifically comment on TURP. In a recent European study,[93] in which patients were randomized to saturation biopsy only or saturation biopsy + TURP, TURP increased the detection of clinically significant cancer. The investigators comment that this strategy has to be balanced against the small increased incidence of urinary retention, emergency readmission, and longer hospital stay.

The role of transperineal biopsy in the repeat setting is debatable. The theoretic advantage of the transperineal route over the transrectal route stems from the direct longitudinal access to the prostate gland, potentially resulting in more efficacious sampling of the peripheral apical region, which seems to be underrepresented in the transrectal route. Several researchers have shown encouraging results with the use of template transperineal biopsies.[94,95] However, this strategy has to be weighed against the need for anesthesia and increased morbidity with such an invasive procedure. Modern imaging studies such as MRI might have a relevant role in visualizing clinically significant cancers to facilitate precise sampling from any suspicious areas.

REPEAT PB AFTER SUSPICIOUS OR POSITIVE INITIAL BIOPSY

Suspicious pathologic findings, including ASAP and high-grade prostatic intraepithelial neoplasia (HGPIN) in previous biopsy may be an indication for repeat PB. ASAP describes a situation in which the pathologist is unable to establish the diagnosis of PCa. The incidence of ASAP ranges between 0.7% and 23.4%, with a median incidence of 4.4%.[87,96] It is an almost certain clinical indication for a rebiopsy, because approximately 40% of patients are found to have cancer, even in the extended biopsy era.[8,97,98] Allen and colleagues[99] reported that the chance of detecting cancer is greatly increased by performing a rebiopsy not only of the atypical site but also of the adjacent contralateral and adjacent ipsilateral areas. In general, a biopsy is performed within 3 to 6 months. Scattoni and colleagues[84] suggest obtaining 14 cores with no TZ biopsies in patients with previous diagnosis of ASAP.

HGPIN at PB is found in between 0% and 24.6% of patients, with a median incidence of 4.7%.[87] It represents a discrete pathologic entity and is a potential precursor lesion to PCa.[100] A single focus of HGPIN does not warrant a repeat biopsy, but controversy persists about whether the presence of multifocal HGPIN truly represents an important risk factor for consideration of a repeat biopsy. Initial reports, based on sextant biopsies, showing a high prevalence of cancers in rebiopsies have not been reproduced in the extended biopsy era.[87] Based on level 2a evidence, the EAU[85] does not recommend repeat biopsy in the presence of HGPIN. However, some investigators suggest that multifocal HGPIN carries a 40% risk of cancer in subsequent biopsies and recommend a repeat biopsy within 1 year.[101,102] Godoy and colleagues[103] have reported a continued risk of PCa development in these patients, regardless of changes in PSA, and proposed a delayed-interval biopsy every 3 years.

Repeat biopsy at 3 to 18 months form diagnosis of low-risk PCa, in patients who opt for AS, has been suggested to reduce misclassification.[104,105] Several investigators[106] found that approximately 1 in 3 patients considered candidates for AS have more significant disease. In addition, in AS protocols, surveillance biopsies, to determine progression, are performed at intervals of every year to every 3 to 4 years.[106] The optimal number and location of biopsies in AS protocols has not been established. The use of other parameters such as PCA3 score and MRI in selecting patients for AS protocols is under study.[107,108]

IMAGE-GUIDED ENHANCEMENTS FOR PB

PB through a center of cancer contains more tissue, which allows more accurate characterization for pathologic interpretation. Thus, modalities that allow for visualization of PCa may aid in image-guided PB. Several technologies are being evaluated, namely color Doppler ultrasonography, MRI, and elastography.[109] An important and obvious limitation of the image-guided PB techniques is that they are operator dependent and require significant radiologic expertise and cooperation with radiologic experts.

COLOR DOPPLER ULTRASONOGRAPHY

PCa is associated with angiogenesis and neovascularization; this is also seen by increase in microvessel density (**Fig. 6**).[110] It is estimated that as a

result of these factors, a disturbed perfusion of malignant tissue compared with normal prostate tissue is present.[111,112] Contrast-enhanced ultrasound (CEUS) imaging was developed to image perfusion.[113,114] Ultrasound contrast agents consist of small encapsulated gas bubbles that can be administered intravenously and remain intravascular. Adding microbubbles as additional reflectors into the blood stream increases the sensitivity of color Doppler and power Doppler imaging. However, these techniques use relatively high ultrasound energy levels and, as a result, a large proportion of the microbubbles are destroyed as they are imaged.[115] During the last few years, new imaging techniques have been developed that enable sensitive microbubble imaging even in microvasculature, with lower destruction rates (low mechanical index imaging). A long list of CEUS techniques is available, from harmonic imaging, using the nonlinear behavior of microbubbles in an ultrasound beam, via pulse inversion techniques, using various pulses to isolate the nonlinear reflections, to even more specific imaging techniques that provide selective imaging techniques that provide selective imaging of the signal reflected by the bubbles, canceling most of the tissue reflections.[116] CEUS imaging has been extensively studied, with 2 main objectives, namely, to increase the diagnostic yield of the biopsy and in addition to detect more clinically significant cancers.

Two studies reported on the value of CEUS and found that targeted biopsies detected as many cancers as systemic biopsies, with fewer than half the number of biopsy cores.[117,118] Linden

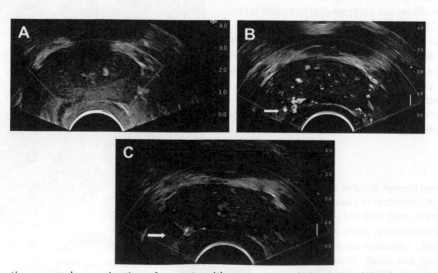

Fig. 6. (A) Routine grayscale examination of prostate with no suspicious lesions seen. (B) Color Doppler examination; increased vascularity noted in right base; which proved to be a Gleason 7 (3 + 4) cancer (arrow). (C) Power Doppler image showing the Gleason 7 cancer at right base (arrow).

and colleagues[119] used CEUS to compare it with systemic biopsy in 60 patients and concluded that the vascularity detail allowed directed biopsy of these areas, with increased detection of PCa. Nelson and colleagues[120] showed a sensitivity of 29% and a specificity of 80% for the CEUS-targeted biopsies. Halpern and colleagues[121] concluded that CEUS improves the sensitivity of PCa detection without substantial loss of specificity. In a recent Chinese study, the sensitivity and negative predictive value of CEUS-targeted biopsies was significantly better than standard biopsy.[122] However, in all studies, CEUS techniques alone would miss many tumors, and researchers suggest targeted biopsies to areas of abnormal flow in addition to systemic biopsies.

Mitterberger and colleagues[117] found that the Gleason score detected by CEUS was higher than that detected by standard biopsy. In a study of 690 men, the mean Gleason score was 6.8 for CEUS versus 5.4 for standard biopsy. Jiang and colleagues[123] correlated findings between CEUS techniques, Gleason score, and microvessel density and found similar results. Halpern and colleagues[124] reported excellent accuracy of CEUS for the detection of high-grade cancer, with greater than 50% biopsy core involvement. This finding may have profound implications in detecting higher-grade cancers and might be particularly useful in patients who opt for AS.

Morelli and colleagues[125] evaluated the ability of a phosphodiesterase type 5 inhibitor vardenafil to increase prostate microcirculation visibility. Analysis of standard technique, contrast, and vardenafil-enhanced CEUS findings by biopsy core showed significantly higher detection rates using vardenafil versus contrast and standard techniques (41.2% vs 22.7% and 8.1%, respectively). Methods to decrease the blood flow related to benign causes and thereby increase the sensitivity of blood flow–directed biopsy techniques have been performed. In a randomized, double-blind, placebo-controlled study, Halpern and colleagues[124] found that pretreatment with dutasteride had no significant impact on the detection of PCa.

MRI

MRI has been shown to have a high degree of accuracy in the detection of clinically significant cancer when compared with RP specimens.[126] When functional parameters, such as dynamic-contrast enhancement, diffusion-weighted imaging, and spectroscopy are used, in addition to standard T1-weighted and T2-weighted sequences, MRI may afford an opportunity for image-guided approach to the prostate.[127] A recent systemic review of MRI-derived targets[128] reported that cancer was detected in 30% of targeted cores versus 7% of systematic cores. MRI lesions can be targeted either within the magnet or by allowing a lesion defined on MRI to be identified on ultrasound during a TRUS-guided procedure. MRI-guided biopsies within the magnet are difficult to perform because of high costs, long intervention time, and poor ergonomics.[129,130] MRI during a TRUS-guided PB setting can be used either visually or with computerized MRI-TRUS image registration.[131,132] Delonchamps and colleagues[133] found that PB combined with MRI-TRUS image registration improved significantly cancer detection over systemic or visually aided PB. Similarly, Pinto and colleagues[134] showed that MRI detected more cancer per core than a standard 12-core biopsy.

ELASTOGRAPHY

Elastography is an ultrasound imaging technique based on the concept that significant differences exist between elastic properties of benign and malignant tissue (**Fig. 7**).[135] It is able to detect the change in reflection of sound waves when manual compression is applied to the tissue. Current studies suggest that using a real-time elastography (RTE) targeted approach, using less than half of the biopsy cores in the EPB approach, results in an equivalent PCa detection rate.[135,136] Nelson and colleagues[120] compared systematic PB and

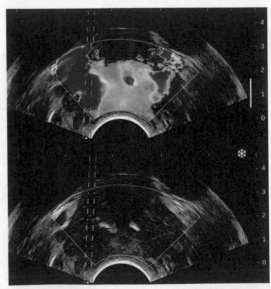

Fig. 7. Gleason 6 cancer right midprostate visualized on elastography (*top panel*) and not detected on routine grayscale imaging. Dotted lines represent projected path of biopsy needle.

targeted biopsies with grayscale, color Doppler, and RTE. Targeted biopsies based on elastography were twice as likely to yield a cancer diagnosis, with a trend toward higher-grade cancers. No abnormality on elastography or other sonographic modality was seen in 53.8% of positive systematic biopsy cores. Brock and colleagues[137] prospectively randomized 353 patients to either undergo RTE and grayscale TRUS. Both groups were comparable in terms of age, PSA, prostate volume, and clinical stage. RTE guidance showed an 11.7% higher detection rate of PCa. Sensitivity for visualizing PCa using RTE was 60.8% compared with 15% using gray scale. Thus, the sensitivity remains low, and a systematic biopsy approach remains mandatory. Shear-wave elastography is an alternative system using acoustic radiation force impulse to generate a shear wave. It has the advantage of being less operator-dependent, because it does not require manual application of pressure and the results are normally presented in absolute numbers. Two small studies were reported, with encouraging results, and the use of this technique continues to evolve.[124,138]

COMPLICATIONS OF PB

Urologic side effects of the procedure (Table 2) include UTI, bleeding (hematuria, bleeding per rectum, or hematospermia) and acute urinary tract obstruction. The increased number of biopsy cores, rates of bacterial resistance,[27] an increase in the use of antiplatelet agents,[139] and a high prevalence of benign prostatic hyperplasia (BPH)[140] have all contributed to increased morbidity associated with TRUS biopsy. Complications associated with PB had a prominent role in the US Preventative Services Task Force 2012 recommendations against PCa screening.[141]

Table 2
Summary of common complications reported form transrectal PB

Complications	%
Hematospermia	37.4
Hematuria >1 d	14.5
Rectal bleeding <2 d	2.2
Prostatitis	1.0
Fever >101.3°F, epididymitis, rectal bleeding >2 d, retention	<1.0
Other complications requiring hospitalization	0.3

Data from EAU Guidelines. Available at: http://www.uroweb.org. Accessed February 21, 2012.

In a large population-based study from Ontario, the probability of being admitted to hospital within 30 days of the procedure increased 4-fold between 1996 and 2005.[25] The overall 30-day mortality was 0.09% and did not change over the study period. When analyzed by cancer status, the 30-day admission rate was 1.9% for patients without cancer versus 0.8% for patients with cancer. The mean time to hospital admission from TRUS biopsy was 5 days. Most hospital admissions were for infection-related complications (71.6%), followed by bleeding-related diagnosis (19.4%) and urinary obstruction–related diagnoses (9.0%). The rates of hospital admissions related to infection increased from 0.6% in 1996 to 3.6% in 2005. This increase is probably related to a multitude of factors, including lack of standardization of antibiotic prophylaxis protocol, use of mechanical bowel preparation, and the emergence of fluoroquinolone-resistant organisms.

The hospital admission rates for patients undergoing repeat biopsy, when normally more cores are obtained, were not higher than those undergoing a first biopsy. Also, studies that compare the sextant pattern and the extended pattern of biopsies showed no significant increase in morbidity.[142,143] There was a small increase in complications related to urinary tract obstruction, which may have resulted from higher prevalence of BPH in an aging population.[140] A steady rate of bleeding-related complications is consistent with findings that men taking low-dose aspirin did not have increased rates of bleeding.[139] The same researchers found that patients of physicians who performed a high volume of biopsies experienced a low 30-day hospital admission rate.

SUMMARY

Grayscale TRUS PB using local anesthesia remains the standard approach to the definitive diagnosis of PCa. Careful patient evaluation and preparation are essential to maximize the results and minimize the complications of the biopsy procedure.

REFERENCES

1. Sigel R, Naishadham D, Jemel A. Cancer statistics, 2012. CA Cancer J Clin 2012;62:10–29.
2. Gomella L, Liu X, Trabulsi E, et al. Screening for prostate cancer: the current evidence and guidelines controversy. Can J Urol 2011;18:5875–83.
3. Stamey T. Making the most out of six systematic sextant biopsies. Urology 1995;45:2–12.
4. Presti JC Jr. Prostate biopsy: how many cores are enough? Urol Oncol 2003;21:361–5.

5. Singh H, Canto E, Shariat S, et al. Improved detection of clinically significant, curable prostate cancer with systematic 12-core biopsy. J Urol 2004;171:1089–92.

6. NCCN guidelines: prostate cancer early detection (v.2.2012). Comprehensive Cancer Network Website. Available at: http://www.nccn.org. Accessed April 28, 2013.

7. Okotie O, Roehl K, Han M, et al. Characteristics of prostate cancer detected by digital rectal examination only. Urology 2007;70:1117–20.

8. Andriole G, Crawford E, Grubb R 3rd, et al. Prostate cancer screening in the randomized Prostate, Lung, Colorectal, and Ovarian Cancer Screening Trial: mortality results after 13 years of follow-up. J Natl Cancer Inst 2012;104:125–32.

9. Schroder F, Hugosson J, Roobol M, et al. Prostate-cancer mortality at 11 years of follow-up. N Engl J Med 2012;366:981–90.

10. Punglia R, D'Amico A, Catalona W, et al. Effect of verification bias on screening for prostate cancer by measurement of prostate-specific antigen. N Engl J Med 2003;349:335–42.

11. Andriole G, Bostwick D, Brawley O, et al. Effect of dutasteride on the risk of prostate cancer. N Engl J Med 2010;362:1192–202.

12. Yanke B, Carver B, Bianco F Jr, et al. African-American race is a predictor of prostate cancer detection: incorporation into a pre-biopsy nomogram. BJU Int 2006;98:783–7.

13. Hemmerich J, Ahmad F, Meltzer D, et al. African American men significantly underestimate their risk of having prostate cancer at the time of biopsy. Psychooncolgy 2013;22(2):338–45.

14. Prensner J, Rubin M, Wei J, et al. Beyond PSA: the next generation of prostate cancer biomarkers. Sci Transl Med 2012;28:127–34.

15. Thompson I, Ankerst D, Chi C, et al. Assessing prostate cancer detection risk: results from the Prostate Cancer Prevention Trial. J Natl Cancer Inst 2006;98:529–34.

16. Roobol M, Steyerberg E, Kranse R, et al. A risk-based strategy improves prostate-specific antigen-driven detection of prostate cancer. Eur Urol 2010;57:79–85.

17. Darwish O, Raj G. Management of biochemical recurrence after primary localized therapy for prostate cancer. Front Oncol 2012;2:48–52.

18. Shandera K, Thibault G, Deshon G Jr. Variability in patient preparation for prostate biopsy among American urologists. Urology 1998;52:644–6.

19. Melekos MD. Efficacy of prophylactic antimicrobial regimens in preventing infectious complications after transrectal biopsy of the prostate. Int Urol Nephrol 1990;22:257–62.

20. Brown R, Warner J, Turner B, et al. Bacteremia and bacteriuria after transrectal prostate biopsy. Urology 1981;18:145–8.

21. Jeon S, Woo S, Hyun J, et al. Bisacodyl rectal preparation can decrease infectious complications of transrectal ultrasound-guided prostate biopsy. Urology 2003;62:461–6.

22. Park DS, Oh JJ, Lee JH, et al. Simple use of the suppository type povidone-iodine can prevent infectious complications in transrectal ultrasound-guided prostate biopsy. Adv Urol 2009;2009: 750598. Available at: http://www.pubmedcentral. nih.gov/articlerender.fcgi?artid=2673474&tool= pmcentrez&rendertype=abstract. Accessed January 21, 2013.

23. Carey J, Korman H. Transrectal ultrasound guided biopsy of the prostate: do enemas decrease clinically significant complications? J Urol 2001;166: 82–5.

24. AbuGhosh Z, Margolick J, Goldenberg S, et al. A prospective randomized trial of povidone-iodine prophylactic cleansing of the rectum prior to transrectal ultrasound-guided prostate biopsy. J Urol 2012;187:438–9.

25. Nam R, Saskin R, Lee Y, et al. Increasing hospital admission rates for urological complications after transrectal ultrasound guided prostate biopsy. J Urol 2010;183:963–7.

26. Pinkhasov G, Lin Y, Palmerola R, et al. Complications following prostate needle biopsy requiring hospital admission or emergency department visits–experience from 1000 consecutive patients. BJU Int 2012;110:369–74.

27. Feliciano J, Teper E, Ferrandino M, et al. The incidence of fluoroquinolone resistant infections after prostate biopsy–are fluoroquinolones still effective prophylaxis? J Urol 2008;179:952–7.

28. Carignan A, Roussy J, Lapointe V, et al. Increasing risk of infectious complications after transrectal ultrasound-guided prostate biopsies: time to reassess antimicrobial prophylaxis? Eur Urol 2012;62: 453–9.

29. Loeb S, Heuvel S, Zhu X, et al. Infectious complications and hospital admissions after prostate biopsy in a European randomized trial. Eur Urol 2012;61: 1110–4.

30. Kapoor D, Klimberg I, Malek G, et al. Single-dose oral ciprofloxacin versus placebo for prophylaxis during transrectal prostate biopsy. Urology 1998; 52:552–8.

31. American Urological Association. Best practice policy statement on urologic surgery antimicrobial prophylaxis. Baltimore (MD): American Urological Association Education and Research; 2007.

32. Adibi M, Hornberger B, Bhat D, et al. Reduction in hospital admission rates due to post-prostate biopsy infections after augmenting standard antibiotic prophylaxis. J Urol 2013;189:535–40.

33. Ho H, Ng L, Tan Y, et al. Intramuscular gentamicin improves the efficacy of ciprofloxacin as an

antibiotic prophylaxis for transrectal prostate biopsy. Ann Acad Med Singap 2009;38:212–6.

34. Liss M, Peeples A, Peterson E. Detection of fluoroquinolone-resistant organisms from rectal swabs by use of selective media prior to a transrectal prostate biopsy. J Clin Microbiol 2011;49: 1116–8.

35. Taylor A, Zembower T, Nadler R, et al. Targeted antimicrobial prophylaxis using rectal swab cultures in men undergoing transrectal ultrasound guided prostate biopsies is associated with reduced incidence of postoperative infectious complications. J Urol 2012;187:1275–9.

36. Paul R, Korineck C, Necking U, et al. Influence of transrectal ultrasound probe on prostate cancer detection in transrectal ultrasound-guided sextant biopsy of the prostate. Urology 2004;64:532–6.

37. Ching C, Moussa A, Li J, et al. Does transrectal ultrasound probe configuration really matter? End-fire versus side-fire probe prostate cancer detection rates. J Urol 2009;181:2077–82.

38. Rom M, Pycha A, Wiunig C, et al. Prospective randomized multicenter study comparing prostate cancer detection rates of end-fire and side-fire transrectal ultrasound probe configuration. Urology 2012;80:15–8.

39. Raber M, Scattoni V, Gallina A, et al. Does transrectal ultrasound probe influence prostate cancer detection in patients undergoing an extended prostate biopsy scheme? Results of a large retrospective study. BJU Int 2011;109:672–7.

40. Bertaccini A, Fandella A, Prayer-Galetti T, et al. Systematic development of clinical practice guidelines for prostate biopsy: a 3-year Italian project. Anticancer Res 2007;27:659–66.

41. Ozden E, Yaman O, Gogus C, et al. The optimum doses of and injection locations for periprostatic nerve blockade for transrectal ultrasound guided biopsy of the prostate: a prospective, randomized, placebo controlled study. J Urol 2003;170: 2319–22.

42. Seymour H, Perry M, Lee-Elliot C, et al. Pain after transrectal ultrasonography-guided prostate biopsy: the advantages of periprostatic local anesthesia. BJU Int 2001;88:540–4.

43. Schostak M, Christoph F, Muller M, et al. Optimizing local anesthesia during 10-core biopsy of the prostate. Urology 2002;60:253–7.

44. Alavi A, Soloway M, Vaidya A, et al. Local anesthesia for ultrasound guided prostate biopsy: a prospective randomized trial comparing 2 methods. J Urol 2001;166:1343–5.

45. Addla S, Adeyoju A, Wemyss-Holden G, et al. Local anesthesia for transrectal ultrasound-guided prostate biopsy: a prospective, randomized, double blind, placebo-controlled study. Eur Urol 2003;43:441–3.

46. Cormio L, Lorusso F, Selvaggio O, et al. Noninfiltrative anesthesia for transrectal biopsy: a randomized prospective study comparing lidocaine-prilocaine cream and lidocaine-ketorolac gel. Urol Oncol 2013;31(1):68–73.

47. Leibovici D, Zisman A, Siegel Y, et al. Local anesthesia for prostate biopsy by periprostatic lidocaine injection: a double-blind placebo controlled study. J Urol 2002;167:563–5.

48. Wu C, Carter H, Naqibuddin M, et al. Effect of local anesthetics on patient recovery after transrectal biopsy. Urology 2001;57:925–9.

49. Ismail T, Janane A, Dakkak Y, et al. The contribution of periapical nerve block in transrectal ultrasound-guided prostate biopsy: results from a prospective randomized trial. African J Urol 2012;18:78–81.

50. Obek C, Ozkan B, Tunc B, et al. Comparison of 3 different methods of anesthesia before transrectal prostate biopsy: a prospective randomized trial. J Urol 2004;172:502–5.

51. Pendleton J, Costa J, Wludyka P, et al. Combination of oral tramadol, acetaminophen and 1% lidocaine induced periprostatic nerve block for pain control during transrectal ultrasound guided biopsy of the prostate: a prospective, randomized, controlled trial. J Urol 2006;176:1372–5.

52. Onur R, Littrup P, Pontes J, et al. Contemporary impact of transrectal ultrasound lesions for prostate cancer detection. J Urol 2004;172:512–4.

53. Toi A, Neill M, Gina A, et al. The continuing importance of transrectal ultrasound identification of prostatic lesions. J Urol 2007;177:516–20.

54. Heidenreich A, Bellmunt J, Bolla M, et al, European Association of Urology. EAU guidelines on prostate cancer. Part 1: screening, diagnosis, and treatment of clinically localized disease. Eur Urol 2011;59: 61–71.

55. Chun F, Epstein J, Ficarra V, et al. Optimizing performance and interpretation of prostate biopsy: a critical analysis of the literature. Eur Urol 2010;58: 851–64.

56. Presti J, Chang J, Bhargava V, et al. The optimal systematic prostate biopsy scheme should include 8 rather than 6 biopsies: results of a prospective clinical trial. J Urol 2000;163:163–6.

57. Eskew L, Bare R, McCullough D, et al. Systematic 5 region prostate biopsy is superior to sextant method for diagnosing carcinoma of the prostate. J Urol 1997;157:199–202.

58. Scattoni V, Raber M, Abdollah F, et al. Biopsy schemes with the fewest cores for detecting 95% of the prostate cancer detected by a 24-core biopsy. Eur Urol 2010;57:1–8.

59. Ficarra V, Novella G, Novra G, et al. The potential impact of prostate volume in the planning of optimal number of cores in the systematic transperineal prostate biopsy. Eur Urol 2005;48:932–7.

60. Ploussard G, Nicolaiew N, Marchand C, et al. Pro-spective evaluation of an extended 21-core biopsy scheme as initial prostate cancer diagnostic strat-egy. Eur Urol, in press.

61. Jones J. Prostate cancer: are we over-diagnosing–or under-thinking? Eur Urol 2008;53:10–2.

62. Eichler K, Hempel S, Wilby J, et al. Diagnostic value of systematic biopsy methods in the investi-gation of prostate cancer: a systematic review. J Urol 2006;175:1605–12.

63. Moussa A, Meshref A, Schoenfield L. Importance of additional "extreme" anterior apical needle bi-opsies in the initial detection of prostate cancer. Urology 2010;75:1034–9.

64. Gore J, Shariat S, Miles B, et al. Optimal combina-tions of systematic sextant and laterally directed bi-opsies for the detection of prostate cancer. J Urol 2001;165:1554–9.

65. Presti JC Jr, O'Dowd G, Miller M, et al. Extended peripheral zone biopsy schemes increase cancer detection rates and minimize variance in prostate specific antigen and age related cancer rates: re-sults of a community multi-practice study. J Urol 2003;169:125–9.

66. Wright J, Ellis W. Improved prostate cancer detec-tion with anterior apical prostate biopsies. Urol On-col 2006;24:492–5.

67. McNeal J, Redwine E, Freiha F, et al. Zonal distribu-tion of prostatic adenocarcinoma. Correlation with histological pattern and direction of spread. Am J Surg Pathol 1998;12:897–906.

68. San Francisco I, DeWolf W, Rosen S, et al. Extended prostate needle biopsy improves concor-dance of Gleason grading between prostate nee-dle biopsy and radical prostatectomy. J Urol 2003;169:136–40.

69. Milan B, Lehr D, Moore C, et al. Role of prostate bi-opsy schemes in accurate prediction of Gleason scores. Urology 2006;67:379–83.

70. Bjurlin M, Carter H, Schellhammer P, et al. Optimi-zation of prostate biopsy in clinical practice: sam-pling, labelling, and specimen processing. J Urol 2013;189(6):2039–46.

71. Boccon-Gibod L, Van der Kwast T, Montironi R, et al, European Society of Uropathology and Euro-pean Society of Pathology Uropathology Working Group. Handling and pathology reporting of pros-tate biopsies. Eur Urol 2004;46:177–84.

72. Iczkowski K, Casella G, Seppala R, et al. Needle core length in sextant biopsy influences prostate cancer detection. Urology 2002;59:698–702.

73. Öbek C, Doğanca T, Erdal S, et al. Core length in prostate biopsy: size matters. J Urol 2012;187:2051–5.

74. Doagn H, Aytac B, Kordan Y, et al. What is the ad-equacy of biopsies for prostate sampling? Urol On-col 2011;29:280–3.

75. Campos-Fernandes JL, Bastien L, Nicolaiew N, et al. Prostate cancer detection rate in patients with repeat extended 21-sample needle biopsy. Eur Urol 2009;55:600–9.

76. Zaytoun O, Moussa A, Gao T, et al. Office based transrectal saturation biopsy improves prostate can-cer detection compared to extended biopsy in repeat biopsy population. J Urol 2011;186:850–4.

77. US Food and Drug Administration. Premarket approval letter for the Progensa PCA3 assay. Avail-able at: http://www.accessdata.fda.gov/cdrh_docs/pdf10/p100033a.pdf. Accessed February 18, 2013.

78. Auprich M, Haese A, Walz J, et al. External valida-tion of urinary PCA3-based nomograms to individ-ually predict prostate biopsy outcome. Eur Urol 2010;58:727–32.

79. Auprich M, Bjartell A, Chun F, et al. Contempo-rary role of prostate cancer antigen 3 in the man-agement of prostate cancer. Eur Urol 2011;60:1045–54.

80. Aubin S, Reid J, Sarno M, et al. PCA3 molecular urine test for predicting repeat prostate biopsy outcome in populations at risk: validation on the placebo arm of dutasteride REDUCE trial. J Urol 2010;184:1947–52.

81. Ploussard G, Haese A, Van Poppel H. The prostate cancer gene 3 (PCA3) urine test in men with previ-ous negative biopsies: does free-to-total prostate-specific antigen ratio influences the performance of the PCA3 score in predicting positive biopsies? BJU Int 2010;106:1143–7.

82. Auprich M, Augustin H, Budaus L, et al. A compara-tive performance analysis of total prostate-specific antigen, percentage free prostate-specific antigen, prostate-specific antigen velocity and uri-nary prostate cancer gene 3 in the first, second and third repeat prostate biopsy. BJU Int 2012;109:1627–35.

83. Scattoni V, Montironi R, Schulman V, et al. Extended and saturation prostatic biopsy in the diagnosis and characterization of prostate cancer: a critical analysis of the literature. Eur Urol 2007;52:1309–22.

84. Scattoni V, Raber M, Capitanio U, et al. The optimal rebiopsy prostatic scheme depends on patient clinical characteristics: results of a recursive parti-tioning analysis based on a 24-core systematic scheme. Eur Urol 2011;60:834–41.

85. Heidenreich A, Aus G, Bolla M, et al. EAU guide-lines on prostate cancer. Eur Urol 2008;53:68–80.

86. Bott S, Young M, Kellet M, et al. Anterior apical can-cer: is it more difficult to diagnose? BJU Int 2002;89:886–9.

87. Epstein J, Herawi M. Prostate needle biopsies con-taining prostatic intraepithelial neoplasia or atyp-ical foci suspicious for carcinoma: implications for patient care. J Urol 2006;175:820–34.

88. Djavan B, Ravery V, Zlotta A, et al. Prospective evaluation of prostate cancer detected on biopsies 1, 2, 3 and 4: when should we stop? J Urol 2001;166: 1679–83.

89. Tan N, Lane B, Li J, et al. Prostate cancers diagnosed at repeat biopsy are smaller and less likely to be high grade. J Urol 2008;180:1325–9.

90. Puppo P, Intoini C, Chun F, et al. Role of transurethral resection of the prostate and biopsy of the peripheral zone in the same session after repeated negative biopsies in the diagnosis of prostate cancer. Eur Urol 2006;49:873–8.

91. Ornstein D, Rao G, Smith D, et al. The impact of systematic prostate biopsy on prostate cancer incidence in men with symptomatic benign prostatic hyperplasia undergoing transurethral resection of the prostate. J Urol 1997;157:880–3.

92. Zigeuner R, Schips L, Lipsky K, et al. Detection of prostate cancer by TURP or open surgery in patients with previously negative transrectal prostate biopsies. Urology 2003;62:883–7.

93. Yates D, Gregory G, Roupert M, et al. Transurethral resection biopsy as a part of saturation biopsy protocol: a cohort study and review of literature. Urol Oncol 2012;187(6):2051–5.

94. Taira A, Merrick G, Galbreath R, et al. Performance of trans-perineal template-guided mapping biopsy in detecting prostate cancer in the initial and repeat biopsy setting. Prostate Cancer Prostatic Dis 2010; 13:71–7.

95. Bott S, Henderson A, Furuno T, et al. Extensive transperineal template biopsies of the prostate: modified technique and results. Urology 2006;68:1037–41.

96. Montironi R, Scattoni V, Mazzucchelli R. Atypical foci suspicious but not diagnostic for malignancy in prostate needle biopsies (also referred to as "atypical small acinar proliferation suspicious for but not diagnostic of malignancy"). Eur Urol 2006; 50:666–74.

97. Abouassaly R, Tan N, Moussa A, et al. Risk of prostate cancer after diagnosis of atypical glands suspicious for carcinoma on saturation and traditional biopsies. J Urol 2008;180:911–4.

98. Chan T, Epstein J. Follow-up of atypical prostate needle biopsies suspicious for cancer. Urology 1999;53:351–5.

99. Allen E, Kahane H, Epstein J. Repeat biopsy strategies for men with atypical diagnosis on initial prostate needle biopsy. Urology 1998;52:803–7.

100. Bostwick D, Monitironi R. Prostatic intraepithelial neoplasia and the origins of prostatic carcinoma. Pathol Res Pract 1995;191:828–32.

101. De Nunzio C, Trucchi A, Miano R, et al. The number of cores positive for high grade prostatic intraepithelial neoplasia on initial biopsy is associated with prostate cancer on second biopsy. J Urol 2009;181:1069–74.

102. Schoenfield L, Jones J, Zippe C, et al. The incidence of high-grade prostatic intraepithelial neoplasia and glands suspicious for carcinoma on first-time saturation needle biopsy, and the subsequent risk of cancer. BJU Int 2007;99:770–4.

103. Godoy G, Huang G, Patel T, et al. Long-term follow-up of men with isolated high-grade prostatic intraepithelial neoplasia followed by serial delayed interval biopsy. Urology 2011;77:669–74.

104. Berglund R, Masterson T, Vora K, et al. Pathological upgrading and up staging with immediate repeat biopsy in patients eligible for active surveillance. J Urol 2008;180:1964–7.

105. Bul M, Van den Bergh R, Rannikko A, et al. Predictors of unfavourable repeat biopsy results in men participating in a prospective active surveillance program. Eur Urol 2012;61:370–7.

106. Dahabreh I, Chung M, Balk E, et al. Active surveillance in men with localized prostate cancer: a systematic review. Ann Intern Med 2012;156:582–90.

107. Ploussard G, Durand X, Xylinas E, et al. Prostate cancer antigen 3 score accurately predicts tumor volume and might help in selecting prostate cancer patients for active surveillance. Eur Urol 2011;59: 442–9.

108. Margel D, Yap S, Lawrentschuk N, et al. Impact of multiparametric endorectal coil prostate magnetic resonance imaging on disease reclassification among active surveillance candidates: a prospective cohort study. J Urol 2012;187:1247–52.

109. Trabulsi EJ, Sackett D, Gomella L. Enhanced transrectal ultrasound modalities in the diagnosis of prostate cancer. Urology 2010;76:1025–33.

110. Fregene T, Khanuja P, Noto A, et al. Tumor-associated angiogenesis in prostate cancer. Anticancer Res 1993;13(6B):2377–81.

111. Sedelaar J, Van Leenders G, Hulsbergen-van de Kaa C, et al. Microvessel density: correlation between ultrasonography and histology of prostate cancer. Eur Urol 2001;40:285–93.

112. Erbersdobler A, Isbam H, Dix K, et al. Prognostic value of microvessel density in prostate cancer: a tissue microarray study. World J Urol 2010;28: 687–92.

113. Feinstein S. The powerful microbubble: from bench to bedside, from intravascular indicator to therapeutic delivery system, and beyond. Am J Physiol Heart Circ Physiol 2004;287:H450–7.

114. Albrecht T, Blomley M, Bolondi L, et al. Guidelines for the use of contrast agents in ultrasound. Ultraschall Med 2004;25:249–56.

115. De Jong N. Mechanical index. Eur J Echocardiogr 2002;3:73–4.

116. Wink M, Frauscher F, Cosgrove D, et al. Contrast-enhanced ultrasound and prostate cancer: a multi-centre European research coordination project. Eur Urol 2008;54:982–93.

117. Mitterberger M, Pingerra G, Horninger W, et al. Comparison of contrast enhanced color Doppler targeted biopsy to conventional systematic biopsy: impact on Gleason score. J Urol 2007;178:464–8.

118. Halpern E, Ramey J, Strup S, et al. Detection of prostate carcinoma with contrast-enhanced sonography using intermittent harmonic imaging. Cancer 2005;104:2373–83.

119. Linden R, Trabulsi E, Forsberg F, et al. Contrast enhanced ultrasound flash replenishment method for directed prostate biopsy. J Urol 2007;178:2354–8.

120. Nelson E, Slotoroff C, Gomella L. Targeted biopsy of the prostate: the impact of color Doppler imaging and elastography on prostate cancer detection and Gleason score. Urology 2007;70:1136–40.

121. Halpern E, McCue P, Aksnes A, et al. Contrast-enhanced US of the prostate with Sonazoid: comparison with whole mount prostatectomy specimens in 12 patients. Radiology 2002;222(2):361–6.

122. Guo Y, Li F, Xie S, et al. Value of contrast-enhanced sonographic micro flow imaging for prostate cancer detection with t-PSA level of 4-10 ng/ml. Eur J Radiol 2012;81:3067–71.

123. Jiang J, Chen Y, Zhu Y, et al. Contrast-enhanced ultrasonography for the detection and characterization of prostate cancer: correlation with microvessel density and Gleason score. Clin Radiol 2012;66:732–7.

124. Zhai L, Polascik T, Foo W, et al. Acoustic radiation force impulse imaging of human prostate: initial in vivo demonstration. Ultrasound Med Biol 2012; 38:50–61.

125. Morelli G, Pagni R, Mariani C, et al. Results of vardenafil mediated power Doppler ultrasound, contrast enhanced ultrasound and systematic random biopsies to detect prostate cancer. J Urol 2011;185:2126–31.

126. Rosenkrantz A, Mendrinos S, Babb J, et al. Prostate cancer foci detected on multiparametric magnetic resonance imaging are histologically distinct from those not detected. J Urol 2012;187:2032–8.

127. Kirkham A, Emberton M, Allen C. How good is MRI at detecting and characterising cancer within the prostate. Eur Urol 2006;50:1163–75.

128. Morre C, Robertson N, Arsnious N. Image-guided prostate biopsy using magnetic resonance imaging-derived targets: a systematic review. Eur Urol 2013;63:125–40.

129. Beyersdorff D, Winkel A, Hamm B, et al. MR imaging-guided prostate biopsy with a closed MR unit at 1.5 T: initial results. Radiology 2005;234:576–81.

130. Hambrock T, Somford D, Hoeks C, et al. Magnetic resonance imaging guided prostate biopsy in men with repeat negative biopsies and increased prostate specific antigen. J Urol 2010;183:520–7.

131. Miyagawa T, Ishikawa S, Kimura T, et al. Real-time virtual sonography for navigation during targeted prostate biopsy using magnetic resonance imaging data. Int J Urol 2010;17:855–60.

132. Schlaier J, Warnat J, Dorenbeck U, et al. Image fusion of MR images and real-time ultrasonography: evaluation of fusion accuracy combining two commercial instruments, a neuronavigation system and a ultrasound system. Acta Neurochir 2004; 146:271–6.

133. Delongchamps N, Peyromaure M, Schull A, et al. Pre-biopsy magnetic resonance imaging and prostate cancer detection: comparison of random and MRI-targeted biopsies using three different techniques of MRI-TRUS image registration. J Urol 2013;189:493–9.

134. Pinto P, Chung P, Rastinehad A, et al. Magnetic resonance imaging/ultrasound fusion guided prostate biopsy improves cancer detection following transrectal ultrasound biopsy and correlates with multiparametric magnetic resonance imaging. J Urol 2011;186:1281–5.

135. Kapoor A, Mahajan G, Sidhu B. Real-time elastography in the detection of prostate cancer in patients with raised PSA level. Ultrasound Med Biol 2011;37:1374–81.

136. Aigner F, Pallwein L, Junker D, et al. Value of real-time elastography in the detection of prostate cancer in men with prostate specific antigen 1.25ng/ml or greater. J Urol 2010;184:913–7.

137. Brock M, Von Bodman C, Palisaar R, et al. The impact of real-time elastography guiding of a systematic prostate biopsy to improve cancer detection rate: a prospective study of 353 patients. J Urol 2012;187:2039–43.

138. Correas J, Khairoune A, Tissier A, et al. Trans-rectal quantitative shear wave elastography: application to prostate cancer: a feasibility study. In: Radiology Congress. 2011. http://dx.doi.org/10.1594/ecr2011/C–1748.

139. Giannarini G, Mogorovich A, Valent F, et al. Continuing or discontinuing low-dose aspirin before transrectal prostate biopsy: results of a prospective randomized trial. Urology 2007;70:501–5.

140. Roehrborn C, Nuckolls J, Wei J, et al. The benign prostatic hyperplasia registry and patient survey: study design, methods and patient baseline characteristics. BJU Int 2007;100:813–20.

141. Moyer V, US Preventive Services Task Force. US Preventive Services Task Force recommendation statement. Ann Intern Med 2012;157:120–34.

142. Paul R, Scholer S, Van Randenborgh H, et al. Morbidity of prostate biopsy for different biopsy strategies: is there a relation to core number and sampling region? Eur Urol 2004;45:450–6.

143. Naughton C, Ornstein D, Smith D, et al. Pain and morbidity of transrectal ultrasound guided prostate biopsy: a prospective randomized trial of 6 versus 12 cores. J Urol 2000;163:163–8.

Office-based Management of Nonmuscle Invasive Bladder Cancer

Joshua J. Meeks, MD, PhD[a], Harry W. Herr, MD[b],*

KEYWORDS

- Bladder cancer • Office-based management • Surveillance • Recurrence • Fulguration

KEY POINTS

- Office-based management of the bladder can be used in low risk-stratified patients to reduce costs and burden of care.
- Smoking cessation and narrow-band imaging may play important underevaluated roles in the future management of bladder cancer.

INTRODUCTION

Bladder cancer is the fifth most common malignancy in the United States, but it is estimated to be the most expensive lifetime cancer due to the high cost of surveillance. In select patients with a history of low-grade and noninvasive tumors, office-based surveillance may be oncologically safe, with significant reductions in cost and complications from operating room transurethral resection (TUR). This article attempts to identify the ideal candidates, as well as management and surveillance strategies of low-grade bladder tumors in the office-based setting.

NATURAL HISTORY OF NONINVASIVE BLADDER CANCER

Over 2.7 million people live with bladder cancer,[1] and over 380,000 incident bladder tumors were identified annually worldwide in 2008,[2] including 73,000 tumors in the United States.[3] In fact, bladder cancer is the fifth most common cancer in the United States. The worldwide age-standardized rate (ASR) for bladder cancer is 10.1 cases per 100,000 men and 2.5 cases per 100,000 women, with a mortality rate of 4 deaths per 100,000 men and 1.1 deaths per 100,000 women.[4] Most bladder tumors identified are nonmuscle invasive (75%–85%). Of nonmuscle invasive bladder tumors, 70% are stage pTa; 20% are stage pT1, and 10% are carcinoma in situ (CIS).[5] The overall rate of recurrence for nonmuscle invasive bladder cancer is 48%,[6] with a range of 31% to 78% at 5 years, ranging from low to high risk.[6,7] In a prospective study of 215 patients from Memorial Sloan-Kettering Cancer Center (MSKCC), low-grade bladder tumors were found to have a recurrence rate of 31% (papilloma), 52% (papillary urothelial neoplasm of low malignant potential [PUNLMP]), and 72% (TaLG), with a median time of recurrence of 72 months for PUNLMP and 18 months for TaLG.[8] Progression occurred in 8% of TaLG patients, with those progressing more likely to have multiple tumors, more frequent recurrences, and require more operative TUR procedures. Progression by grade occurred in 3% of cases, and progression by

Disclosures: None.
Funding: Dr Herr is supported by the Sidney Kimmel Center for Prostate and Urologic Cancers.
Conflicts: None.
[a] Department of Urology, Northwestern University, Feinberg School of Medicine, 303 East Chicago Avenue, Tarry 16-703, Chicago, IL 60611, USA; [b] Department of Surgery, Urology Service, Sidney Kimmel Center for Prostate and Urologic Cancers, Memorial Sloan-Kettering, 353 East 68th Street, New York, NY 10065, USA
* Corresponding author.
E-mail address: herrh@mskcc.org

Urol Clin N Am 40 (2013) 473–479
http://dx.doi.org/10.1016/j.ucl.2013.07.004
0094-0143/13/$ – see front matter © 2013 Elsevier Inc. All rights reserved.

urologic.theclinics.com

stage (T1) occurred in 5% of cases. Progression was heralded by conversion from negative to positive cytology in 71% of cases (12/17).[8] Risk factors for progression include >1 tumor (2-fold increase),[9] recurrence at 3-month cystoscopy,[8,10,11] prior recurrence rate of >1 recurrence per year,[12] and size of tumor >3 cm.[13,14] No patients with PUNLMP or papillomas progressed.[8] Thus, low-grade bladder cancer has a low risk of progression despite a high rate of recurrence.

COST OF MANAGEMENT OF LOW-GRADE BLADDER CANCER

Depending on the model and breadth of features included, bladder cancer has been estimated as the most expensive cancer to health care systems, with a mean cost to Medicare of $96,000 to $187,000 per patient in 2001.[15] In the United States, the total estimated cost in 2006 was $206 billion, with predicted productivity loss of $17.9 billion, and cancer-related morbidity of $110 billion.[16] The majority of the cost for bladder cancer is hospital-based transurethral resection of a bladder tumor (TURBT), estimated to be responsible for 71% of the cost of bladder cancer in the United Kingdom.[17] In a single-institution study, the mean cost per patient with bladder cancer from a period of 1991 to 1999 was $65,158 measured at MD Anderson. The main expense per patient was due to admission ($16,778, 26%) and surgical procedures ($15,781, 24%), with the remaining costs due to surveillance.[18] These prices could be dramatically reduced if patients were managed in the office setting. In a comparison of outpatient TUR (estimated to cost between $2666 and $2113), office fulguration was estimated at only $1167. Routine use of office-based fulguration could mitigate the role of single-dose intravesical therapy after TURBT. Single instillation of postoperative chemotherapy decreases recurrence rates by up to 13%, with possible complications including chemical cystitis. Using Markov state transitional modeling, the cost of office-based fulguration was compared with inpatient TURBT.[19] The cost for outpatient fulguration without perioperative chemotherapy was $1115.21, compared with $3436.34 for inpatient TUR. Using sensitivity analysis, the authors found that with a recurrence rate of >14%, the use of repeated office fulgurations was more cost-effective than perioperative intravesical chemotherapy instillation.

IDENTIFICATION OF PATIENTS FOR OFFICE-BASED MANAGEMENT OF BLADDER CANCER

The critical factor to determine the suitability of office-based management of bladder cancer is an accurate assessment of risk of progression. Although the initial identification of bladder cancer occurs in the office, the authors recommend outpatient TUR with examination under anesthesia for complete and accurate staging. Based on TUR pathology, tumors amenable to office-based management are papillomas, PUNLMP, and TaLG tumors. The main concern with office-based management is missing progression to higher stage or grade, which would warrant greater resection and/or intravesical therapy. No prospective trials have determined the best candidates for office-based fulguration. Donat and colleagues[20] described successful management of low-grade tumors with no recurrence within 6 months of their initial TUR. All tumors were smaller than 0.5 cm, with a negative urine cytology. The risk of progression in this group is approximately 8%.[8] Using data from 2596 patients from 7 European Organisation for Research and Treatment of Cancer (EORTC) trials, risk for individual patients can be calculated. The Donat criteria would suggest a yearly progression risk of 1%, and by 5 years, a progression of 6% (intermediate risk of progression based on http://www.eortc.be/tools/bladdercalculator/).[6] Thus, patients with a risk score of 6 or less would be potential candidates for office-based management.

One of the most important elements of office-based management is the accurate visual diagnosis of papillary or low-stage and -grade tumors. Urologists were able to predict low-grade and -stage tumors using flexible cystoscopy in 93% of cases with 99% accuracy if cytology was included in a study of 144 tumors.[21] In a larger study of over 500 patients, only 5% of tumors were inaccurately categorized as noninvasive by flexible cystoscopy.[22] Yet, series from other institutions suggest that urologists have a lower accuracy to predict grade, with only 26 of 49 (53%) predicted accurately by cystoscopy.[23] Thus, the correct determination of risk by nomograms and visual observation plays a pivotal role in choosing patients for office-based fulguration. The experience of the urologist is a critical factor for successful outpatient management of low-grade papillary bladder tumors.

EFFECTIVENESS AND TOLERABILITY OF OFFICE-BASED MANAGEMENT

Herr described the use of office-based cystoscopy with fulguration in 69 patients with both high- and low-grade lesions, some of which demonstrated invasion.[24] Of the 32% of patients who required TUR, 5 had CIS, and 3 had muscle invasion. Office-based fulguration was the only intervention in 68% of patients, with 30% of patients requiring repeat treatment. In a prospective study of 267 patients carefully selected (as per the Donat criteria), office-based fulguration was the only intervention required in 60% of patients,[20] with a median follow-up of 6.8 years and 2.2% dying of bladder cancer. Patients who underwent TUR (higher risk) had no difference in progression compared with cystodiathermy, suggesting appropriate risk-based management. In a series of 91 patients treated with office-based fulguration with local anesthetic, 12% found it painful, but 90% of procedures were completed within 5 minutes, with none lasting longer than 10 minutes.[25] At 15 weeks, 59% of patients had no recurrence, and only 6% of patients had recurrence at the site of treatment. Wedderburn and colleagues[26] described 103 patients managed with cystodiathermy, with an overall recurrence rate of 49% and 12% recurring at or near the site of treatment. When rated for discomfort, an average visual analog pain scale of mild or negligible was reported by 80% of patients. These data suggest that in carefully selected patients, office-based cystodiathermy can be performed safely and comfortably with reasonable recurrence outcomes.

WATCHFUL WAITING OF IDENTIFIED BLADDER TUMORS

Some patients with small or low-grade bladders tumors may be watched without the need for TUR or cystodiathermy after identification of new tumors. Soloway and colleagues[27] described observation of 32 patients with a mean duration of 10.8 months, and patients undergoing an average of 1.8 interval cystoscopies between treatments (range of 1–5). Importantly, the authors described a tumor growth rate of 1.77 mm per month, with a progression rate of 6.7%. Gofrit and colleagues[28] described the active surveillance of 38 tumors in 28 patients, with surveillance halted for tumor size (9 patients), increased number (19 patients), or hematuria. All tumors were Ta on TUR. The authors noted that if the initial tumor was smaller than 5 mm, the growth rate was significantly less than if the tumor was >5 mm. Pruthi and colleagues[29] described the expectant management of 22 patients with low-grade bladder tumors. Over 25 months, 8 patients had no growth of identified tumors; 9 patients had minimal growth, and 5 patients had moderate growth. Sixty-eight percent of patients required no intervention; 14% required office cystodiathermy, and 18% required TUR. Only 9% of patients had progression, half (1 patient) of whom had stage progression. Thus, watchful waiting may be a strategy to consider in patients with significant comorbidities, on blood thinning agents, and having small tumors of <0.5 cm.

FREQUENCY AND TIMING OF FOLLOW-UP AND TUMOR SURVEILLANCE

No prospective randomized trials have demonstrated sufficient level of evidence to support a specific surveillance protocol for the management of noninvasive bladder tumors. The goals of surveillance would be to minimize the cost and psychological burden of surveillance, tempered by prudent follow-up to prevent growth of tumors necessitating inpatient TUR. From watchful waiting studies, it has been noted that small tumors (<5 mm) may be observed for almost 10 months without intervention.[28] Yet, to prevent an operative TUR, one could argue that repeated cystodiathermy may be prudent at decreased intervals. Thus, cystoscopic tumor surveillance (from the National Comprehensive Cancer Network [NCCN] 2013) is recommended at 3 months and then subsequently at increasing intervals.[30] The European Association of Urology (EAU) recommends a cystoscopy at 3 months, then 9 months, then yearly for 5 years for low-risk tumors.[4] Many urologists manage low-risk tumors similar to higher-risk tumors and perform cystoscopy every 3 months for the first 2 years, every 6 months for 2 years after, and yearly thereafter. Clearly this is an area of future clinical research to determine the appropriate follow-up interval for low-grade tumors to minimize cost and intervention but not increase risk of bulky recurrence.

VOIDED BIOMARKERS FOR SURVEILLANCE

The use of prognostic biomarkers could potentially play a critical role in the management of patients with low-grade bladder cancer. Invasive procedures, such as cystoscopy, could potentially be avoided if a biomarker reliably had a high negative predictive value. There are several biomarkers approved for surveillance by the US Food and Drug Administration. Voided cytology has a long-documented role in the identification of high-grade bladder cancer and can be used to identify patients who require further intervention.[31] The sensitivity ranges from 13% to 75% (median 35%); specificity ranges from 75% to 95% (median 94%).[32] Although a positive cytology is a predictor of high-grade bladder cancer, atypical and suspicious cytologies are more troubling to the urologist without a clear indication for intervention. Limitations of cytology include interobserver variability and artifact associated with fixation. NMP22 is a point-of-care test with a sensitivity ranging from 47% to 100% (median 54%), and a specificity ranging from 55% to 98% (median 78%).[33] The Urovysn fluorescence in-situ hybridization (FISH) has a sensitivity of 70% to 86% (median79%) and a specificity ranging from 66% to 93% (median 70%).[34] BTAstat is a point-of-care marker that can be tested at home by the patient, with a sensitivity of 29% to 74%(median 58%) and specificity of 56% to 86% (median 73%).[35] There are currently no markers that reliably outperform cystoscopy for detection of a bladder cancer recurrence, or have been demonstrated to be more accurate in prospective trials.[32] In a study of patients undergoing cystoscopic surveillance for bladder cancer, 75% described anxiety related to missing cancer from voided markers and desired a test with 95% sensitivity to identify a bladder recurrence to forgo cystoscopy.[36]

ROUTINE IMAGING FOR SURVEILLANCE

Progression of low-grade bladder cancer to upper tract or extravesical tumors occurs at at a frequency of 40% at 15 years, including upper tract and prostate involvement.[37] In low-grade disease, this risk of upper tract progression was 8%, with a median time to development of 29 months.[8] The EAU recommends no upper tract surveillance for low-risk tumors but yearly surveillance for high-risk bladder cancer.[4] The rate of upper tract progression increases yearly, and although routine surveillance should increase detection, only 29% of new upper tract tumors were detected by axial imaging in asymptomatic patients,[38] with the remainder presenting with symptomatic recurrence.

ANTIBIOTICS, PROPHYLAXIS, AND DRUG RESISTANCE

Asymptomatic bacteria is commonly found in elderly patients, and those instrumented for malignancy may be at an increased risk for symptomatic infection.[39] Patients with bladder cancer will undergo many cystoscopies during their lifetime, and unsupervised use of antibiotics to treat colonization rather than infection, even when given for procedural prophylaxis, may result in multidrug bacterial resistance. Routine use of antibiotics is recommended by the American Urological Association (AUA) best practice guideline after cystoscopy performed for bladder cancer surveillance.[40] This recommendation is based largely on best practice. A retrospective study of patients receiving cystoscopy without antibiotic prophylaxis identified a febrile infection rate of 3.5% in patients with infected urine or 1% in patients having uninfected urine.[41] A randomized trial of antibiotics versus no

antibiotics with flexible cystoscopy was halted early due to a low infection rate in the untreated cohort of 0.85%.[42] These data suggest that despite a best practice statement, prudent antibiotic stewardship may lead to decreased prophylaxis use in asymptomatic patients undergoing cystoscopy and will reduce costs.

LIFESTYLE MODIFICATION

One of the most important lifestyle changes the urologist can contribute to the overall health of patients and potentially decrease the rates of bladder tumor recurrence is counseling for smoking cessation. Duration and intensity of smoking are directly correlated to bladder cancer recurrence in patients with noninvasive bladder cancer.[43] Patients report poor knowledge regarding the association with smoking and their bladder cancer, and most describe increased readiness to quit if they knew their bladder cancer was possibly caused by smoking (5-fold greater wish to quit than controls without cancer).[44] The urologist may play a more active role in smoking cessation in the future. Urologists who spent 5 minutes involved in smoking cessation had a 4.6-fold increased rate of smoking cessation and a 7.5-fold increased rate if nicotine replacement was utilized.[45] At 10 years after quitting, smoking cessation decreases the risk of disease recurrence.[46]

Many studies have attempted to determine the utility of supplements to decrease the high rates of bladder cancer recurrence. Despite promising retrospective data on vitamin A, no prospective studies have demonstrated a benefit in decreasing rates of bladder cancer recurrence.[47] Vitamin E and selenium were not demonstrated to improve prevention of bladder cancer in large population-based trials.[48] The probiotic Lactobacillus casei (LC) decreases mutagen and carcinogen production by flora of the gut from ground beef and may potentially decrease the risk of cancer recurrence.[49] Habitual ingestion of Lactobacillus species has been shown to decrease development of bladder cancer in a retrospective case–control series from Japan.[50] In a randomized study of patients with superficial bladder cancer, patients randomized to receive epirubicin instillation plus LC had a significantly lower rate of recurrence at 3 years compared with those receiving epirubicin alone (74% vs 60%, $P=.02$), with no difference in rates of progression or survival.[51]

NARROW-BAND IMAGING

Narrow-band imaging (NBI) is an optical technology that employs filtering of white light into 2 narrow bands (440–460 nm and 540–560 nm) that are absorbed by hemoglobin, resulting in visual detection of increased vascularity with tumors. NBI cystoscopy increases detection of tumors resulting in decreased rates of recurrence of superficial bladder tumors.[52] Unlike other forms of fluorescent-based imaging, NBI does not require instillation of a precursor reagent and only requires a special filter for flexible cystoscopy in the office. In a study of 143 patients, NBI had a greater detection rate for identifying tumors (98% vs 89%, $P=.002$), with similar false-positive detection rates.[53] The major drawback with all forms of fluorescent cystoscopy is the high false-positive rate (36%), resulting in increased number of unneeded TURs.[54] Other drawbacks of NBI include user variability in interpretation of cancer, a learning curve to interpret NBI imaging, and cost of equipment purchase. Herr and Donat followed 126 patients with low-grade tumors using NBI flexible cystoscopy and compared tumor recurrence over a 3-year period in which white-light imaging was used for surveillance. In their study, NBI surveillance resulted in significantly lower rates of tumor recurrence (93% vs 62%, $P=.001$).[55] Randomized trials are underway to determine the impact of NBI-assisted treatments on bladder tumor recurrence rates.

SUMMARY

As more is learned about the biology and natural history of bladder cancer, office-based management is becoming more widely used for low-grade and -stage lesions. Clinical decision making should be based on risk stratification. Low-risk patients can be safely followed on a semiannual or even yearly basis. Patients with high-risk tumors require more stringent cystoscopic surveillance, cytology, and yearly upper tract imaging. Smoking cessation is an invaluable tool to decrease rates of recurrence, and new technology may aid in detection of recurrence.

REFERENCES

1. Ploeg M, Aben KK, Kiemeney LA. The present and future burden of urinary bladder cancer in the world. World J Urol 2009;27:289.
2. Ferlay J, Shin HR, Bray F. GLOBOCAN 2008 v2.0, Cancer Incidence and Mortality Worldwide: IARC CancerBase No. 10 [Internet]. Lyon (France): International Agency for Research on Cancer; 2010. Available at: http://globocan.iarc.fr. Accessed May 29, 2013.
3. Howlader N, Noone AM, Krapcho M, editors. SEER Cancer Statistics Review, 1975-2010. Bethesda (MD): National Cancer Institute; 2013. Available at: http://seer.cancer.gov/csr/1975_2010/. based on November 2012 SEER data submission, posted to the SEER web site. Available at: http://seer.cancer.gov/statfacts/html/urinb.html. Accessed May 29, 2013.
4. Babjuk M, Oosterlinck W, Sylvester R, et al. EAU guidelines on non-muscle-invasive urothelial carcinoma of the bladder, the 2011 update. Eur Urol 2011;59:997–1008.
5. Kirkali Z, Chan T, Manoharan M, et al. Bladder cancer: epidemiology, staging and grading, and diagnosis. Urology 2005;66:4.
6. Sylvester RJ, vanderMeijden AP, Oosterlinck W, et al. Predicting recurrence and progression in individual patients with stage Ta T1 bladder cancer using EORTC risk tables: a combined analysis of 2596 patients from seven EORTC trials. Eur Urol 2006;49:466.
7. Holmäng S, Hedelin H, Anderström C, et al. Recurrence and progression in low grade papillary urothelial tumors. J Urol 1999;162:702.
8. Herr HW, Donat SM, Reuter VE. Management of low grade papillary bladder tumors. J Urol 2007;178:1201.
9. Prout GR Jr, Barton BA, Griffin PP, et al. Treated history of noninvasive grade 1 transitional cell carcinoma. The National Bladder Cancer Group. J Urol 1992;148:1413.
10. Dalesio O, Schulman CC, Sylvester R, et al. Prognostic factors in superficial bladder tumors. A study of the European Organization for Research on Treatment of Cancer: Genitourinary Tract Cancer Cooperative Group. J Urol 1983;129:730.
11. Parmar MK, Freedman LS, Hargreave TB, et al. Prognostic factors for recurrence and followup policies in the treatment of superficial bladder cancer: report from the British Medical Research Council Subgroup on Superficial Bladder Cancer (Urological Cancer Working Party). J Urol 1989;142:284.
12. Schulman CC, Robinson M, Denis L, et al. Prophylactic chemotherapy of superficial transitional cell bladder carcinoma: an EORTC randomized trial comparing thiotepa, an epipodophyllotoxin (VM26) and TUR alone. Eur Urol 1982;8:207.
13. Kurth KH, Schroder FH, Tunn U, et al. Adjuvant chemotherapy of superficial transitional cell bladder carcinoma: preliminary results of a European organization for research on treatment of cancer. Randomized trial comparing doxorubicin hydrochloride, ethoglucid and transurethral resection alone. J Urol 1984;132:258.
14. Millán-Rodríguez F, Chéchile-Toniolo G, Salvador-Bayarri J, et al. Primary superficial bladder cancer risk groups according to progression, mortality and recurrence. J Urol 2000;164:680.

15. Botteman MF, Pashos CL, Redaelli A, et al. The health economics of bladder cancer: a comprehensive review of the published literature. Pharmacoeconomics 2003;21:1315.

16. Sievert KD, Amend B, Nagele U, et al. Economic aspects of bladder cancer: what are the benefits and costs? World J Urol 2009;27:295.

17. Sangar VK, Ragavan N, Matanhelia SS, et al. The economic consequences of prostate and bladder cancer in the UK. BJU Int 2005;95:59.

18. Rao PK, Jones JS. Routine perioperative chemotherapy instillation with initial bladder tumor resection: a reconsideration of economic benefits. Cancer 2009;115:997.

19. Green DA, Rink M, Cha EK, et al. Cost-effective treatment of low-risk carcinoma not invading bladder muscle. BJU Int 2013;111:E78.

20. Donat SM, North A, Dalbagni G, et al. Efficacy of office fulguration for recurrent low grade papillary bladder tumors less than 0.5 cm. J Urol 2004;171:636.

21. Herr HW, Donat SM, Dalbagni G. Correlation of cystoscopy with histology of recurrent papillary tumors of the bladder. J Urol 2002;168:978.

22. Oosterlinck W, Kurth KH, Schröder F, et al. A plea for cold biopsy, fulguration and immediate bladder instillation with epirubicin in small superficial bladder tumors. Data from the EORTC GU Group Study 30863. Eur Urol 1993;23:457.

23. Cina SJ, Epstein JI, Endrizzi JM, et al. Correlation of cystoscopic impression with histologic diagnosis of biopsy specimens of the bladder. Hum Pathol 2001;32:630.

24. Herr HW. Outpatient flexible cystoscopy and fulguration of recurrent superficial bladder tumors. J Urol 1990;144:1365.

25. Davenport K, Keeley FX, Timoney AG. Audit of safety, efficacy, and cost-effectiveness of local anaesthetic cystodiathermy. Ann R Coll Surg Engl 2010;92:706.

26. Wedderburn AW, Ratan P, Birch BR. A prospective trial of flexible cystodiathermy for recurrent transitional cell carcinoma of the bladder. J Urol 1999; 161:812.

27. Soloway MS, Bruck DS, Kim SS. Expectant management of small, recurrent, noninvasive papillary bladder tumors. J Urol 2003;170:438.

28. Gofrit ON, Pode D, Lazar A, et al. Watchful waiting policy in recurrent Ta G1 bladder tumors. Eur Urol 2006;49:303.

29. Pruthi RS, Baldwin N, Bhalani V, et al. Conservative management of low risk superficial bladder tumors. J Urol 2008;179:87.

30. Clark PE, Agarwal N, Biagioli MC, et al. NCCN Clinical Practice Guidelines in Oncology, Bladder cancer, Version 1. 2013. Available at: http://www.nccn.org/professionals/physician_gls/pdf/bladder.pdf. Accessed May 29, 2013.

31. Brown FM. Urine cytology. It is still the gold standard for screening? Urol Clin North Am 2000; 27:25.

32. vanRhijn BW, vanderPoel HG, vanderKwast TH. Urine markers for bladder cancer surveillance: a systematic review. Eur Urol 2005;47:736.

33. Grossman HB, Soloway M, Messing E, et al. Surveillance for recurrent bladder cancer using a point-of-care proteomic assay. JAMA 2006;295:299.

34. Sarosdy MF, Schellhammer P, Bokinsky G, et al. Clinical evaluation of a multi-target fluorescent in situ hybridization assay for detection of bladder cancer. J Urol 2002;168:1950.

35. Kinders R, Jones T, Root R, et al. Complement factor H or a related protein is a marker for transitional cell cancer of the bladder. Clin Cancer Res 1998;4: 2511.

36. Yossepowitch O, Herr HW, Donat SM. Use of urinary biomarkers for bladder cancer surveillance: patient perspectives. J Urol 2007;177:1277.

37. Herr HW. The natural history of a T1 bladder cancer: life-long tumour diathesis. BJU Int 1999;84: 1102.

38. Sternberg IA, Paz GE, Chen LY, et al. Upper tract imaging surveillance is not effective in diagnosing upper tract recurrences in patients followed for non-muscle-invasive bladder cancer. J Urol 2013. [Epub ahead of print].

39. Nicolle LE, Bradley S, Colgan R, et al. Infectious Diseases Society of America guidelines for the diagnosis and treatment of asymptomatic bacteriuria in adults. Clin Infect Dis 2005;40:643–54.

40. Wolf JS, Bennett CJ, Dmochowski RR, et al. Best practice policy statement on urologic surgery antimicrobial prophylaxis. J Urol 2008;179:1379–90.

41. Herr HW. Outpatient urological procedures in antibiotic-naive patients with bladder cancer with asymptomatic bacteriuria. BJU Int 2012;110:E658.

42. Wilson L, Ryan J, Thelning C, et al. Is antibiotic prophylaxis required for flexible cystoscopy? A truncated randomized double-blind controlled trial. J Endourol 2005;19:1006.

43. Rink M, Xylinas E, Babjuk M, et al. Impact of smoking on outcomes of patients with a history of recurrent nonmuscle invasive bladder cancer. J Urol 2012;188:2120.

44. Bassett JC, Gore JL, Chi AC, et al. Impact of a bladder cancer diagnosis on smoking behavior. J Clin Oncol 2012;30:1871.

45. Bjurlin MA, Cohn MR, Kim DY, et al. Brief smoking cessation intervention: a prospective trial in the urology setting. J Urol 2013;189:1843.

46. Rink M, Furberg H, Zabor EC, et al. Impact of smoking and smoking cessation on oncologic outcomes in primary non-muscle-invasive bladder cancer. Eur Urol 2013;63:724.

47. Hung RJ, Zhang ZF, Rao JY, et al. Protective effects of plasma carotenoids on the risk of bladder cancer. J Urol 2006;176:1192.

48. Lotan Y, Goodman PJ, Youssef RF, et al. Evaluation of vitamin E and selenium supplementation for the prevention of bladder cancer in SWOG coordinated SELECT. J Urol 2012;187:2005.

49. Hayatsu H, Hayatsu T. Suppressing effect of *Lactobacillus casei* administration on the urinary mutagenicity arising from ingestion of fried ground beef in the human. Cancer Lett 1993;73:173.

50. Ohashi Y, Nakai S, Tsukamoto T, et al. Habitual intake of lactic acid bacteria and risk reduction of bladder cancer. Urol Int 2002;68:273.

51. Naito S, Koga H, Yamaguchi A, et al. Prevention of recurrence with epirubicin and lactobacillus casei after transurethral resection of bladder cancer. J Urol 2008;179:485.

52. Cauberg EC, Kloen S, Visser M, et al. Narrow band imaging cystoscopy improves the detection of non-muscle-invasive bladder cancer. Urology 2010;76:658.

53. Chen G, Wang B, Li H, et al. Applying narrow-band imaging in complement with white-light imaging cystoscopy in the detection of urothelial carcinoma of the bladder. Urol Oncol 2013;31:475.

54. Herr HW. Low risk bladder tumors–less is more! J Urol 2008;179:13.

55. Herr H, Donat M, Dalbagni G, et al. Narrow-band imaging cystoscopy to evaluate bladder tumours–individual surgeon variability. BJU Int 2010;106:53.

Office-Based Stone Management

Shubha De, MD[a], Manoj Monga, MD[b],*,
Bodo Knudsen, MD, FRCS(C)[c]

KEYWORDS

- Kidney stone • Anesthetic • Sedation • Endoscopy • Surgery • Lithotripsy

KEY POINTS

- A working knowledge of local anesthetics and conscious sedation protocols is important, as many surgical kidney-stone procedures can be performed without general anesthetic.
- Preoperative urinalysis and culture should be routine for patients undergoing genitourinary surgical manipulation, and overt urinary tract infections should receive a full treatment course of culture-specific antibiotics.
- Shockwave lithotripsy can be performed effectively with conscious sedation.
- If a fragment is known to be left behind or is detected on imaging, knowing its significance will help guide management.
- Postoperative protocols for imaging and second-look nephroscopy are surgeon specific, and can range from no imaging/intervention to routine computed tomography and/or nephroscopy.
- Ureteroscopy has become an indispensable tool for the urologist for both the diagnosis and treatment of benign and malignant urologic conditions.
- Patient selection remains a critically important consideration when determining whether to proceed with ureteroscopy and laser lithotripsy under conscious sedation in an ambulatory setting.

As hospital resources are becoming strained, ambulatory surgical centers and day hospitals are being increasingly utilized. For the urologist, a working knowledge of local anesthetics and conscious sedation protocols are important, as many surgical kidney-stone procedures can be performed without general anesthesia (GA). With any anesthesia, the key goal is to maximize patient comfort while minimizing respiratory depression and avoiding prolonged sedation. When using these medications, a working knowledge of emergency reversal, ventilation (bag mask/laryngeal mask airway/intubation), and cardiopulmonary resuscitation is recommended.

GENERAL CONSIDERATIONS

Endoscopic procedures are typically considered to cause mild to moderate pain when performed under local or sedative anesthetic. Modern rigid and flexible endoscopic equipment is more user friendly and better tolerated by patients. A study from Jeong and colleagues[1] compares various modalities of stone surgery under local anesthetic using a 10-point visual analog scale (VAS). Shock-wave lithotripsy (SWL) reported the most pain (6.62/10); retrograde stenting with rigid cystoscopy (4.48/10), semirigid ureteroscopy + lithotripsy (with preprocedural intramuscular midazolam) (3.18/10), and rigid cystoscopy (3.08/10) all

Disclosures: Dr De: No disclosures; Dr Monga: Consultant/Research support - Cook, Bard, Richard Wolf, Fortec, Olympus; Dr Knudsen: Consultant - Boston Scientific, Olympus Surgical; Skills lab instructor - Cook Urological.
[a] Endourology, The Cleveland Clinic, 9500 Euclid Avenue, Q10-1, Cleveland, OH 44195, USA; [b] Stevan Streem Center for Endourology & Stone Disease, The Cleveland Clinic, 9500 Euclid Avenue, Q10-1, Cleveland, OH 44195, USA; [c] Department of Urology, Ohio State University, Columbus, OH, USA
* Corresponding author.
E-mail address: mongam@ccf.org

Urol Clin N Am 40 (2013) 481–495
http://dx.doi.org/10.1016/j.ucl.2013.07.007
0094-0143/13/$ – see front matter © 2013 Elsevier Inc. All rights reserved.

caused mild to moderate pain scores. As such, short-acting intravenous opiates and benzodiazepines can be used; however, with proper preoperative counseling, many patients can tolerate selected stone surgery without GA.

Covered in more detail elsewhere, the protocol of the authors' center involves a 6-hour preoperative fast (2 hours for clear fluids) for most procedures that would be considered moderate sedation/analgesia. At this level patients can purposefully respond to verbal commands while maintaining airway patency and spontaneous respirations. Vital signs are taken before, and every 10 minutes (or less) during the procedure in conjunction with continuous oxygen saturations and respiratory-rate measurements, and electrocardiogram tracings (if cardiac risk factors are present). Commonly used medications include benzodiazepines, and short-acting opioids are given parentally. Intravenous access is established for each patient, and bolus doses are preferred, titrating to the level of discomfort and anxiety.

Postprocedural observation is mandatory for a minimum of 60 minutes, and dedicated nursing staff assesses vital signs, sedation, and pain scores before discharge. Patients are instructed in advance that they will not be able to drive and that someone must be present with them at home over the following 24 hours.

Selection for conscious sedation requires a careful assessment of the patient's medical history and surgical issues. Severe systemic disease, chronic obstructive pulmonary disease, coronary artery disease, congestive heart failure, or difficult airways should all trigger anesthesia's involvement in any planned procedure. The patient's pain tolerance, history of narcotic use, anxiety levels, and specific anatomy should be weighed during consideration for a procedure under sedation. Movement secondary to pain during extracorporeal SWL (ESWL) may reduce efficacy. Similarly, movement during ureteroscopy (URS) could lead to a ureteric perforation, resulting in significant morbidities.

Antibiotics

Preoperative urinalysis and culture should be routine for patients undergoing genitourinary (GU) surgical manipulation. Overt urinary tract infections should receive a full treatment course of culture-specific antibiotics and, if possible, procedures should be delayed until urine cultures are negative.

According to the American Urological Association (AUA) recommendations for preprocedural antibiotics, cystoscopy with GU manipulation warrants prophylaxis for 24 hours or less, or it should be tailored to risk factors. Fluoroquinolones or trimethoprim/sulfamethoxazole as first-line recommendations are well suited for ambulatory surgery; prescriptions given in advance allow oral doses to be taken by patients 60 minutes preprocedure. Alternative antimicrobials are aminoglycosides with or without ampicillin, first-generation or second-generation cephalosporins, or amoxicillin/clavulanate. Percutaneous surgery also warrants antibiotic prophylaxis of up to 24 hours, with first-line antibiotics including first-generation or second-generation cephalosporins and aminoglycosides (with metronidazole or clindamycin). Second-line agents include ampicillin/sulbactam or fluoroquinolones. Updated in 2008, endocarditis guidelines by the American Heart Association state that prophylaxis for routine GU procedures is not necessary.[2]

The 2008 AUA recommendation for prophylaxis for all patients undergoing ESWL was recently revisited.[3] A meta-analysis of 9 randomized controlled trials involving 1364 patients failed to demonstrate reductions in positive urine cultures, urinary tract infections, or febrile episodes.[4] A large prospective trial analyzing 389 patients (with only 2% receiving prophylaxis) identified 1 post-SWL urinary tract infection, no cases of urosepsis, and 11 (2.8%) patients with asymptomatic positive urine cultures.[5] Therefore, with little evidence of benefit, only those with risk factors (advanced age, anatomic abnormalities, poor nutritional status, smoking history, steroid use, immunodeficiency, externalized catheters, colonized urine, distant coexistent infection, and prolonged hospitalization) are now recommended for routine prophylaxis.

CYSTOSCOPY AND STENT INSERTION

Ambulatory cystoscopy can be performed in various settings, including regular procedure beds or dedicated cystoscopy suites with lithotomy-positioning aids with fluoroscopic units and monitors. Undertaken for both the diagnosis and treatment of urolithiasis, procedures can be performed under local anesthetic, regional blocks, or conscious sedation. Flexible cystoscopy, or rigid cystoscopy in women, is considered the least bothersome, and is typically carried out with only topical xylocaine jelly.

Ambulatory ureteral studies can be performed under local or sedative anesthetic, because retrograde/antegrade contrast studies and ureteral stent insertions or changes are procedurally similar to performance under GA. This procedure may precede SWL in patients with a solitary kidney or large stones. The more complicated procedures, or those involving ureteric manipulation, require careful patient selection and attention to preprocedural pain levels, anxiety, and complicating anatomic or pathologic factors.

Both digital and fiberoptic flexible cystoscopes are available. Modern digital scopes have been shown in several head-to-head comparisons to be favored for their color differentiation in shades of red, contrast, resolution, and fine focusing at varying distances.[6]

Stent Size and Diameter

In determining the ureteric length, Kawahara and colleagues[7] prospectively measured the ureters of 151 patients using a 5F ureteric catheter. Multiple regression analysis of surrogate measurements for ureteric length identified that the distance from renal vein to ureterovesical junction (UVJ) on axial computed tomography (CT) imaging correlated the most strongly with actual ureteric length. In this study, height and obesity were less strongly associated with ureteric length, as was also seen by Paick and colleagues,[8] who compared patients' characteristics with intravenous urography imaging. These measurements can easily be performed by noting the slice thickness on the CT study (1, 3, or 5 mm typically), then counting the slices from the renal vein to the UVJ, and multiplying by slice thickness. If, however, a significant amount of tortuosity or redundancy is present, this method will underestimate the length needed.

The authors use 7F double-J ureteric stents, although studies have shown that the diameter of stents does not contribute to symptomology. Distal migration was found more commonly in 4.7F stents than in 6F stents, with no symptomatic or physiologic differences noted otherwise.[9] If performing stent insertions under local anesthetic, pain has been noted when resistance is met at an impacted stone or high-grade obstruction.[10] If this is suspected, a thinner stent may be preselected, along with verbal instructions as to what the patient may feel when negotiating these areas. However, at times smaller stents composed of softer material may buckle or "accordion" when they reach an impacted stone. In this scenario, a larger or stiffer stent may actually slide by the stone more easily, owing to the increased torsional rigidity.

Analgesia

Inadequate analgesia has been associated with poorer compliance with follow-up flexible cystoscopy in the management of superficial bladder cancer.[11] Regular lubrication or lidocaine jelly can be used to aid in scope insertion. Single-application prefilled disposable syringes help lubricate and dilate the urethra while providing topical analgesia to the patient. Penile clamps are used by some to stop backflow while increasing the dwell time for the topical anesthetic to take effect.

A meta-analysis from 2009, comparing 4 randomized trials measuring pain during flexible cystoscopy, showed a significant improvement in moderate pain levels when using 2% lidocaine jelly.[12] Three of the 4 studies showed no difference, yet a significant advantage was found when patients were pooled with a fourth, larger study. Another meta-analysis including 3 additional studies with less severe pain thresholds also failed to demonstrate a clear advantage.[13]

Intravesical lidocaine instillation has also been described as both a therapeutic and a diagnostic tool. Used to help differentiate patients with chronic bladder pain from those with pelvic pain, it has been used by some centers to supplant hydrodistention.

Watching the procedure on the video monitor has shown mild improvements in perceived pain levels and, rarely, worsened discomfort.[9,14,15] Kobayashi and colleagues[16] comment that improved outcomes in their patients were noted if verbal instructions were given to patients, based on when the scope was being inserted and when they were about to traverse the membranous urethra.

Male Versus Female

The short urethra of females makes rigid cystoscopy more accessible, and potentially less painful, than in men. A study comparing VAS pain measures during cystoscopy in women showed similar ratings between flexible (1.4/10) and rigid cystoscopes (1.6/10).[17] Older women may have less sensation, but more friable and delicate mucosal surfaces.[18] Vaginal atrophy can lead to lacerations and bleeding if care is not used in manipulation. The urethral meatus can also be difficult to locate and intubate in postmenopausal women. Atrophy leads to the meatus being displaced posterior to the pubis, requiring blind intubation using the rigid sheath and the obturator (or flexible scope) to reduce trauma.

In men, a significant reduction in postprocedural symptomatology was found 1 week after local anesthetic and flexible cystoscopy (33%), compared with rigid cystoscopy under GA (76%).[19] Of patients who have had previous rigid cystoscopy under GA, only 11% preferred it to flexible cystoscopy under local anesthesia.[20]

Procedure

When rigid cystoscopy is performed on women selecting the sheath of smallest diameter, using adequate lubrication with minimal bladder distention are important in minimizing pain. Room-temperature irrigation, warmed skin-preparation solution, proper draping, and fluid drainage maintain patient comfort and thus reduce anxiety levels. Draping for sterility while protecting patient modesty and ensuring irrigation drains away from the patient will improve comfort and minimize movement. Water-based lubricant is instilled at the meatus before scope insertion to provide urethral dilation and comfortable passage. To minimize discomfort, the authors enter the bladder with the assistance of the blunt obturator and use the 70° lens to visualize the entire bladder with minimal torque.

Women may be placed in lithotomy (for rigid) or frog-leg position for flexible cystoscopy. If hip pain or contractures limit articulation, padding may be used to support the knees in a frog-leg position, or the most flexible leg can be bent (with the surgeon moving to that side of the bed). Both legs can also simply be adducted, or low lithotomy may be more comfortable for some. The meatus can be visualized using the light from the scope to help illuminate the area. If not seen, palpation can help locate its position (typically deviating posteriorly with atrophic vaginitis) while using the other hand to introduce the scope tip. The female urethra angles anteriorly, and can be visualized best when coming out of the bladder with irrigation fully open.

In men the foreskin is retracted and the penis is gripped laterally just proximal to the coronal sulcus, and held on stretch at 45°. The scope tip is introduced after saline irrigation has bled the air out of the system, keeping the lumen centered as the scope is advanced. At the level of the external sphincter, a verbal warning that a pinching sensation may be experienced is important.[16] One study documented that a transient increase in irrigation pressure (by squeezing the irrigation bag) hydrodistends the sphincter, decreasing pain (3.0–1.38/10) when passing a flexible scope through the membranous urethra.[21] Once past the sphincter, anterior flexion allows passage through the prostatic urethra and into the bladder.

A systematic evaluation of the bladder will keep any abnormality organized, especially if multiple lesions are present. Dividing the bladder into anterior, posterior, right/left lateral, and trigone will help organize findings for communication with the patient and documentation. Full retroflexion of the scope will help evaluate the median lobe and the bladder neck. Testing deflection before insertion of the scope will help ensure the scope is not damaged, and confirms which direction of angulation has the greatest deflection. If a high bladder neck precludes the scope being deflected adequately to assess the trigone, rotating the entire scope 180° to have maximal deflection posteriorly may help improve visualization.

Stent Insertion

Most retrograde double-J stent insertions in North America are currently done under GA using fluoroscopic guidance. Stent insertions can also be done under conscious sedation (CS) or local anesthetic, and is well tolerated in many patients.

Acutely obstructing stones may also be stented under local anesthetic, as described in a retrospective review of 46 patients. Rigid or flexible cystoscopy was used to introduce a Sensor guide wire (Boston Scientific) up to the level of the kidney, then a retrograde pyelogram performed through a 5F open-ended catheter. A 6F double-J was then placed (without tether), and postprocedural radiographs were used for confirmation of position. Failures· (5 under local anesthetic) were due to inability to position a wire or stent because of stenotic ureteric orifice or impacted stones, and inability to find the ureteric orifice, while 1 procedure was terminated owing to the patient's discomfort. One stent was malpositioned under GA yet, even accounting for these discrepancies in failure, the cost was 3 times greater on average in the GA group ($30,000 vs $11,000).[10]

Jin and colleagues[22] compared ureteric catheter placement via rigid and flexible cystoscopy (under local anesthetic), finding the latter to afford better comfort in men (VAS: 7.2/10 vs 3.5/10) and lower gross hematuria rates (8.6% vs 25%), with no difference in procedural times. There was no significant difference in the number of successful intubations or in pain levels experienced by women. Though not equivalent to stent insertion, this study does highlight the role of flexible cystoscopy in minimizing morbidity while facilitating intubation of the ureteric orifice.

Stenting without fluoroscopy has also been described, and is often required in situations where patient transfer or radiography are not available (ie, the intensive care unit). A retrospective analysis of a nonfluoroscopy stent-placement technique was found to have equal outcomes and complications in comparison with standard stent placement.[23] In this study, stent placement without fluoroscopy was performed after ureteroscopic stone removal, when the length of the ureter can be measured from the ureteropelvic junction to the UVJ. This distance is then measured on the stent from the proximal curl, and marked on the distal aspect. The wire is then back-loaded through a cystoscope and the stent inserted until the mark has advanced into the ureteric orifice. The wire is then withdrawn 10 cm, and the cystoscope backed out until it is 1 cm distal to the bladder neck. The stent is then released when the most distal tip is visualized, and placement is confirmed by assessing the curl directly.

This technique is only applicable when there is no ureteric obstruction, and length of the ureter is measured with a ureteroscope. This procedure can be helpful in reducing radiation doses in those with significant previous exposures, younger patients, and pregnant women. For most patients, using fluoroscopy while minimizing exposures will facilitate proper stent placement without having to subject the patient to ureteroscopy. As an alternative, ultrasonography can be used to monitor the placement of the guide wire, followed by monitoring the coiling of the renal end of the ureteral stent.[24]

Post–Stent Insertion Symptomatology

Discomfort after stent insertion and understanding of the procedure may be poorly addressed; for this reason written material can help alleviate patients' uncertainties, potentially minimizing the need for emergency phone calls and assessments.[25] The use of as-needed medications can help significantly reduce flank pain and lower urinary tract symptoms caused by refluxing urine and stent irritation. Nonsteroidal anti-inflammatories (NSAIDs), anticholinergics, pyrimidine, and α-blockers can be used alone or in combination.

A randomized placebo-controlled trial comparing pyrimidine and extended-release oxybutynin showed no difference in bothersome symptoms in stented patients between the medication and placebo arms[26]; however, the sample size of this study was small. α-Blockers have been used to help relax ureteric smooth muscle contractions and trigonal spasms. Several studies have prospectively examined the use of α-blockers in stented patients and their effects on urinary tract symptoms, quality of life, and pain.[27–35] Two meta-analyses have been performed, including up to 12 trials, all of which showed significant improvements in the Ureteral Stent Symptom Questionnaire and pain scores.[36,37]

Recently a randomized controlled trial comparing tamsulosin (0.2 mg daily), solifenacin (5 mg daily), a combination of both, or no

medication was performed. International Prostate Symptom Score and pain scores were used, and combination therapy significantly improved both irritative and obstructive symptoms.[38]

SHOCK-WAVE LITHOTRIPSY
Anesthetic Considerations

GA, epidurals, paravertebral blocks, CS, and topical analgesia have all been used in ambulatory ESWL. The first 3 modalities require involvement of and monitoring by dedicated anesthesia staff, and have varying lengths of recovery.[39] Epidural blocks tend to have longer lag times than modern short-acting anesthetic agents.[40] Subcutaneous and intramuscular injection of short-acting (lidocaine) and long-acting (ropivacaine) local analgesics have been studied, and show improvements in pain if administered over the correct area of shock-wave focus, sparing patients the need for systemic agents.[41]

Specific lithotripsy units and characteristics of patient (body habitus, spinal deformations, anxiety, baseline pain tolerance, and so forth) will dictate the pain experienced. Type and position of stones, renal anatomy, and the need for adjunctive procedures (stenting, ureteroscopy, and so forth) must be considered when triaging for GA versus CS. The Hounsfield units (HFU) of stones on unenhanced CT scans may also help predict which patients are better suited for SWL than for endoscopic treatment. In a study reviewing the outcomes of 50 patients with stones smaller than 1 cm undergoing SWL, it was found that stones with HFU greater than 900 had significantly worse stone-free rates than those with HFU of less than 500.[42]

Several studies have implicated that the modality of anesthesia may affect SWL outcomes. Lee and colleagues[43] showed outcome differences were greatest in upper pole stones; however, there was no difference in stones 10 mm or smaller with use of either GA or CS. Zommick and colleagues[44] found equivalent efficacies, while GA was slower and required less fluoroscopy time. Though somewhat contradicted by other retrospective series, one has to consider that modality may play a role in the final outcome of stone treatment.[45]

Topical lidocaine/prilocaine cream (EMLA) has been investigated, and has decreased intraoperative analgesic sedation, improved fragmentation, and decreased patient movement, although it is not effective enough to mitigate the use of intravenous sedation.[46,47] A 3-armed study investigating pain control using preoperative NSAIDs versus morphine versus EMLA showed no significant differences in pain score, and no increased risk of hematoma or hematuria.[48] NSAIDs are commonly used for renal colic, and, lacking gastrointestinal side effects, COX-2 inhibitors may carry a renoprotective effect after SWL, as demonstrated by Park and colleagues[49] in a mouse model. A meta-analysis of 3 randomized controlled trials using NSAID analgesia in modern ESWL therapy showed significant pain reduction equivalent to that seen with opiates.[50]

Several randomized trials investigating a combination of auditory and visual distraction during lithotripsy have noted improvements in the extent of pain and distress of patients.[51–53] Providing self-selected music and/or video has been shown to reduce anxiety, pain scores, and analgesic requirements. Music can be facilitated by providing headphones, isolating the patient from the ambient noise of the lithotripsy suite (even before entry), along with a portable video monitor on an adjustable stand. Once positioned on the lithotripsy table, adjusting the monitor prevents neck strain, and subsequent movement is avoided. Simply providing ear plugs has also been shown to reduce the amount of propofol required during SWL.[54]

Each lithotripter will have unique peak pressures, focal area at skin level, and focal zones, in addition to settings required to fragment stones (number of shocks, energy settings, and duration of treatment). Just as important as understanding the equipment settings is ensuring efficient delivery of the shock waves (SW), which can be significantly affected by coupling issues. To ensure maximal energy transfer from the treatment head to the patient, coupling the two involves using a gel or oil medium. This medium should be similar in density to soft tissue, without air bubbles, yet viscous enough to adhere to both body and treatment head. A study quantifying the air-bubble content of coupling media found that maximal phantom stone fracture was provided by a silicone-based lubricant, and ultrasound gel in which the bubbles had been removed. With media including more air, the efficacy of the SW diminished.[55] When the surface area of the air bubbles was quantified, 2% coverage of the treatment head by bubbles reduced stone breakage by 20% to 40%.[56]

To effectively deliver a shock wave from the treatment head to the stone, the pulse has to travel through fairly homogeneous materials. Heavier coupling agents such as petroleum jelly may negatively affect wave transmission.[57] Ensuring initial and continued contact with the treatment head preserves a maximally air-free transition. When a patient moves, breaking the seal and recoupling without readministering the medium decreases peak pressures by 37% and decreases energy transmission 57%, in turn requiring more shocks for the same stone. Applying liberal amounts of gel to the treatment head and raising the unit to meet the patient's back will initially ensure minimal formation of air bubbles.[56] The patient should be positioned with care before coupling; however, if there is a need for repositioning or the patient decouples, the application process should be repeated.

Imaging

Fluoroscopic guidance during lithotripsy is standard for most units, although in-line ultrasound probes are now becoming readily available. The urologist should be aware of the radiation risk, and take an active role in minimizing exposures. Judicious use of radiation time, positioning the intensifier closer to the patient, standing away from the fluoroscopy head, using last-image hold, and reducing the pulse rate from 30 frames per second (FPS) to 15 fps help reduce total radiation exposure. In addition to surgeon experience,[58] employing experienced technologists has also been shown to improve outcomes while reducing fluoroscopic time.[59]

Radioopaque stones in the kidney and ureter are located just as for any endoscopic procedure; however, F2 is defined by rotating the C-arm to judge the stone's 3-dimensional positioning. This action can be taken purely fluoroscopically or in conjunction with ultrasonography, which may be used to further reduce radiation (ie, in children) or for radiolucent stones. Without ultrasonography, intravenous contrast can be given safely as a bolus or drip infusion to identify filling defects, or retrograde pyelography can be performed.[60,61]

Complications

Anesthetic modality has not changed the risk of complications from SWL. Although there is a theoretically reduced risk of complications of GA from avoiding intubation, no study has been large enough to demonstrate such trends. Hematoma, hematuria, flank pain, skin bruising, ureteric obstruction, urinary tract infection, and sepsis are all possible. Rates of perinephric hematoma range from 1% to 8% with current-generation lithotripters, and a case-matched review of 6172 SWL treatments showed intraoperative hypertension and anticoagulation/antiplatelet use to significantly increase its risk.[62] Almost all can be managed conservatively, without requiring transfusions or additional procedures.

SWL Settings

In controlling the rate and energy levels, several strategies have shown benefits in efficacy and morbidity. In attempts to improve shock-wave delivery, modern machines have increased power ranges, higher peak pressures, and smaller focal zones. Although this has led to greater patient comfort with less focused energy at the skin level, greater hematoma rates and lower stone-free rates have been noted in comparison with the earlier Dornier HM3 lithotripter.[63] Delivering the fastest rate at the highest power for the maximal number of shocks[64] may intuitively improve fragmentation, anesthetic times, and energy delivered, but does not necessarily improve outcomes.

Energy

Priming kidneys with a lower energy level (12 kV) for 100 to 500 shocks, before delivering the balance of 2000 SW at full power (24 kV), was shown to have protective effects with regard to hemorrhagic lesions when tested in porcine models.[63] Whether these priming shocks are given with a 3-minute pause or over a period of approximately 4 minutes, they confer the same benefits, resulting in subsequent treatment-dosed SW being less damaging.[65]

Several clinical studies have approached stepwise protocols for SWL in terms of stone comminution, complications, and functional renal outcomes. The first randomized trial allocated 25 patients to 3000 shocks of escalating energy (starting at 11 kV, increasing by 1 kV every 500 SW to 13 kV), compared with a fixed protocol (13 kV).[66] Stone-free rates were slightly improved, with smaller fragments being produced by energy escalation, and with no differences in complication rates. In 2010, 45 patients underwent escalating (500 SW at 14 kV, then 1000 SW at 16 kV, then 1000 SW at 18 kV) or fixed-energy protocols (2400 SW at 18 kV) with gated rates between 60 and 80 shocks per minute (spm) using the Dornier DoLi-50 lithotripter.[67] Although patients received less total energy in the stepwise arm, they showed better stone fragmentation on 1-month follow-up radiography, and renal injury (assessed by urinary β2-microglobulin and β2-macroglobulin excretion) was significantly reduced, with no significant differences in complication rates.

Rate

In addition to optimizing energy the rate has been studied, generally showing better results with slower shock-wave rates. This finding may be due to faster rates leading to decreased wave transmission, decreased negative pressure components, and less efficient formation of cavitation bubbles.[68,69]

Assessing the conventional 120 spm in comparison with 60 spm, a randomized trial showed improved successful fragmentation for stones larger than 10 mm (44% vs 10.8% fragments <4 mm).[70] For all stones, stone density predicted successful fragmentation, whereas for those larger than 10 mm, density, stone size, patient age, and 60 spm were all significant predictors. No differences in pain, complications, or urinary markers for renal injury were noted, although there was an increase in fluoroscopic time. This rate decrease effectively doubles the treatment time, as a similar number of shocks were delivered in both arms. Several other protocols have been tested, showing that slower rates improve fragmentation, reducing the need for auxiliary procedures without increasing complications. A case-controlled study[71] compared rates of 70 spm and 100 spm, with stepwise energy increases (for both groups) and follow-up imaging at 6 months. The slow-rate group required fewer total shocks in this study (3045 vs 4414; $P<.001$), had improved stone-free rates (67% vs 25.25%; $P<.001$), and had reduced retreatment rates (21.6% vs 45%; $P = .013$). Hospital Costing Department information determined a 50% cost reduction in the slower-rate group (£497 vs £1002, $P = .001$).

SECOND-LOOK PERCUTANEOUS NEPHROLITHOTOMY

Percutaneous nephrolithotomy (PCNL) is now the preferred procedure in patients with large renal stone burdens. Performed mostly under GA in the prone position, stone-free rates from 40% to 95% have been reported, depending on many factors relating to the patient's anatomy, stone burden, stone composition, and surgical expertise.[72]

Ideally a CT scan is available for surgical planning to assess stone burden, renal anatomy, and adjacent structures. Before completion, visual and fluoroscopic survey of all calyces, renal pelvis, and ureter minimizes the risk of leaving significant fragments. However, this is not always possible because of bleeding and poor visualization, hemodynamic instability under GA, sepsis, and so forth. In these cases residual fragments may not be fully appreciated, and even if identified may not be immediately extractable.

If surgery is terminated before completion, or if one is uncertain of the size, number, or location of remaining fragments, postoperative imaging is helpful. Kidney/ureter/bladder radiographs or CT studies are commonly used on postoperative day 1, whereas ultrasonography is technically difficult because of in-field dressings and drainage tubes.

Natural History of Residual Fragments After PCNL

If a fragment is known to be left behind or is detected on imaging, knowing its significance will help guide management. In a study by Raman and colleagues,[73] postoperative CT scans showed residual fragments in 8% of their PCNL cases; 47% of fragments were lower pole, 32% intrapolar, 24% upper pole, and 18% pelvic/ureteric stones. Sixty percent of fragments were smaller than 2 mm and 79% were smaller than 5 mm. All of these patients were treated conservatively, and over the following 32 months 43% required medical care, 61% of whom underwent surgical intervention. Factors predicting fragment-related events were fragments larger than 2 mm and location within the pelvis or ureter.

Assessing economics of expectant management and second-look PCNL, fragments smaller than 2 mm did not warrant routine second looks, as the added cost of the procedure (US $2475) outweighed the cost of expectant management ($690). Stones 4 mm or larger had higher associated costs with expectant management ($4672) owing to the increased percentage of patients who required medical attention/secondary procedures, making second-look nephroscopy economically advantageous in these patients.[74]

Given the belief that any residual fragments in children are significant risks for future stones, Roth and colleagues[75] reported that stone-free goals may be accomplished with second-look and third-look nephroscopy. Stone-free rates were 46% after initial PCNL, 86% after the second look, and 97% after third-look nephroscopy. Children, however, had all procedures completed under GA, and 2 patients required a second placement of renal access.

Postoperative Drainage

On deciding to terminate a case that may require a second-look nephroscopy, it is important to determine whether the same access is adequate. If so, it is imperative that this tract be maintained until the second-look procedure is possible. If the tract is maintained, ureteric access allows straightforward placement of a safety wire. Clinical situations may dictate one's choice of drainage tubes. Brisk bleeding may necessitate a large-bore catheter for balloon tamponade while multiple accesses may allow for placement of a loop nephrostomy tube. Nephroureteral catheters (with both bladder and renal pelvis curls) may be used to help minimize accidental displacement and maintain ureteric access. If external drainage is not necessary, a straight 5F ureteric catheter may be advanced antegradely to the distal ureter, suturing the free end at skin level and tucking the excess under a dressing. As long as a clear tract exists from skin to collecting system, the size of the nephrostomy tube does not affect the accommodation of a nephroscope if the second-look procedure is performed within several days.[76]

Intraoperative/Postoperative Imaging

At the completion of each case the scope should be removed, and on high magnification the kidney should be observed fluoroscopically, manipulating the sheath to ensure it is not obscuring any fragments. If there were initially stones in the calyx entered, the sheath should be backed out under direct vision while inspecting for fragments.

Postoperative protocols for imaging and second-look nephroscopy are surgeon specific, and can range from no imaging/intervention (especially in tubeless techniques) to routine CT and/or nephroscopy. CT scans provide information on residual stone burden, hematoma formation, and renal anatomy. Stone dust may be overcalled by CT, and timing may be important because fragments found immediately after surgery may wash out over time.[77] Therefore, it is important to correlate preoperative and postoperative imaging with intraoperative knowledge of what was fragmented and what may have been left behind. The negative predictive value of fluoroscopy + endoscopy is 100% for fragments 4 mm or larger, 88% for fragments from 2 to 4 mm, and 73% for the smallest fragments. Consequently, more than a quarter of cases that were deemed stone-free at the time of surgery had fragments 4 mm or smaller.[78]

The radiation dose is an important consideration, and should be considered for each patient based on intraoperative findings, gender, age, total number of previous scans, and patient preference. Once a CT scan is performed, the stone burden should be considered based on its risk of passage, possible future need for surgical intervention, risk for future stone growth, patient preference, and technical feasibility via URS, PCNL, or SWL. Routine CT scans can avoid second-look procedures, as only 80% of cases whereby the surgeon believed there were residual stones had stones confirmed on CT. This finding implies that routine CT in patients thought to have residual fragments may reduce second-look procedures in 20% of cases.[78]

Timing

Second-look procedures have been typically performed between 48 and 72 hours postoperatively, the average length of stay being 3.7 days.[75,79] Postponing a second look until hematuria resolves will optimize visibility. If a patient is febrile or shows signs of sepsis, a second procedure should be delayed for 24 hours until the patient is stable and afebrile. Patients with indwelling nephrostomy tubes who are discharged home and brought back after several weeks will have mature tracts; however, unless a large-bore tube is in place, dilation of these tracts will likely be required.

Preprocedure Preparation

In attempting second-look nephroscopy consent should be obtained, clearly outlining any complications that may be encountered. Common morbidities include bleeding/hematuria, infection, discomfort/pain with manipulation, conversion to GA, and need for additional procedures. Hydrothorax is also possible in supracostal access, and may necessitate the placement of a chest tube.

There is no standard approach to second-look nephroscopy; although most surgeons position the patient prone or flank, a posterior approach to patients sitting upright has been described. A Foley catheter is required because of the quick accumulation of irrigation. Scout images and nephrostograms can be acquired to highlight radioopaque stones, renal anatomy, and filling defects. Residual clots may cause filling defects, and retained contrast or sand may appear as radioopaque densities on fluoroscopy, requiring visual inspection. If postoperative imaging is sufficient and residual stones are straightforward with a ureteric-access catheter in place, fluoroscopy can potentially be omitted. In these cases careful inspection of each calyx should be performed, and all stone fragments removed must correlate with post-PCNL imaging to ensure completeness.

Depending on the type of nephrostomy tube present, a safety wire is inserted to the level of the bladder if possible, or curled in the renal pelvis. This maneuver is easily performed when nephroureteral catheters, reentry Malecot nephrostomy tubes, or open-ended ureteric catheters are placed during initial surgery. If only renal drainage is present, a combination of Bentson guide wires (Cook Medical) and straight/angled Glide wires (Boston Scientific) can be used in addition to Kumpe (Cook Medical) or straight/angled Torque catheters (Boston Scientific). Fluoroscopy is then used to guide the wire down to the bladder, and the free end is fixed to the drapes. If a mature tract is present a safety wire may not be necessary to enter the kidney; however, to prevent loss of access while maintaining the ability to place a stent or nephrostomy tube quickly, the authors use a safety wire when working in the upper tract.

Other equipment to have on hand includes an assortment of tipless baskets based on residual stone size. A flexible cystoscope is the main scope used during most second looks, and a flexible ureteroscope can be used for nephroscopy and anterograde ureteroscopy. A Holmium laser with a 200-and 365-μm fiber should be present, in case fragments are too large to be pulled out in one piece. A 365-μm fiber will be adequate for the flexible cystoscope, but is too large for flexible ureteroscopy. Using a semirigid ureteroscope next to, or even through the nephrostomy tube has been described, but requires fragments to be relatively small and in a straight line from the entered calyx.[80] A rigid nephroscope, graspers, and dilation instruments (balloon or rigid) should be available, yet will rarely be used under CS. Stents and nephrostomy tubes predicted to be needed at completion should be present to minimize delays in case closure.

With the nephrostomy tube removed, redilation and sheath placement are rarely required when using a flexible nephroscope. Irrigation is initially maintained at approximately 60 mm H_2O, then adjusted based on visualization. The flexible scope can be introduced next to a safety wire or over a second wire. Once in the collecting system, clots may be present and adherent to mucosa and stones. Hooking up suction tubing to the instrument port allows intermittent irrigation and suction as necessary. Irrigating and grasping clots with endoscopic baskets may reveal associated fragments that are simultaneously removed.

Sheath insertion is not always necessary, but may be helpful in select situations. If the tract is difficult to navigate with a flexible instrument and multiple passes are required, a 24F sheath may be used. Bleeding from the tract will reduce visualization, and inserting the largest sheath size tolerated will minimize blood in the field while maximizing drainage. A reported series of routine second-look nephroscopy without sheaths discovered that 5% of supracostal accesses resulted in hydrothorax requiring chest-tube insertions. This situation prompted the investigators to routinely use sheaths in all supracostal nephroscopies.[79]

Small stones can be removed via extraction of endoscopic baskets. Nitinol tipless baskets allow for negotiation within tight spaces. Time to extraction has been shown to be quickest for stones smaller than 5 mm using the Halo basket (Sacred Heart Medical), and for larger stones using the Zerotip basket (Microvasive).[81] Care should be taken to ensure the stones are seated securely in the basket, ensuring they are not lost within the tract during extraction. When a sheath is not used, fragments remaining in subcutaneous or perirenal tissue could become a source of chronic irritation and infection, and may confuse future imaging.

Laser litholapaxy can be performed during ambulatory nephroscopy. Under CS, involuntary movements, along with renal excursion secondary to respirations, may lead to a challenging environment, increasing the risk of mucosal injury and perforation. Starting at 6.4 W (0.8 J/0.8 Hz) using a flexible nephroscope and 365-μm fiber (or a 200-μm fiber if severe angulation is required), the goal is to fracture large pieces until they are removable by basket.

"Popcorning" fragments is difficult in this setting, as it requires steady laser positioning near a stone to cause fragments to bounce and make repeated contact with the laser. However, if stones are within a large hydronephrotic calyx with a narrow infundibulum, popcorning these stones can be helpful, as fragments are trapped and pieces need to be fairly small to be pulled through the infundibulum. Incision or dilation of stenotic infundibulum during an ambulatory procedure is not recommended, owing to the risk of bleeding and pain.

Gentle anterograde flexible ureteroscopy with laser litholapaxy and basket extraction may also be performed. Several studies have shown that patients tolerate retrograde semirigid and flexible ureteroscopy under local or sedative analgesia without increased morbidity or decreased rate of efficacy.[82,83] If a large volume of stone is present and manipulated during the session, antegrade ureteroscopy will ensure the ureter is stone free. Sand and small fragments can be washed down to the bladder using the ureteroscope. If gravity irrigation is used for nephroscopy and stones are not fragmented, or if the ureter is previously stented, the risk is reduced on wash down. In cases involving steinstrasse or large ureteric stones, GA should be considered during second-look procedures.

Placement of a ureteric stent and nephrostomy tube at the completion of second look are facilitated by having a safety wire in place, although most patients may not need either. Antegrade stenting is best performed with fluoroscopy (to assess the distal curl) and through or beside a flexible nephroscope. If performed through the scope the wire has to be back-loaded into the working channel, and pushers supplied with stents are not of adequate length. In these situations a 5F open-ended catheter can be used to advance the stent to the correct position while confirming that the curl is in the renal pelvis. Stent graspers may be needed if the stent is not placed in the correct position. Advancing the stent alongside the flexible nephroscope can be tricky, as it can be challenging to stabilize the wire and stent if they buckle without a working sheath.

URETEROSCOPY

Ureteroscopy has become an indispensable tool for the urologist for the diagnosis and treatment of both benign and malignant urologic conditions. Although the bulk of ureteroscopy is still performed in an operating-room setting under GA, a role for office and ambulatory procedures with either local anesthesia only, or combined local anesthesia with moderate sedation, in select patients has developed. In these patients the ambulatory setting may provide more convenient care in a cost-effective environment that is easy to access.

Diagnostic Procedures

Jones and Streem[84] first reported office-based cystoureteroscopy using a flexible cystoscope in a select group of patients who had undergone a prior distal ureterectomy and had a patulous neo-orifice. Only intraurethral lidocaine was used, and patients tolerated the procedure well. Visibility was deemed excellent.

Subsequently Reisiger and colleagues[85] reported their experience with anesthesia-free ureteroscopy in the office in the surveillance of patients who had undergone prior endoscopic treatment of upper-tract urothelial cell carcinoma. Of note, these patients had all undergone prior "unroofing" of this distal ureter, which facilitated passage of the ureteroscope in the office.[86] These procedures were performed in the office and were well tolerated by the patients, with 65 of 67 (97%) having a complete survey of the collecting systems including the lower pole. Fluoroscopy was not used, but a prior retrograde pyelogram served as a template of the collecting system. The investigators note that initially they selected patients who had significant anesthetic risk factors for the office-based procedure, but with increasing experience it was offered to a wider range of patients in an effort to reduce cost, time, and inconvenience to patients. Office-based upper-tract surveillance seems a viable option for patients with a history of transitional cell carcinoma.

Ureteral Stones

Indications and technique

Patient selection remains a critically important consideration when determining whether to proceed with ureteroscopy and laser lithotripsy under CS in an ambulatory setting. Patients with a history of sleep apnea, history of difficult intubation, American Society of Anesthesiologists (ASA) physical class score of III or higher, and chronic narcotic use are typically managed with general or regional anesthesia in the operating room.

In men, primarily distal stones are considered for ambulatory procedure under CS, whereas in women mid and distal stones are considered. Although no strict cutoff in terms of size is used, clinical judgment is necessary in selecting patients. In general, solitary stones 8 mm or smaller are considered.

Hosking and Bard[87] first reported the treatment of small (≤5 mm) distal ureteral stones under intravenous sedation with fentanyl and midazolam in 1996. Using a small 6F rigid ureteroscope, they were able to basket-extract the stones successfully in 67 of 70 patients (68 patients had distal stones and 2 were in either the middle or upper third) in a safe fashion. A follow-up study in 2003 compared ureteroscopic stone removal with ESWL, both under CS, for the management of distal ureteral stones.[88] The investigators reported that women tolerated distal URS equally with ESWL, whereas men showed a preference toward ESWL. However, treatment success was higher with URS, at 95% versus only 72% in the ESWL group. In an environment where ESWL had primarily been used for these patients, this technique now provided an attractive, cost-effective alternative.

Subsequent work has demonstrated that ureteroscopy with pneumatic or laser lithotripsy can be safely performed under CS. Rao and colleagues[89] administered diclofenac sodium (75 mg) and promethazine hydrochloride (12.5 mg) 30 minutes before the procedure, then sedated patients with a combination of fentanyl and midazolam at the initiation of the ureteroscopy with lithotripsy. Of their patients, 87.10% deemed the procedure acceptable and only 4.84% reported the procedure as painful. Success rates were highest for distal stones at 97.30%, with 86.66% for upper and 80% for mid-ureteral stones.

Anesthetic considerations

At the authors' institution (The Ohio State University Wexner Medical Center), physicians administering moderate conscious sedation must be first accredited by the institution. This process involves completing a hands-on airway course, demonstrating competencies through computer-based learning modules, and being Advanced Cardiovascular Life Support (ACLS) certified. Nurses, also ACLS certified, administer the medications as directed by the physician and monitor the patient during the procedure. Monitoring includes continuous pulse oximetry, cardiac rate and rhythm assessment, intermittent blood pressure monitoring, and assessment of the relative degree of patient comfort. Patients are administered promethazine hydrochloride, 12.5 mg intravenously, in the preoperative holding area to reduce nausea at the time of the procedure. Oxygen via nasal prongs is used during the duration of the procedure. Once positioned in the procedure area and the surgical time-out is completed, the patient is sedated with a combination of fentanyl and midazolam. Typically 2 mg midazolam and 100 µg fentanyl are used to start the procedure. The patient's response to this dose is evaluated. If the patient is not adequately sedated, or if discomfort is noted during the procedure, additional aliquots of 50 µg fentanyl and 1 mg midazolam are administered. A maximum of 500 µg fentanyl and/or 5 mg midazolam are used. The ratio of fentanyl to midazolam is somewhat individualized. For patients who report primarily pain, a greater ratio of fentanyl to midazolam is used; conversely, if patient anxiety is the primary concern, the ratio of fentanyl to midazolam is reversed. After the procedure is complete, patients are monitored in the postprocedure recovery area for approximately 1 hour until discharge criteria are met.

Technical considerations

Once the patient is adequately sedated, a flexible cystoscope is used to pass a hydrophilic guide wire up the ureter on the affected side. Fluoroscopy is used to confirm the guide-wire placement and the cystoscope is removed. The bladder is then emptied with a 16F straight catheter. An 8F to 10F coaxial dilator is then carefully passed and used to dilate the distal ureteral orifice. Often, a distal stone can be felt as the dilator passes up to it. The 8F to 10F coaxial dilator is then removed. A 7F or smaller semirigid ureteroscope is then carefully passed via the urethra into the bladder and into the distal ureter. The combination of the dilation with the 8F to 10F dilator and the 7F (or smaller) ureteroscope make balloon dilation rarely necessary. The ureteroscope is then carefully advanced alongside the guide wire until the stone is reached. If there is difficulty reaching the stone, such as from ureteral edema, a second hydrophilic guide wire can be passed through the working channel of the ureteroscope to help guide the scope to the target. Once the stone is reached, the guide wire in the working channel is removed. If the stone is very small, basket extraction with a nitinol stone basket may be performed; however, if there is any concern that the stone is too large to easily extract, the authors strongly recommend first fragmenting it with a Holmium:YAG laser. An optical fiber of 365 μm core size is loaded through the working channel and the stone is targeted. Pulse-energy settings of 0.6 J at 6 Hz are used initially and then increased slightly up to 1.0 J at 10 Hz, depending on how hard the stone is. Higher pulse-energy settings increase the degree of stone retropulsion, so using as low a setting as possible that effectively fragments the stone is recommended.[90] Once the fragments are broken into pieces small enough to extract, the nitinol basket is used to pull the fragments out of the ureter. To limit the risk of trauma to the urethra from passing the semirigid ureteroscope in and out, the majority of the fragments are deposited in the bladder. On the last pass, a fragment is captured and removed, and sent for biochemical stone analysis.

The authors do not routinely place stents after uncomplicated semirigid ureteroscopy. After the ureteroscope is removed, a retrograde pyelogram is performed through a 5F open-ended catheter. Pulse fluoroscopic images are obtained. If there is no extravasation and if contrast appears to be draining briskly down to the bladder, a stent is not placed. However, if the procedure has been complicated, such as from an impacted stone, perforation, ureteral injury from the laser, or other similar concerns, a stent should be placed at the completion of the procedure.

At present, the authors' practice is to treat most upper ureteral and renal stones in the operating room. With the use of a ureteral access sheath and liberal basketing of stone fragments, the use of a GA is preferred.

REFERENCES

1. Jeong BC, Park HK, Kwak C, et al. How painful are shockwave lithotripsy and endoscopic procedures performed at outpatient urology clinics? Urol Res 2005;33:291–6.

2. Nishimura RA, Carabello BA, Faxon DP, et al. ACC/AHA 2008 guideline update on valvular heart disease: focused update on infective endocarditis: a report of the American College of Cardiology/American Heart Association Task Force on Practice Guidelines Endorsed by the Society of Cardiovascular Anesthesiologists, Society for Cardiovascular Angiography and Interventions, and Society of Thoracic Surgeons. J Am Coll Cardiol 2008;52:676–85.

3. Wolf S, Bennett CJ, Dmochowski RR, et al. Best practice policy statement on urologic surgery antimicrobial prophylaxis (2008), Updated February 2012. AUA best practice guidelines (2012). Available at: http://www.auanet.org/content/media/antimicroprop08.pdf. Accessed August 1, 2013.

4. Aaronson D, Li P, Forouzeh Z. Antibiotic prophylaxis for shock wave lithotripsy in patients with sterile urine before treatment may be unnecessary: a systematic review and meta-analysis. J Urol 2012. http://dx.doi.org/10.1016/j.juro.2012.08.211.

5. Honey RJ, Ordon M, Ghiculete D, et al. A prospective study examining the incidence of bacteriuria and urinary tract infection post-shockwave lithotripsy with targeted antibiotic prophylaxis. J Urol 2012. http://dx.doi.org/10.1016/j.juro.2012.12.063.

6. Borin JF, Abdelshehid CS, Clayman RV. Comparison of resolution, contrast, and color differentiation among fiberoptic and digital flexible cystoscopes. J Endourol 2006;20:54–8.

7. Kawahara T, Ito K, Terao H, et al. Which is the best method to estimate the actual ureteral length in patients undergoing ureteral stent placement? Int J Urol 2012;19:634–8.

8. Paick SH, Park HK, Byun SS, et al. Direct ureteric length measurement from intravenous pyelography: does height represent ureteric length? Urol Res 2005;33:199–202.

9. Erturk E, Sessions A, Joseph JV. Impact of ureteral stent diameter on symptoms and tolerability. J Endourol 2003;17:59–62.

10. Sivalingam S, Tamm-Daniels I, Nakada SY. Office-based ureteral stent placement under local anesthesia for obstructing stones is safe and efficacious. Urology 2013. http://dx.doi.org/10.1016/j.urology.2012.10.021.

11. Schrag D, Hsieh LJ, Rabbani F, et al. Adherence to surveillance among patients with superficial bladder cancer. J Natl Cancer Inst 2003;95:588–97.

12. Aaronson DS, Walsh TJ, Smith JF, et al. Meta-analysis: does lidocaine gel before flexible cystoscopy provide pain relief? BJU Int 2009;104:506–9 [discussion: 509–10].

13. Patel AR, Jones JS, Babineau D. Lidocaine 2% gel versus plain lubricating gel for pain reduction during flexible cystoscopy: a meta-analysis of prospective, randomized, controlled trials. J Urol 2008;179:986–90.

14. Cornel EB, Oosterwijk E, Kiemeney LA. The effect on pain experienced by male patients of watching their office-based flexible cystoscopy. BJU Int 2008;102:1445–6.

15. Patel AR, Jones JS, Angie S, et al. Office based flexible cystoscopy may be less painful for men allowed to view the procedure. J Urol 2007;177: 1843–5.

16. Kobayashi T, Kamoto T, Ogawa O. Re: office based flexible cystoscopy may be less painful for men allowed to view the procedure: A. R. Patel, J. S. Jones, S. Angie and D. Babineau J Urol 2007; 177: 1843-1845. J Urol 2007;178:2703–4.

17. Gee JR, Waterman BJ, Jarrad DF, et al. Flexible and rigid cystoscopy in women. JSLS 2009;13: 135–8.

18. van der Aa MN, Steyerberg EW, Sen EF, et al. Patients' perceived burden of cystoscopic and urinary surveillance of bladder cancer: a randomized comparison. BJU Int 2008;101:1106–10.

19. Denholm SW, Conn IG, Newsam JE, et al. Morbidity following cystoscopy: comparison of flexible and rigid techniques. Br J Urol 1990;66:152–4.

20. Flannigan GM, Gelister JS, Noble JG, et al. Rigid versus flexible cystoscopy. A controlled trial of patient tolerance. Br J Urol 1988;62:537–40.

21. Gunendran T, Briggs RH, Wemyss-Holden GD, et al. Does increasing hydrostatic pressure ('bag squeeze') during flexible cystoscopy improve patient comfort: a randomized, controlled study. Urology 2008;72:255–8 [discussion: 258–9].

22. Jin X, Li Z, Luo XO, et al. Feasibility and safety evaluation of retrograde inserting of ureteric catheter via flexible cystoscope. Zhonghua Yi Xue Za Zhi 2008;88:1687–9 [in Chinese].

23. Brisbane W, Smith D, Schlaifer A, et al. Fluoro-less ureteral stent placement following uncomplicated ureteroscopic stone removal: a feasibility study. Urology 2012;80:766–70.

24. Fabrizio MD, Gray DS, Feld RI, et al. Placement of ureteral stents in pregnancy using ultrasound guidance. Tech Urol 1996;2:121–5.

25. Joshi HB, Newns N, Stainthorpe A, et al. The development and validation of a patient-information booklet on ureteric stents. BJU Int 2001;88:329–34.

26. Norris RD, Sur RD, Springhart WP, et al. A prospective, randomized, double-blinded placebo-controlled comparison of extended release oxybutynin versus phenazopyridine for the management of postoperative ureteral stent discomfort. Urology 2008;71:792–5.

27. Beddingfield R, Pedro RN, Hinck B, et al. Alfuzosin to relieve ureteral stent discomfort: a prospective, randomized, placebo controlled study. J Urol 2009;181:170–6.

28. Nazim SM, Ather MH. Alpha-blockers impact stent-related symptoms: a randomized, double-blind, placebo-controlled trial. J Endourol 2012;26: 1237–41.

29. Damiano R, Autorino R, De Sio M, et al. Effect of tamsulosin in preventing ureteral stent-related

30. Mokhtari G, Shakiba M, Ghodsi S, et al. Effect of terazosin on lower urinary tract symptoms and pain due to double-J stent: a double-blind placebo-controlled randomized clinical trial. Urol Int 2011;87:19–22.

31. Kuyumcuoglu U, Eryildirim B, Tuncer M, et al. Effectiveness of medical treatment in overcoming the ureteral double-J stent related symptoms. Can Urol Assoc J 2012;6:E234–7.

32. Wang CJ, Huang SW, Chang CH. Effects of specific alpha-1A/1D blocker on lower urinary tract symptoms due to double-J stent: a prospectively randomized study. Urol Res 2009;37:147–52.

33. Navanimitkul N, Lojanapiwat B. Efficacy of tamsulosin 0.4 mg/day in relieving double-J stent-related symptoms: a randomized controlled study. J Int Med Res 2010;38:1436–41.

34. Martov AG, Marsimov VA, Ergakov DV, et al. Tamsulosin administration for prophylaxis and treatment of stent-related symptoms. Urologiia 2010;3–8 [in Russian].

35. Park SC, Jung SW, Lee JW, et al. The effects of tolterodine extended release and alfuzosin for the treatment of Double-J stent-related symptoms. J Endourol 2009;23:1913–7.

36. Lamb AD, Vowler SL, Johnston R, et al. Meta-analysis showing the beneficial effect of α-blockers on ureteric stent discomfort. BJU Int 2011;108:1894–902.

37. Yakoubi R, Lemdani M, Monga M, et al. Is there a role for α-blockers in ureteral stent related symptoms? A systematic review and meta-analysis. J Urol 2011;186:928–34.

38. Lim KT, Kim YT, Lee TY, et al. Effects of tamsulosin, solifenacin, and combination therapy for the treatment of ureteral stent related discomforts. Korean J Urol 2011;52:485–8.

39. Jamieson BD, Mariano ER. Thoracic and lumbar paravertebral blocks for outpatient lithotripsy. J Clin Anesth 2007;19:149–51.

40. Richardson MG, Dooley JW. The effects of general versus epidural anesthesia for outpatient extracorporeal shock wave lithotripsy. Anesth Analg 1998; 86:1214–8.

41. Madbouly K, Alshahrani S, Al-Omair T, et al. Efficacy of local subcutaneous anesthesia versus intramuscular opioid sedation in extracorporeal shockwave lithotripsy: a randomized study. J Endourol 2011;25:845–9.

42. Pareek G, Aremanakas NA, Fracchia JA. Hounsfield units on computerized tomography predict stone-free rates after extracorporeal shock wave lithotripsy. J Urol 2003;169:1679–81.

43. Lee C, Weiland D, Ryndin I, et al. Impact of type of anesthesia on efficacy of Medstone STS lithotripter. J Endourol 2007;21:957–60.

44. Zommick J, Leveillee R, Zabbo A, et al. Comparison of general anesthesia and intravenous sedation-analgesia for SWL. J Endourol 1996;10:489–91.

45. Sorensen C, Chandhoke P, Moore M, et al. Comparison of intravenous sedation versus general anesthesia on the efficacy of the Doli 50 lithotriptor. J Urol 2002;168:35–7.

46. Tiselius HG. Cutaneous anesthesia with lidocaine-prilocaine cream: a useful adjunct during shock wave lithotripsy with analgesic sedation. J Urol 1993;149:8–11.

47. Gallego Vilar D, Garcia FG, Di Capua SC, et al. Topical EMLA for pain control during extracorporeal shock wave lithotripsy: prospective, comparative, randomized, double-blind study. Urol Res 2012;40:575–9.

48. Issa MM, El-Galley R, McNamara DE, et al. Analgesia during extracorporeal shock wave lithotripsy using the Medstone STS lithotriptor: a randomized prospective study. Urology 1999;54:625–8.

49. Park HK, Lee HW, Lee KS, et al. Preventive effects of COX-2 inhibitor, celecoxib on renal tubular injury induced by shock wave lithotriptor. Urol Res 2010; 38:223–8.

50. Mezentsev VA. Meta-analysis of the efficacy of non-steroidal anti-inflammatory drugs vs. opioids for SWL using modern electromagnetic lithotripters. Int Braz J Urol 2009;35:293–7 [discussion: 298].

51. Yilmaz E, Ozcan S, Basar M, et al. Music decreases anxiety and provides sedation in extracorporeal shock wave lithotripsy. Urology 2003;61: 282–6.

52. El-Hassan H, McKeown K, Muller AF. Clinical trial: music reduces anxiety levels in patients attending for endoscopy. Aliment Pharmacol Ther 2009;30: 718–24.

53. Marsdin E, Noble JG, Reynard JM, et al. Audiovisual distraction reduces pain perception during shockwave lithotripsy. J Endourol 2012;26:531–4.

54. Tharahirunchot S, Tatiyapongpinij S, Uerpairojkit K. Effect of noise block using earplugs on propofol sedation requirement during extracorporeal shock wave lithotripsy. J Med Assoc Thai 2011; 94(Suppl 2):S103–7.

55. Jain A, Shah TK. Effect of air bubbles in the coupling medium on efficacy of extracorporeal shock wave lithotripsy. Eur Urol 2007;51:1680–6 [discussion: 1686–7].

56. Pishchalnikov YA, Neucks JS, VonDerHaar RJ, et al. Air pockets trapped during routine coupling in dry head lithotripsy can significantly decrease the delivery of shock wave energy. J Urol 2006; 176:2706–10.

57. Cartledge JJ, Cross WR, Lloyd SN, et al. The efficacy of a range of contact media as coupling agents in extracorporeal shockwave lithotripsy. BJU Int 2001;88:321–4.

58. Chen WC, Lee YH, Chen MT, et al. Factors influencing radiation exposure during the extracorporeal shock wave lithotripsy. Scand J Urol Nephrol 1991;25:223–6.

59. Elkoushy MA, Morehouse DD, Anidjar M, et al. Impact of radiological technologists on the outcome of shock wave lithotripsy. Urology 2012; 79:777–80.

60. Pearle MS, McClennan BL, Roehrborn CG, et al. Bolus injection v drip infusion contrast administration for ureteral stone targeting during shockwave lithotripsy. J Endourol 1997;11:163–6.

61. Buchholz NP, Van Rossum M. Shock wave lithotripsy treatment of radiolucent ureteric calculi with the help of contrast medium. Eur Urol 2001;39:200–3.

62. Razvi H, Fuller A, Nott L, et al. Risk factors for perinephric hematoma formation after shockwave lithotripsy: a matched case-control analysis. J Endourol 2012;26:1478–82.

63. Willis LR, Evan AP, Connors BA, et al. Prevention of lithotripsy-induced renal injury by pretreating kidneys with low-energy shock waves. J Am Soc Nephrol 2006;17:663–73.

64. Bierkens AF, Hendrikx AJ, de Kort VJ, et al. Efficacy of second generation lithotriptors: a multicenter comparative study of 2,206 extracorporeal shock wave lithotripsy treatments with the Siemens Lithostar, Dornier HM4, Wolf Piezolith 2300, Direx Tripter X-1 and Breakstone lithotriptors. J Urol 1992; 148:1052–6 [discussion: 1056–7].

65. Handa RK, McAteer JA, Connors BA, et al. Optimising an escalating shockwave amplitude treatment strategy to protect the kidney from injury during shockwave lithotripsy. BJU Int 2012;110: E1041–7.

66. Demirci D, Sofikerim M, Yalcin E, et al. Comparison of conventional and step-wise shockwave lithotripsy in management of urinary calculi. J Endourol 2007;21:1407–10.

67. Lambert EH, Walsh R, Moreno MW, et al. Effect of escalating versus fixed voltage treatment on stone comminution and renal injury during extracorporeal shock wave lithotripsy: a prospective randomized trial. J Urol 2010;183:580–4.

68. Choi MJ, Coleman AJ, Saunders JE. The influence of fluid properties and pulse amplitude on bubble dynamics in the field of a shock wave lithotripter. Phys Med Biol 1993;38:1561–73.

69. Pishchalnikov YA, McAteer JA, Williams JC Jr. Effect of firing rate on the performance of shock wave lithotriptors. BJU Int 2008;102:1681–6.

70. Burmeister MA, Brauer P, Wintruff M, et al. A comparison of anaesthetic techniques for shock wave lithotripsy: the use of a remifentanil infusion alone compared to intermittent fentanyl boluses combined with a low dose propofol infusion. Anaesthesia 2002;57:877–81.

71. Koo V, Beattie I, Young M. Improved cost-effectiveness and efficiency with a slower shock-wave delivery rate. BJU Int 2010;105:692–6.

72. Delvecchio FC, Preminger GM. Management of residual stones. Urol Clin North Am 2000;27:347–54.

73. Raman JD, Bagrodia A, Gupta A, et al. Natural history of residual fragments following percutaneous nephrostolithotomy. J Urol 2009;181:1163–8.

74. Raman JD, Bagrodia A, Bensalah K, et al. Residual fragments after percutaneous nephrolithotomy: cost comparison of immediate second look flexible nephroscopy versus expectant management. J Urol 2010;183:188–93.

75. Roth CC, Donovan BO, Adams JM, et al. Use of second look nephroscopy in children undergoing percutaneous nephrolithotomy. J Urol 2009;181:796–800.

76. Knudsen BE. Second-look nephroscopy after percutaneous nephrolithotomy. Ther Adv Urol 2009;1:27–31.

77. Portis AJ, Laliberte MA, Holtz C, et al. Confident intraoperative decision making during percutaneous nephrolithotomy: does this patient need a second look? Urology 2008;71:218–22.

78. Portis AJ, Laliberte MA, Drake S, et al. Intraoperative fragment detection during percutaneous nephrolithotomy: evaluation of high magnification rotational fluoroscopy combined with aggressive nephroscopy. J Urol 2006;175:162–5 [discussion: 165–6].

79. Pearle MS, Watamull LM, Mullican MA. Sensitivity of noncontrast helical computerized tomography and plain film radiography compared to flexible nephroscopy for detecting residual fragments after percutaneous nephrostolithotomy. J Urol 1999;162:23–6.

80. Goel A, Aron M, Hemal AK, et al. Simple method of residual stone retrieval through the nephrostomy catheter after PCNL: point of technique. Int Urol Nephrol 2002;34:183–4.

81. Lukasewycz S, Skenazy J, Hoffman N, et al. Comparison of nitinol tipless stone baskets in an in vitro caliceal model. J Urol 2004;172:562–4.

82. Abdel-Razzak OM, Bagley DH. Clinical experience with flexible ureteropyeloscopy. J Urol 1992;148:1788–92.

83. Livadas KE, Varkarakis IM, Skolarikos A, et al. Ureteroscopic removal of mildly migrated stents using local anesthesia only. J Urol 2007;178:1998–2001.

84. Jones JS, Streem SB. Office-based cystoureteroscopy for assessment of the upper urinary tract. J Endourol 2002;16:307–9.

85. Reisiger K, Hruby G, Clayman RV, et al. Office-based surveillance ureteroscopy after endoscopic treatment of transitional cell carcinoma: technique and clinical outcome. Urology 2007;70:263–6.

86. Kerbl K, Clayman RV. Incision of the ureterovesical junction for endoscopic surveillance of transitional cell cancer of the upper urinary tract. J Urol 1993;150:1440–3.

87. Hosking DH, Bard RJ. Ureteroscopy with intravenous sedation for treatment of distal ureteral calculi: a safe and effective alternative to shock wave lithotripsy. J Urol 1996;156:899–901 [discussion: 902].

88. Hosking DH, Smith WE, McColm SE. A comparison of extracorporeal shock wave lithotripsy and ureteroscopy under intravenous sedation for the management of distal ureteric calculi. Can J Urol 2003;10:1780–4.

89. Rao MP, Kumar S, Dutta B, et al. Safety and efficacy of ureteroscopic lithotripsy for ureteral calculi under sedoanalgesia—a prospective study. Int Urol Nephrol 2005;37:219–24.

90. Sea J, Jonat LM, Chew B, et al. Optimal power settings for Holmium:YAG lithotripsy. J Urol 2012;187:914–9.

Office-Based Anesthesia for the Urologist

Ursula Galway, MD[a],*, Raymond Borkowski, MD[b]

KEYWORDS

- Office-based anesthesia • Office-based surgery • Patient safety • Non–operating-room anesthesia
- Preoperative evaluation • Postoperative nausea and vomiting • Postoperative analgesia
- Recovery from anesthesia

KEY POINTS

- Advances in surgical techniques coupled with the development of faster-acting, safer anesthetics allow for more invasive procedures to be performed in an office setting.
- Economic demands to decrease health costs and patients' preference for the nonhospital setting also have contributed to the growth of office-based surgery (OBS), and will continue to fuel its growth in the future.
- It is imperative that we continue to strive to hold the OBS centers to the same standards as ambulatory and hospital settings with regard to patient safety.
- Anesthesia for OBS should be such that the patient recovers quickly with few side effects or pain, and has a timely discharge.

INTRODUCTION

Office-based anesthesia (OBA) is defined as the provision of anesthesia services in an operating or procedure room that is not accredited as an Ambulatory Surgery Center (ASC) by the state in which it operates and is integrated into the day-to-day operations of a physician's office[1]; that is, anesthesia and surgery are being performed in an office setting.

Office-based surgery (OBS) is on the increase. In 2005, 25% (10 million) of all elective procedures performed in the United States were performed in an office setting, twice the number seen in 1995.[2]

Urologic procedures are expected to increase by 35% in the United States as the population older than 65 years increases[3]; at present they make up 5% of all ambulatory procedures.[4]

Current office-based urologic procedures include flexible cystoscopy, transrectal prostate biopsy, urethral dilation, urethral meatotomy, vasectomy, varicocele repair, stone removal, circumcision, transurethral surgery of the bladder, and transurethral needle ablation of prostate lesions.[1]

The growth of OBS can be attributed to advances in surgical techniques, associated with less postoperative pain coupled with the development of rapid-acting, safer anesthetics allowing for more complex procedures to be performed in an office-based facility. In addition, the economic demands to decrease health costs and patient preference for the nonhospital setting have contributed to its growth. The advantages of an office setting consist of a more personal, less intimidating environment for patients, ease of scheduling, lower

Disclosure: Please note that the design and conduct of the work was performed by all the authors. The article has been written, read, and approved by all of the authors; and the material has not been published, whole or in part, nor is it being sent for consideration for publication elsewhere. Neither Dr Ursula Galway nor Dr Raymond Borkowski have any relationship with a commercial company that has a direct financial interest in the subject matter or materials discussed in this article, or with a company making a competing product.
^a Department of Anesthesiology, Cleveland Clinic Lerner College of Medicine of Case Western Reserve, Cleveland Clinic, E/31, 9500 Euclid Avenue, Cleveland, OH 44195, USA; ^b Department of Anesthesiology, Cleveland Clinic, E/31, 9500 Euclid Avenue, Cleveland, OH 44195, USA
* Corresponding author.
E-mail address: galwayu@ccf.org

urologic.theclinics.com

costs, increased privacy, and decreased nosocomial infections.[5] Patients' perception that procedures performed in the office setting are less invasive and, thus, safer, has also stimulated interest in OBS.[6] A survey performed by Coyle and colleagues[7] found that patients report an overwhelming satisfaction with OBA. Identified predictors of satisfaction were lack of pain and nausea, the ability to remember discharge instructions, and having no memory of the procedure. Identified predictors of dissatisfaction were anxiety, pain, vomiting, and inadequate depth of anesthesia.

OBA is not for every provider or patient, nor is OBS appropriate for every surgeon. Because of the remote location of the office setting, proper selection of patients and procedures is imperative. All types of anesthesia ranging from local, monitored anesthesia care (MAC), regional anesthesia, and general anesthesia (GA) can be performed in the office setting. The main priority of OBA is to minimize pain, postoperative nausea and vomiting (PONV), and postprocedure drowsiness, to ensure patient safety and satisfaction, and to provide a speedy discharge home. The disadvantage of office-based procedures lies with patient safety, owing to a lack of uniform oversight and regulation. In addition, the anesthesiologist may have to practice without backup, consultation, or clinical assistance.[8] It is therefore imperative that the surgeon, anesthesiologist, and office staff ensure that the location where the OBA is being administered is safe.

Despite the rapid growth of OBS, it still remains unregulated in many states, and adherence to safety standards may not be uniform. This article focuses on the requirements for setting up a safe office-based practice, patient selection, and anesthetic management for OBS. The degree of evidence in literature in relation to office-based procedures and complications is not as extensive as that on ambulatory and day-case hospital-based surgery. Ambulatory surgery paradigms can be used for guidance in patient selection and management for OBS. Thus, mention is made herein of ambulatory and hospital-based day surgeries in the hope of extrapolating some of their management rationale to office-based procedures. It is safe to assume that patients who does not meet criteria for a procedure at an ambulatory facility should not be considered for OBS.

FACILITY CONSIDERATIONS AND ACCREDITATION

Despite the growing popularity of OBA and concerns about its safety, there is still relatively little oversight. Whereas ASCs are tightly regulated, OBS is limited in its regulatory oversight. Lack of regulatory oversight may lead to OBS being performed in an environment with limited or outdated equipment, inadequate emergency resources, and insufficient policies. The skill level of the person providing anesthesia care may range from a board-certified anesthesiologist or certified registered nurse anesthetist (CRNA) to a surgeon with little or no anesthesia training. At present, only 25 states have issued guidelines to meet safety standards, 14 states require hospital transfer plans for emergency situations, and 9 states require reporting of complications.[9–11] Eleven states now require accreditation through 1 of several agencies to evaluate the office-based practice setting.[11]

The 3 major organizations for accreditation for OBS facilities are the Joint Commission on Accreditation of Healthcare Organizations (JCAHO), The Accreditation Association for Ambulatory Healthcare (AAAHC), and the American Association for Accreditation of Ambulatory Surgery Facilities (AAAASF). These organizations differ in their requirements for reporting of adverse events and peer-review process, credentialing and privileging of practitioners without hospital privileges, and enforcement. Accreditation with these associations is voluntary in most states; however, most third-party payers will not reimburse the OBS facility for procedures performed in a nonaccredited office.[10] The Federation of State Medical Boards issued guidelines in 2002 outlining recommended policies and procedures for physicians performing OBS. The American Medical Association (AMA) has also issued 10 core principles for establishing safety standards in offices, and these standards have been endorsed by state medical boards (**Box 1**).[12] In addition, several professional societies (American Society of Plastic Surgeons, American Society for Anesthetic Plastic Surgery, American College of Surgeons, American Society of Anesthesiologists [ASA]) have issued guidelines and recommendations for improving safety in ambulatory surgery or OBS/OBA.

The establishment, construction, accreditation, and operation of an OBS facility should be in accordance with the local, state, and federal laws.[9] From an anesthesia standpoint the ASA has developed guidelines for OBA (**Table 1**).[13] The ASA states that the anesthesiologist "must satisfactorily investigate areas taken for granted in the hospital or ambulatory surgical facility such as governance, organization, construction and equipment as well as policies and procedures including fire, safety, drugs, emergencies, staffing, training and unanticipated patient transfers." The anesthesiologist must adhere to these guidelines and communicate with the surgeon and staff the need to adhere to these safety guidelines.[13]

- Patient informed consent should be obtained.

- Guidelines and regulation for OBS should be developed according to levels of anesthesia as defined by the ASA.

- Physicians should use the ASA patient selection classification in considering patient selection for surgery.

- Physicians should have proper qualifications such as board certification.

- Physicians should have hospital-admitting privileges or emergency transfer agreement.

- Facilities should be accredited.

- There should be a policy in place for adverse event reporting and peer review process.

- There should be a peer-review process for physician privileging, or a physician may show competence by maintaining core privileging at a licensed hospital or ASC.

- There should be at least 1 physician trained in ACLS/ATLS or PALS immediately available with appropriate equipment. BLS is mandatory for everyone else in direct patient contact.

- Those administering sedation/GA should be appropriately trained.

Abbreviations: ACLS, advanced cardiac life support; ATLS, advanced trauma life support; BLS, basic life support; GA, general anesthesia; OBS, office-based surgery; PALS, pediatric advanced life support.

Adapted from American Medical Association. Office based surgery core principles. Chicago: American Medical Association; 2003. Available at: http://www.ama-assn.org/ama1/pub/upload/mm/370/obscorepri nciples.pdf. Accessed March 1, 2013.

The facility should have a medical director who is ultimately responsible for the facility, the personnel, and observation of all local, state, and federal laws, codes, and regulations. A formal policy and procedure manual should be available to address issues such as provider qualifications, records, documents, quality improvement, professional liability, handling of controlled medications, and policy for clinical care issues. All health care providers should hold a valid license. The anesthesiologist should ensure that the local state and federal regulations concerning the use of controlled medications are followed. A fire safety plan should be in effect, and emergency evacuations rehearsed. The anesthesiologist should ensure the proper storage, ventilation, and backup of operating-room gases. Anesthesiologists should also ensure that the equipment used is fully supported by the manufacturer or qualified service personnel and that backup electrical power is available, along with emergency lighting and protection against electric shocks or hazards. All elements of infection control should be properly practiced.[13,14]

MONITORING AND EQUIPMENT

The ASA OBA guidelines state that there should be appropriate anesthesia equipment that is maintained and current, along with basic anesthesia monitoring. Monitoring is expected to be of hospital standard. **Box 2** describes the ASA statement on equipment for anesthesia in non–operating-room locations.[15] **Box 3** describes the basics of anesthesia monitoring.[16]

PROCEDURE SUITABILITY

Clearly not all procedures are suited to the office. In general, procedures should be of short enough duration and complexity to allow patient recovery and discharge from the facility.[13] The American Society of Plastic Surgeons has recommended that surgical procedures not exceed 6 hours and that all procedures be completed by 3 PM. Procedures more than 6 hours long may be associated with the development of hypothermia and increased risk for deep venous thrombosis.[17] Surgical procedures involving major blood loss, intractable pain, or immobility severe enough to interfere with routine activities of daily living, as well as major intra-abdominal, intrathoracic, or intracranial surgeries, are unsuitable for the office setting.[1,18]

PATIENT SAFETY IN OFFICE-BASED SURGERY

The statistics on morbidity and mortality in OBS are difficult to analyze and compare because of a lack of standard definitions and, thus, of adverse events. In addition, data that are available are conflicting.

Coldiron and colleagues[19] reviewed OBS incidents in Florida over a 7-year period and found 31 reported deaths, 18 associated with cosmetic procedures and 13 associated with medically necessary procedures. Some of these procedures occurred with and some without a licensed anesthesia provider. Seventy-eight percent of the deaths reported occurred following the use of GA for the OBS procedure.

Vila and colleagues[20] reviewed all adverse events reported to the Florida Board of Medicine from 2000 to 2002, and found that the risk of death was 10 times higher in doctors' offices than in ASCs. The

Table 1
American Society of Anesthesiology (ASA) guidelines for office-based anesthesia

Administration and Facility	Clinical Care
Quality of Care	Patient and Procedure Selection
The facility should have a medical director and governing body that establishes policy and is responsible for the facility and its staff	The anesthesiologist should be satisfied that the procedure to be undertaken is within the scope of the facility and the health care practitioners
Policy and procedures should be written and reviewed on an annual basis	The procedure should allow for the patient to be discharged that day
All applicable local, state, and federal regulations should be observed	Patients at too high risk should be referred to an appropriate facility
Health care providers should hold a valid license	Perioperative Care
All operating-room personnel who provide clinical care should be qualified to do so	The anesthesiologist should adhere to the basic standards of preanesthesia care, basic anesthesia monitoring, and postanesthesia care, and guidelines for ambulatory anesthesia and surgery according to the ASA
The anesthesiologist should participate in ongoing quality improvement and risk-management activities	The anesthesiologist should be physically present during the intraoperative period and immediately available until discharge
The basic human rights of patients should be recognized	Patient discharge is the physician's responsibility and should be documented in the medical record
Facility and Safety	Personnel with training in advanced resuscitative techniques (eg, ACLS, PALS) should be immediately available until all patients are discharged home
Facilities should comply with all federal, state, and local laws pertaining to fire, building construction and occupancy, accommodations for the disabled, occupational safety and health, and disposal of medical waste and hazardous waste	Monitoring and Equipment
Correct compliance with laws regarding controlled drugs	See statement on non–operating-room anesthesia locations (see **Table 3**)
	See standards for basic anesthesia monitoring (see **Table 4**)
	Emergencies and Transfers
	All facility personnel should be appropriately trained in and regularly review the facility's written emergency protocols
	There should be written protocols for cardiopulmonary emergencies and other internal and external disasters such as fire
	The facility should have medications, equipment, and written protocols available to treat malignant hyperthermia when triggering agents are used
	The facility should have a written protocol in place for the transfer of patients to a prespecified alternative care facility when extended or emergency services are needed

Based on American Society of Anesthesiologists. Guidelines for office-based anesthesia. Last affirmed October 2009. Available at: http://www.asahq.org/For-Members/Standards-Guidelines-and-Statements.aspx. Accessed March 1, 2013; with permission. A copy of the full text can be obtained from ASA, 520 Northwest Highway, Park Ridge, Illinois 60068-2573.

investigators ascribed this to lack of observance to regulatory controls in doctors' offices.

Domino[21] published results of a review of the ASA closed claims database to compare adverse events after OBA with anesthesia in the ASC setting. The severity of injury for office-based

claims was found to be greater than for ambulatory anesthesia claims. Sixty-four percent of the office-based claims concerned death, versus only 21% of ambulatory anesthesia claims. More than 46% of office-based claims were a result of adverse respiratory events in the recovery period that

---

Box 2
ASA statement on equipment for anesthesia in non–operating-room locations

1. A reliable source of oxygen adequate for the length of the procedure and a backup supply of at least an E cylinder should be present.

2. An adequate source of suction should be present.

3. Scavenging system for scavenging waste anesthetic gases should be present.

4. The following should be present: (a) a self-inflating hand resuscitator bag; (b) adequate anesthesia drugs, supplies, and equipment for the intended anesthesia care; (c) standard ASA monitors; (d) a well-maintained anesthesia machine if inhalation anesthesia is to be administered.

5. Sufficient electrical outlets including an emergency power supply should be present. Also present should be an isolated electric power or electric circuits with ground fault circuit interrupters, if anesthetizing area is deemed a wet location.

6. There should be adequate illumination of the patient, anesthesia machine, and monitoring equipment. In addition, a form of battery-powered illumination should be immediately available.

7. There should be sufficient space to accommodate equipment and personnel and to allow access to the patient.

8. An emergency cart with a defibrillator, emergency drugs, and other equipment adequate to provide cardiopulmonary resuscitation should be present.

9. There should be adequate staff trained to support the anesthesiologist and a reliable means of 2-way communication to request assistance.

10. All applicable building and safety codes and facility standards should be observed.

11. Appropriate postanesthesia management should be provided. In addition to the anesthesiologist, adequate numbers of trained staff and appropriate equipment should be available to safely transport.

Based on American Society of Anesthesiologists. Guidelines for office-based anesthesia. Last affirmed October 2009. Available at: http://www.asahq.org/For-Members/Standards-Guidelines-and-Statements.aspx. Accessed March 1, 2013; with permission. A copy of the full text can be obtained from ASA, 520 Northwest Highway, Park Ridge, Illinois 60068-2573.

---

were judged to be preventable with the use of better monitoring.

Morelo and colleagues[22] demonstrated a disturbing trend. During ASC procedures, 62% of injuries resulted in temporary nondisabling injuries and 21% in death. However, during office procedures 21% of injuries were temporary and nondisabling but 64% resulted in death. Moreover, 46% of injuries occurring in the office were considered preventable, as opposed to only 13% in an ASC. The adverse events that occurred in the office included respiratory (50%), cardiovascular (8%), equipment related (8%), drug related (25%), and blunt needle trauma.

Other studies, however, found that there is no difference in the rates of death and adverse events on comparing office-based procedures with ASC procedures.[23,24]

PATIENT SELECTION FOR AMBULATORY SURGERY

Just as not all procedures are suitable for the office setting, neither are all patients well suited for OBS.

The staff surgeon should be aware of exclusions for OBA, screen the patient for suitability, and forward pertinent health information to the anesthesiologist for review before the day of surgery. Often the anesthesiologist meets the patients for the first time on the morning of surgery, so it is incumbent on the surgeon to ensure that the patient is appropriate for OBA and has undergone appropriate preoperating testing and evaluation. In general, the most suitable patients for OBS are those classified as ASA 1 and 2; however, patients of ASA 3 and 4 may be accepted if their disease states are compensated (**Box 4**).[25] Most recent recommendations and national surveys do not mention ASA grade as an exclusion criterion for office-based surgery.[26,27] There is general consensus that patients of ASA 4 are at high risk for OBS.[28] However, this does not mean that OBS is contradicted, rather that the medical conditions degree of stabilization needs to be stringently assessed and the procedure in question thoroughly considered before accepting the patient for OBS.

One must take into consideration patients' chronic disease states and whether they are

---

Box 3
Standards for basic anesthesia monitoring

1. Qualified anesthesia personnel shall be present in the room throughout the conduct of all general anesthetics, regional anesthetics, and monitored anesthesia care.

2. During all anesthetics, the patient's oxygenation shall be continually evaluated.

   - During administration of GA using an anesthesia machine, the concentration of oxygen in the patient's breathing system shall be measured by an oxygen analyzer with a low oxygen concentration limit alarm in use.

   - During all anesthetics, pulse oximetry shall be used.

3. During all anesthetics, the patient's ventilation shall be continually evaluated.

   - Patients receiving GA shall have continual monitoring of expired carbon dioxide.

   - Alarms to detect and disconnect end-tidal CO_2 should be used.

   - During regional anesthesia (with no sedation) or local anesthesia (with no sedation), the adequacy of ventilation shall be evaluated by continual observation of qualitative clinical signs. During moderate or deep sedation, the adequacy of ventilation shall be evaluated by continual observation of qualitative clinical signs and monitoring for the presence of exhaled carbon dioxide.

4. During all anesthetics, the patient's circulation shall be continually evaluated.

   - Patients receiving anesthesia shall have the electrocardiogram continuously displayed from the beginning of anesthesia until preparing to leave the anesthetizing location.

   - Blood pressure and heart rate shall be determined every 5 minutes.

5. During all anesthetics, the patient's temperature shall be continually evaluated.

   - Patients receiving anesthesia shall have temperature monitored when clinically significant changes in body temperature are intended, anticipated, or suspected.

Based on American Society of Anesthesiologists. Standards for basic anesthesia monitoring. Last amended October 2010. Available at: http://www.asahq.org/For-Members/Standards-Guidelines-and-Statements.aspx. Accessed March 1, 2013; with permission. A copy of the full text can be obtained from ASA, 520 Northwest Highway, Park Ridge, Illinois 60068-2573.

Box 4
ASA physical class

ASA Physical Status 1: A normal healthy patient

ASA Physical Status 2: A patient with mild systemic disease

ASA Physical Status 3: A patient with severe systemic disease

ASA Physical Status 4: A patient with severe systemic disease that is a constant threat to life

ASA Physical Status 5: A moribund patient who is not expected to survive without the operation

ASA Physical Status 6: A declared brain-dead patient whose organs are being removed for donor purposes

Based on American Society of Anesthesiologists. ASA physical status classification system. Available at: http://www.asahq.org/Home/For-Members/Clinical-Information/ASA-Physical-Status-Classification-System. Accessed March 1, 2013; with permission. A copy of the full text can be obtained from ASA, 520 Northwest Highway, Park Ridge, Illinois 60068-2573.

---

compensated and stabilized. Patients with uncontrolled medical problems or those severe enough to require hospitalization after surgery are unacceptable.

Urologic patients harbor the widest range of ages from infants to the elderly. Compared with the "average" patient undergoing surgery, however, they tend to be older and have more comorbid disease states. More than one-third of urologic patients have severe systemic disease, a higher prevalence than that seen in other specialties.[29] Exclusions to OBA are listed in **Box 5**.[17,18,30] **Box 6** lists conditions that have been associated with adverse outcomes in ambulatory surgery.[31]

PREOPERATIVE EVALUATION

The preoperative evaluation should start with a thorough history and physical examination including health history, identification of comorbidities, social and family history, allergies, medications, review of systems, and anesthetic history. The physical examination should include

---

Box 5
Exclusions to OBA

- Unstable ASA 3 or 4
- Myocardial infarction (MI) in past 6 months
- Severe cardiomyopathy or congestive heart failure (CHF)
- Uncontrolled hypertension (HTN)
- Brittle diabetes
- Active multiple sclerosis
- Acute substance abuse
- History of malignant hyperthermia (MH) or strong family history of MH
- Severe morbid obesity (body mass index [BMI] >35 kg/m²)
- Morbid obesity (BMI>30 kg/m²) with poorly controlled comorbidities
- Severe obstructive sleep apnea or chronic obstructive pulmonary disease
- Pacemaker/automatic implantable cardioverter-defibrillator
- End-stage renal disease
- Sickle-cell anemia
- Dementia
- Patient on transplant list
- Recent stoke within 3 months
- Psychologically unstable
- Myasthenia gravis
- Lack of adult escort
- Difficult airway
- Acute illness
- Poorly compensated or incompletely evaluated systemic disease

Adapted from Refs.[17,18,30]

Box 6
Conditions shown to be associated with adverse outcomes in ambulatory surgery

- Congestive heart failure: 12% prolongation of postoperative stay
- Hypertension: 2-fold increase in risk of intraoperative cardiovascular events
- Asthma: 5-fold increase in the risk of postoperative respiratory events
- Smoking: 4-fold increase in the risk of postoperative respiratory events
- Obesity: 4-fold increase in the risk of intraoperative and postoperative respiratory events
- Gastroesophageal reflux: 8-fold increase in the risk of intubation-related adverse events

Adapted from Chung F, Mezei G. Adverse events in ambulatory anesthesia. Can J Anaesth 1999;46 (5 Pt 2):21; with permission.

---

therapies, some of which will undoubtedly be in the office setting.

Chronic medical conditions are more prevalent in the elderly. In patients 70 years or older, hypertension (HTN) is present in 45% to 50%, coronary artery disease (CAD) in 3% to 40%, diabetes in 12% to 15%, and chronic obstructive pulmonary disease (COPD) in 7% to 9%.[34] In a cohort study spanning over 5 years incorporating 1.2 million hospital-based outpatient surgeries, age greater than 85 years was one of the strongest predictors of hospital admission and death within 7 days of surgery.[35] Fleisher and colleagues[24] studied 564,267 patients older than 65 undergoing

vital signs, general appearance, height, weight, and examination of the cardiac and respiratory systems.[17] An airway examination should be performed and documented to include the Mallampati score and assessment of state of dentition, mouth opening, and thyromental distance, and range of motion of the neck. The patient should be informed of nil-by-mouth instructions and anesthetic options (**Table 2**),[32] and of the need to have a responsible adult available at the time of discharge.

Elderly Patients

Between 2005 and 2020 the elderly population is expected to increase by more than 53%,[33] which will result in the growth and demand for surgical

---

Table 2
Guidelines for fasting before surgery

Food Material	Minimum Fasting Time (h)
Clear liquids (water, pulp-free juice, black coffee, carbonated beverages)	2
Breast milk	4
Infant formula/nonhuman milk	6
Light meal (toast)	6
Fried, fatty foods	8

Adapted from American Society of Anesthesiologists Task Force on Preoperative Fasting. Practice guidelines for preoperative fasting and the use of pharmacologic agents for the prevention of pulmonary aspiration: application to healthy patients undergoing elective procedures. Anesthesiology 1999;90:899; with permission.

hospital day-case surgery, ASC, and physician OBS. Age greater than 85 years, prior inpatient hospital admission within 6 months, and surgery at a physician's office identified those patients who were at greater risk of inpatient hospital admission or death within 7 days. The cardiovascular and respiratory response to anesthetics is altered in the elderly by age-induced alterations in pharmacodynamics and kinetics. Chung and Mezei[31] found that the frequency of intraoperative adverse events increased linearly with increasing age, whereas the frequency of postoperative adverse events decreased.

However, elderly patients are at risk for cognitive dysfunction and confusion after surgery, and therefore may benefit from the secure, family environment of an office facility. Canet and colleagues[36] hypothesized that day surgery that minimizes the impact of surgery on daily activities and reduced separation from the home environment may be beneficial to the elderly. Improvements in anesthetic technique now allow patients to return to their baseline state as a result of newer medications with a shorter half-life and quicker elimination. This factor is particularly important in the elderly.

In conclusion, although perioperative complication rates are higher in the elderly, age itself is not a contraindication to OBS. However, elderly patients do require a more thorough preoperative evaluation and management of comorbidities.

Pediatrics

The minimum age in OBA for an otherwise healthy infant has not been established; however, it has been suggested to restrict selection of infants older than approximately 6 months and exclude ex-premature infants because of the risk of apnea. Obviously the personnel who care for children need to be Pediatric Advanced Life Support certified, and the facility needs to have age-appropriate equipment available.[14]

Obesity

Obesity is defined as an excess of body weight 20% greater than ideal body weight, or a body mass index (BMI; calculated as weight in kilograms divided by height in meters squared, ie, kg/m^2) of greater than 30. The obese population poses several issues with regard to ambulatory surgery and OBA. Hypertension, congestive heart failure, respiratory abnormalities, and diabetes are more common in the obese. The prevalence of cardiovascular disease in the obese population is 37%.[37] In addition, approximately 5% of morbidly obese patients have obstructive sleep apnea

(OSA).[38] Obese patients have been shown to have a significantly increased risk of intraoperative and postoperative respiratory events, including bronchospasm and desaturation caused by decreased functional residual capacity.[31] Difficult intubation is more common in the obese population. Patients with a BMI greater than 35 or a BMI greater than 30 with other comorbidities are contraindicated for OBS.

Pulmonary

As mentioned earlier, asthma and COPD both increase the risk of perioperative complications. Patients should be well stabilized before considering OBA. Patients with asthma and COPD should be questioned on the severity of their symptoms, and medication use including steroids and any aggravating factors. Inhalers should be used as usual, and the patient instructed to bring them on the day of surgery. If the patient has worsening symptoms or poorly controlled COPD/asthma, the office is not an appropriate location for surgery.

In general, patients should stop smoking before surgery. Smoking increases airway reactiveness, inhibits ciliary motility, causes poor wound healing, and increases the rate of complications after surgery.

The evaluating physician should inquire about signs associated with OSA such as snoring, chronic fatigue, and daytime somnolence. The prevalence of OSA is estimated to be 2% in women and 4% in men.[39]

Serious long-term effects include an increase in sympathetic tone caused by chronic hypercarbia and hypoxia, which can lead to ischemic heart disease, hypertension, tachyarrhythmias, deterioration in cognitive function, pulmonary hypertension, cor pulmonale, congestive heart failure, cardiovascular accident/stroke, and sudden death.[40]

Patients with OSA, owing to their airway anatomy, are at a higher risk of experiencing airway obstruction during sedation. The upper airway abnormalities associated with OSA can be the same as those that lead to difficult airway management and intubation. Snoring and OSA were found to be independent risk factors for difficult mask ventilation.[41] Difficult intubation was found to occur 8 times more often in OSA patients than in control patients.[42]

The prevalence of OSA is increasing, most likely as the prevalence of obesity and increased testing for OSA occurs. There is insufficient evidence in the literature to offer guidance as to which OSA patients can be cared for in the office.

However, the ASA has published practice guidelines for the perioperative management of patients with OSA. The task force stated that patients with documented OSA may be candidates for OBS if they do not require continuous positive airway pressure, will undergo a minimally invasive procedure, and have limited need for narcotic analgesia.[39]

Neurologic

The evaluating physician should inquire about neurologic diseases such as previous stroke, multiple sclerosis, muscular disorders such as myasthenia gravis, and seizures. Antiseizure medications should be continued throughout the perioperative period. The patients' baseline functional and neurologic status should be documented. Patients with severe neurologic illnesses, uncontrolled seizures, or recent stroke are not candidates for OBA.

Renal

Chronic kidney disease can arise from numerous systemic diseases, HTN and diabetes being 2 common causes. Although patients with chronic kidney disease may be candidates for OBA, dialysis patients are not suitable for OBA.

Hepatic

Common causes of liver disease include cancer, alcohol abuse, infections such as hepatitis C, or autoimmune conditions. Patients with end-stage liver disease, ascites, coagulopathies, and encephalopathy are not candidates for OBA.

Diabetes

With regard to major surgery, diabetes has been associated with an increased risk of perioperative cardiac, respiratory, and infectious complications.[43] However, despite the increased risk of complications in diabetics undergoing major surgery, it is not an independent predictor of morbidity and mortality following day-case hospital and ASC surgery.[44] The comorbidities associated with diabetes such as difficult airway from stiff joint syndrome (decreased mobility of the atlantoaxial joint), silent myocardial infarction (MI), autonomic neuropathy, decreased ventricular compliance, gastroparesis, abnormal blood pressure, and decreased wound healing should be strongly considered before accepting a patient for OBA. In addition, the duration of the operative procedure, anesthesia, and the disrupted meal schedule, along with potential postoperative emesis, could lead to labile blood sugar levels. Intraoperative blood glucose monitoring should occur every 1 to 2 hours.[45] Only stable, well-controlled diabetics should be considered for OBA.

The history should include the type of diabetes (1 or 2), medications (insulin or oral medications), blood sugar control, and the presence of complications and associated disease states arising from diabetes. Patients should be given instructions on how to manage their diabetic medications before surgery (**Table 3**).[45]

Cardiovascular Disease

A thorough cardiac history should be obtained. Patients with an MI within the previous 6 months, severe cardiomegaly, congestive heart failure

Table 3
Preoperative diabetic instructions

Medication	Day Before Surgery	Day of Surgery
Oral hypoglycemics	Continue oral hypoglycemic medications	Hold oral hypoglycemic medications
Insulin	Continue to take usual dose of insulin If prone to nocturnal or morning hypoglycemia, decrease nighttime dose by 20%–30%	Take 75%–100% morning dose of long-acting insulin (Lantus, Levemir) Take 50%–75% morning dose of intermediate-acting insulin (NPH, Lente, Ultralente) 70/30 mixed: replace with intermediate-acting insulin and take 50%–75% of morning insulin dose Short-acting insulin should not be taken
Insulin pump	Continue as usual	Continue basal rate

Adapted from Joshi GP, Chung F, Vann MA, et al, Society for Ambulatory Anesthesia. Society for Ambulatory Anesthesia consensus statement on perioperative blood glucose management in diabetic patients undergoing ambulatory surgery. Anesth Analg 2010;111(6):1382; with permission.

(CHF), or uncontrolled HTN, or patients who have a pacemaker or automatic implantable cardioverter-defibrillator are not candidates for OBA. All cardiac medications should be documented, including those with which the patient is advised to continue on the day of surgery.

The patients' functional class in metabolic equivalents (METS) should also be evaluated. The basal oxygen requirement by the body in its resting state is approximately 3.5 ml/O_2/kg/min in a 40-year-old 70-kg male. This quantity has been designated as 1 metabolic equivalent (MET). The ability to take care of oneself, activities of daily living, is equal to 1 MET. The ability to walk up a flight of stairs or walk up a hill is equal to 4 METS. The ability to perform at least 4 METS of activity indicates a good functional status, thus making the presence of severe underlying ischemic heart disease less likely.

Surgical risk in cardiac patients has been attributed to the type of surgery. High-risk surgery (aortic and major vascular procedures) has a greater than 5% risk of cardiac complications, intermediate-risk surgery (head and neck, orthopedic, intraperitoneal, and so forth) has a 1% to 5% risk of cardiac complications, and low-risk surgery (superficial procedures, biopsies, endoscopy) has a less than 1% risk of cardiac complications.[46] Most office-based procedures would be considered low-risk surgeries.

As per the ACC/AHA 2007 guidelines on the preoperative cardiac workup for noncardiac surgery, patients undergoing low-risk surgery, regardless of their functional capacity, need not undergo any further cardiac testing. However, if patients show signs and symptoms of an active cardiac condition (**Table 4**), further evaluation is required before they undergo any procedure, even a low-risk one.[46] These patients clearly are unsuited to OBA.

Patients who have undergone coronary artery bypass grafting and are asymptomatic have been shown to have a low rate of adverse cardiac events.[34] Patients with cardiac stents pose another problem. If a patient has undergone revascularization of a coronary artery with a stent, serious consideration must be given as to whether antiplatelet (aspirin and clopidogrel) medication can be stopped. Premature discontinuation of antiplatelet medication can lead to an acute stent thrombosis, leading to Q-wave MI.[47] The period of time a patient must be on dual antiplatelet medication differs depending on the type of stent placed.

Patients undergoing balloon angioplasty need to wait 2 to 4 weeks to allow vessel healing before undergoing elective surgery. Those with bare-metal stents need to undergo 4 to 6 weeks of dual antiplatelet therapy to allow endothelialization of the stent. Patients with drug-eluting stents need to complete 12 months of dual antiplatelet therapy to allow for endothelialization of the stent before undergoing elective surgery. If clopidogrel must be stopped for surgery, aspirin should be continued during the perioperative period and clopidogrel restarted as soon as is safe.[47]

In a survey by Mukerji and colleagues,[48] almost half of the urologists surveyed stated they would stop clopidogrel irrespective of its indication, and 40.7% never consulted a cardiologist before stopping clopidogrel.

Table 4
Active cardiac conditions (ACC/AHA)

Unstable coronary syndromes	Unstable angina Acute MI: 7 d Recent MI: 7–30 d
Decompensated CHF	
Significant arrhythmias	High-grade AV block Mobitz 2 AV block Third-degree AV block Symptomatic ventricular arrhythmias Supraventricular arrhythmias including AF with HR >100 beats/min Symptomatic bradycardia New ventricular tachycardia
Severe valvular disease	Severe AS: mean pressure gradient >40 mm Hg, valve area <1 cm^2 or symptomatic Symptomatic MS

Abbreviations: AF, atrial fibrillation; AS, aortic stenosis; AV, atrioventricular; CSF, congestive heart failure; HR, heart rate; MI, myocardial infarction; MS, mitral stenosis.

Adapted from Fleisher LA, Beckman JA, Brown KA, et al. ACC/AHA 2007 guidelines on perioperative cardiovascular evaluation and care for noncardiac surgery. Circulation 2007;116(17):e424; with permission.

Patients with mild CHF should be carefully evaluated before deciding to treat them in the office setting. Patients with aortic stenosis are not candidates for OBA unless only for the most minor noninvasive procedure.

Gastrointestinal

The patient should be questioned on symptoms of acid reflux, dyspepsia, gastroparesis, and regurgitation. Signs and symptoms of reflux increase the risk of aspiration. Patients at high risk for aspiration (severe uncontrolled gastroesophageal reflux disease, gastroparesis, and so forth) are not candidates for OBA.

Prior Anesthetic History

A history of difficult intubation, PONV, poor pain control, and postoperative delirium or combativeness should be ascertained preoperatively. The patient should also be questioned regarding personal or family history of serious adverse anesthetic problems such as malignant hyperthermia or pseudo–cholinesterase deficiency.

Allergies and Social Habits

A history of alcohol intake, smoking, and illegal drug use should be obtained. These patients may be at risk for unexpected withdrawal symptoms following surgery, and have an increased tolerance to anesthetic agents and pain medications. Chronic drug or alcohol abusers are not candidates for OBA.

Medications

All medications and their dosages should be documented. Patients should be instructed on which medications need to be stopped before surgery and which medications need to be continued on the day of surgery (**Table 5**).[49] Management of patients on warfarin should be discussed with their primary physician or cardiologist.

PREOPERATIVE LABORATORY TESTING

At present there are no guidelines for preoperative testing in the OBS setting.[1] Often physicians order tests, as they wish to see what the patients' baseline values are. However, laboratory testing should be directed by findings on history and physical examination. Testing should not be ordered based on age. Although older patients are more likely to have abnormalities on testing, these tests are not as predictive of complications as is information gained from the history and physical.

In 2002 the ASA created a task force to develop a practice guideline for routine preoperative tests. The ASA encouraged that testing be based on information obtained from medical records, patient interview, physical examination, and type and invasiveness of planned procedure. Routine laboratory tests are not good screening devices and should not be used to screen for disease. Patients undergoing minimally invasive procedures may not need tests, and healthy patients do not need testing. A test should only be ordered if its result

---

Table 5
Medication instructions before surgery

Medications to be Taken on the Day of Surgery	Medications to be Held on the Day of Surgery	Herbals and Vitamins	Anticoagulants
β-Blockers	Oral hypoglycemic agents	Vitamin E 10–14 d before surgery	Aspirin: hold for 7 d
Asthma medications	Diuretics	Multivitamins 10–14 d before surgery	Clopidogrel: hold for 5 d (7 d if planning neuraxial block)
Antihypertensives (except ACE inhibitors and diuretics)	ACE inhibitors	Herbals 7 d before surgery	Dabigatran: hold for 3 d
Antiseizure medications	Angiotensin 2 antagonists		Prasugrel: hold for 7 d
Narcotic pain medications			Pletal: hold for 2 d (4 d if planning neuraxial block)
H2 and proton-pump inhibitors			NSAIDs: hold for 3 d (some NSAIDs need to be held longer, eg, Mobic 5 d, Feldene 11 d)
Cholesterol-lowering drugs.			
Cardiac medications			

Abbreviations: ACE, angiotensin-converting enzyme; NSAIDs, nonsteroidal anti-inflammatory drugs.
Data from Muluk V, Macpherson DS, Cohn SL, et al. Perioperative medication management. Available at: http://www.uptodate.com/contents/perioperative-medication-management. Accessed March 1, 2013.

will influence management. In general, test results within 6 months are acceptable if the patient's medical history has not changed. If the patient's condition has changed in the interim, laboratory tests within 2 weeks are more favored. Repetition of laboratory work should be avoided.[50]

Pregnancy Testing

If a patient is found to be pregnant, an elective procedure will more than likely be canceled. A history and physical examination are inadequate to determine early pregnancy. Therefore, all premenopausal women of childbearing age who have not had tubal ligation or hysterectomy should have a preoperative pregnancy test.

Complete Blood Count

A complete blood count should be considered in patients who have a history of anemia, recent chemotherapy, or cardiovascular or renal disease.

Renal Function and Electrolytes

Blood urea nitrogen, creatinine, and electrolytes should be tested in patients with chronic liver disease, kidney disease, and diabetes, and also in patients who are on medications (diuretics, digoxin, angiotensin-converting enzyme inhibitors, and so forth) that may result in electrolyte or renal function abnormalities.

Blood Glucose

Blood glucose should be ordered for all patients with diabetes. It can also be considered in patients on chronic steroid use, as this may alter blood glucose homeostasis.

Prothrobin Time/Activated Partial Thromboplastin Time/International Normalized Ratio

If a patient is currently using anticoagulants such as warfarin or intravenous heparin, a prothrombin time/activated partial thromboplastin time (aPTT)/ international normalized ratio (INR) should be drawn. Clopidogrel and enoxaparin do not cause any derangements in laboratory values. Neuraxial block for surgery (spinal/epidural or nerve block) is not an indication for aPTT and INR testing unless the patient was recently on anticoagulants.

Liver Function Tests

Liver function tests are generally ordered for patients with cirrhosis, alcohol abuse, or malnutrition. However, these conditions alone would preclude the patient from having OBA.

Chest Radiography

A thorough history and physical examination should direct the physician toward ordering a chest radiograph (CXR). The available evidence is not compelling enough to suggest that a CXR is indicated in asymptomatic patients older than 50 years who have no risk factors. Patients with significant risk factors for postoperative pulmonary complications, patients with active pulmonary disease, or those with abnormal lung sounds on physical examination may warrant a preoperative CXR irrespective of age; however, they are unlikely to be candidates for OBA. Patients with COPD, smokers, patients with stable cardiac disease, and patients with recent but resolved upper respiratory tract infections do not necessarily need a CXR.

Electrocardiography

When deciding whether to order an electrocardiogram (ECG), a history of cardiovascular or respiratory disease and type and invasiveness of surgery should be considered. ECG abnormalities may be more numerous in older patients. Patients older than 70 years have a 75% chance of having at least 1 abnormality. However, this may not be predictive of postoperative complications.[51] Age alone should not be a criterion for ordering a preoperative ECG. According to the ACC/AHA 2007 guidelines, an ECG is not indicated for asymptomatic patients undergoing low-risk surgery or for patients who do not have any clinical risk factors who may be undergoing intermediate-risk surgery (Box 7).[46]

TYPES OF ANESTHESIA

Sedation in the office traditionally has been provided by the surgeon or proceduralist. There is a general consensus that OBS procedures using traditional doses of local anesthesia (LA) with oral

---

Box 7
Clinical risk factors

- History of coronary artery disease
- History of compensated or prior heart failure
- History of cerebrovascular disease
- Chronic renal insufficiency
- Diabetes (insulin requiring)

Adapted from Fleisher LA, Beckman JA, Brown KA, et al. ACC/AHA 2007 guidelines on perioperative cardiovascular evaluation and care for noncardiac surgery. Circulation 2007;116(17):e427; with permission.

sedation can sometimes be accomplished without a licensed anesthesia provider. Sedation administered by surgeons for procedures has been well documented in the literature. However, the fine line between conscious and deep sedation is ever evident. Published reports of patients receiving 300 µg fentanyl with 10 mg midazolam by a surgeon for office-based urologic procedures without the use of pulse oximetry or capnography may be abhorrent to an anesthesiologist, but was the practice in some offices.[52] Complex procedures and patients with comorbidities probably warrant the presence of an anesthesiologist in an OBS setting.[1] There are many ways to administer anesthesia in the office-based setting, from LA only to minimal/moderate sedation, moderate to deep sedation, to GA. For certain procedures, regional or neuraxial anesthesia may be provided.

Local Anesthesia

The use of local infiltration of LA coupled with some degree of sedation is often enough for office-based procedures. LA provides excellent analgesia for the procedure and postoperative pain control. One advantage of local infiltration is the elimination of PONV as a potential complication.

Sedation

Sedation and analgesia comprise a continuum of states ranging from minimal sedation to GA. The ASA define the continuum of depth of sedation as shown in **Box 8**.[53] Because sedation is a continuum, it is not always possible to predict how a patient will respond. Those intending to produce a given level of sedation should be able to rescue patients whose level of sedation becomes deeper than intended. Rescue implies airway management, returning to the previous level of sedation and halting the procedure until the patient returns to the required depth of sedation.

Monitored Anesthesia Care

The term MAC is defined by the ASA as "a specific anesthesia service for a diagnostic or therapeutic procedure"; that is, sedation performed and supervised by a qualified anesthesia provider.[54] Many procedures performed in the office setting are amenable to MAC with or without supplemental LA administered by the surgeon. Performing MAC requires attentiveness to the entire procedure, as the depth of sedation needs to be tailored to the ever-changing level of surgical stimulation. Therefore, MAC is an anesthesiology service that uses the anesthesia providers' expertise

---

Box 8
ASA definition of continuum of sedation

- *Analgesia/Minimal Sedation (Anxiolysis)*. A drug-induced state during which patients respond normally to verbal commands. Although cognitive function and coordination may be impaired, ventilatory and cardiovascular functions are unaffected.

- *Moderate Sedation/Analgesia (Conscious Sedation)*. A drug-induced depression of consciousness during which patients respond purposefully to verbal commands, either alone or accompanied by light tactile stimulation. No interventions are required to maintain a patent airway, and spontaneous ventilation is adequate. Cardiovascular function is usually maintained. Moderate sedation is often provided by non–anesthesia-trained doctors to sedate patients for procedures.

- *Deep Sedation/Analgesia*. A drug-induced depression of consciousness during which patients cannot be easily aroused but respond purposefully following repeated or painful stimulation. The ability to independently maintain ventilatory function may be impaired. Patients may require assistance in maintaining a patent airway, and spontaneous ventilation may be inadequate. Cardiovascular function is usually maintained.

- *General Anesthesia*. A drug-induced loss of consciousness during which patients are not arousable, even by painful stimulation. The ability to independently maintain ventilatory function is often impaired. Patients often require assistance in maintaining a patent airway, and positive-pressure ventilation may be required because of depressed spontaneous ventilation or drug-induced depression of neuromuscular function. Cardiovascular function may be impaired.

Based on American Society of Anesthesiologists. Guidelines for office-based anesthesia. Last affirmed October 2009. Available at: http://www.asahq.org/For-Members/Standards-Guidelines-and-Statements.aspx. Accessed March 1, 2012; with permission. A copy of the full text can be obtained from ASA, 520 Northwest Highway, Park Ridge, Illinois 60068-2573.

---

to safely sedate a patient for a procedure, be it minimal, moderate, deep, or GA.[54]

A surgeon, anesthesiologist, or patient may prefer MAC over GA because of perceived lighter doses of medications, quicker recovery, and improved safety. The ASA closed claims database shows that although there are fewer MAC than GA claims (121 vs 1519), 40% of the MAC claims were for death or permanent brain injury. Injuries from

MAC arose from oversedation leading to hypoxia as a result of respiratory depression.[55] This percentage is similar to that of GA. Deciding between MAC and GA depends on the surgery being performed, the comfort level of the surgeon and anesthesiologist, and patient preference.

General Anesthesia

GA may be necessary for the procedure or patient/surgeon preference. The anesthetic technique chosen should allow rapid recovery to baseline functions with little PONV, have a high safety profile, and be cost effective. Patients on chronic pain medications, those with anxiety disorders, or those who have tremors may not be able to lie still even with the use of MAC, in which case GA is warranted.

The advantages of GA include patient immobility and control of the airway. Disadvantages included the potential for coughing on emergence, PONV, higher doses of intravenous medications, a longer recovery period, and postoperative disorientation. Maintenance of anesthesia can be accomplished with volatile inhaled anesthetic, total intravenous anesthesia (TIVA), or a balanced anesthesia technique.

The compact size and portability of an intravenous infusion pump have made TIVA a popular choice for small offices because it minimizes the need for bulky anesthesia equipment, a scavenging system, and a malignant hyperthermia (MH) cart. However, if succinylcholine is to be used, MH supplies need to be available on site.[14] TIVA usually comprises a propofol infusion with a benzodiazepine and an opioid. Often, short-acting narcotic infusions such as remifentanil or alfentanil are used. A propofol infusion provides the advantage of being of quick onset and offset, rapidly titratable, and with little PONV. If inhalation anesthetics are to be used, recovery from an insoluble agent such as desflurane, which are more quickly eliminated when discontinued in comparison with more soluble agents such as sevoflurane or isoflurane, should be considered for maintenance of anesthesia.[56]

General Anesthesia with Laryngeal Mask Airway Versus General Anesthesia with Endotracheal Tube

After the induction of GA, an endotracheal tube or a laryngeal mask airway (LMA) can be used to secure the airway.

The LMA will provide the ability to either mechanically ventilate the patient or allow the patient to breathe spontaneously. It does not adequately protect from the aspiration of gastric content. An LMA causes less cardiovascular response than an endotracheal tube on insertion, and allows for a smoother emergence from anesthesia with less coughing. In a study by Higgins and colleagues[57] the use of an LMA for a general anesthetic was associated with a postoperative sore throat in 18% of patients, compared with a rate of 45% in patients who received an endotracheal tube.

An endotracheal tube ensures airway protection from aspiration of stomach contents and secretions. However, it is associated with a greater cardiovascular response during insertion and removal. In addition, because of airway reflexes it is more likely to produce a cough on emergence from anesthesia, leading to an increase in intra-abdominal pressure and possible suture-line failure. An endotracheal tube, for the most part, requires neuromuscular blockade for insertion, whereas an LMA does not.

Regional Anesthesia

Little has been written on the use of regional anesthesia, neuraxial blockade (spinal or epidural), or peripheral nerve block in the office setting. The advantages of regional anesthesia include the avoidance of GA and its potential side effects, a reduction in medications needed for anxiolysis or sedation, and adequate postoperative pain relief leading to reduced recovery time. Potential disadvantages include the risk of LA toxicity and potential nerve damage.

Placement of peripheral nerve blocks has trended toward the use of ultrasound guidance for block placement. This technique allows for direct visualization of the nervous and vascular structures, and continual observation of placement of the needle tip, allowing LA to be directly deposited in the correct areas and its spread observed. However, not all anesthesiologist are equipped with the skill set required to perform blocks under ultrasound guidance, and it may be technically difficult to perform blocks without an assistant. Therefore a single anesthesiologist working in an office setting may not be able to offer this type of anesthesia.

The selection of LA to be used depends on the desired duration of action and degree of motor blockage in addition to the onset time and safety profile. Frequently used LA includes lidocaine and mepivacaine, which are associated with a quick onset but a shorter duration of action. Bupivacaine is associated with a longer onset and duration of action, but has more severe cardiovascular side effects if injected intravascularly. Ropivacaine has a longer duration of action than lidocaine or mepivacaine, with a safer side-effect profile than bupivacaine.

LA toxicity can occur with the intravascular administration of any local anesthetic. If amide LAs are being used, the practitioner should consider having 20% lipid infusion (Intralipid) available to reverse local anesthetic toxicity should intravascular injection occur.[58]

POSTOPERATIVE NAUSEA AND VOMITING

One of the undesirable outcomes of anesthesia is PONV. Postoperatively these symptoms can lead to increased length of stay in the postanesthesia care unit (PACU), expanded nursing care, and decreased patient satisfaction. It has been shown that 0.1% to 0.2% of unanticipated postoperative hospital admissions occur as a result of severe PONV. In addition, adverse events such as aspiration, suture dehiscence, or even esophageal rupture have been attributed to PONV symptoms. Untreated PONV occurs in 20% to 30% of the general surgical population and in up to 70% to 80% of high-risk patients.[59]

Risk factors for PONV can be divided into 3 groups: patient, anesthetic, and surgical.

Patient factors, which are considered to be independent predictors of PONV, include female gender, nonsmoking status, and a history of PONV or motion sickness. Use of volatile anesthetics, nitrous oxide, and opioids has all been shown to be associated with an increased incidence of PONV. Surgical risk factors include the type of surgery being performed as well as the duration of surgery. Gynecologic, abdominal, and laparoscopic surgery has the highest incidence of PONV, and it has been shown that each 30-minute increase in the duration of surgery increases the risk of PONV by 60%.[59]

The onset of PONV symptoms can be decreased by reducing or avoiding the risk factors previously stated and the administration of prophylactic medications. One method of reduction of baseline factors can be achieved by changing the type of anesthesia or anesthetic agents used. The risk of PONV is 9 times less in those receiving regional anesthesia than in those receiving GA; thus, if feasible, regional anesthesia should be used instead of GA. Because volatile anesthetics and nitrous oxide have been shown to increase the occurrence of PONV, the use of an alternative technique, TIVA with propofol, should be considered. The minimization of intraoperative and postoperative opioids, minimization (<2.5 mg) or avoidance of neostigmine, and adequate hydration have also been shown to decrease the incidence of PONV.[59]

Universal PONV prophylaxis is not cost effective. Apfel and colleagues[60] devised risk stratification for administration of antiemetic prophylaxis based on a risk score (**Table 6**). Risk factors included female gender, prior history of PONV or motion sickness, nonsmoking, and postoperative opioids. The greater the number of risk factors present, the higher the incidence of PONV. Low-risk patients with a risk score of 0 to 1 should receive no prophylaxis. Moderate-risk patients with a risk score of 2 should receive monotherapy prophylaxis. High-risk patients with a risk score of 3 to 4 should receive combination therapy with 2 to 3 agents from different classes, and a TIVA performed as the primary anesthetic.[59]

ANTIEMETIC OPTIONS FOR PROPHYLAXIS OF PONV

Gan and colleagues[59] and The American Society for Ambulatory Anesthesia have issued guidelines for the management of PONV (**Fig. 1**). There are many different options of antiemetic prophylaxis (**Table 7**).[61] Classes include serotonin ($5-HT_3$) antagonists, butyrophenones, phenothiazines, anticholinergics, steroids, antihistamines, and some other alternative antiemetics such as propofol. The authors generally use dexamethasone at the beginning of the case coupled with a $5-HT_3$ antagonist at the end of the procedure as prophylaxis. When no prophylactic medication has been given perioperatively, a $5-HT_3$ antagonist is the recommended first line treatment option. A scopolamine patch can also be placed preoperatively, best placed on the evening before or at least 4 hours before surgery.[62] Metoclopramide has been proved to be ineffective against PONV.[59] Aprepitant is a new NK1 receptor

Table 6	
Simplified risk score for prediction of PONV (Apfel score)	
Number of Risks Present	**Risk of PONV (%)**
0	10
1	21
2	39
3	61
4	79

Risk factors include female gender, history of PONV or motion sickness, opioid use and nonsmoker.

Adapted from Apfel CC, Laara E, Koivuranta M, et al. A simplified risk score for predicting postoperative nausea and vomiting: conclusions from cross-validations between 2 centers. Anesthesiology 1999;91(3):697; with permission.

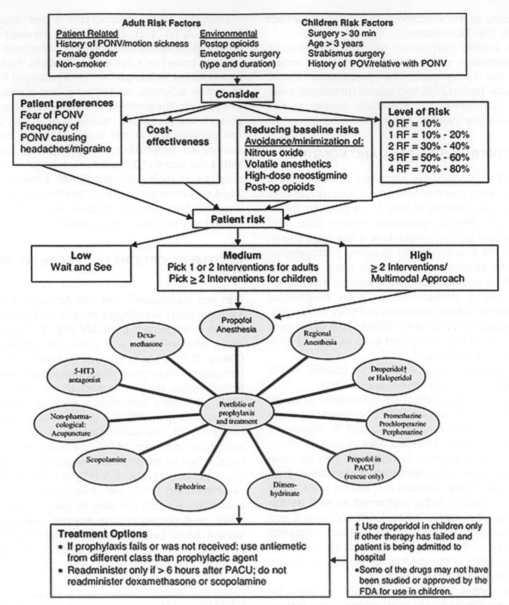

Fig. 1. Algorithm for management of postoperative nausea and vomiting (PONV). (*From* Gan TJ, Meyer TA, Apfel CC, et al. Society for ambulatory anesthesia guidelines for the management of postoperative nausea and vomiting. Anesth Analg 2007;105(6):1619; with permission.)

antagonist antiemetic used for the prevention of chemotherapy-induced nausea and vomiting.

RESCUE THERAPY

If the initial agent is ineffective, a second medication from a different class should be administered. Droperidol and 5-HT$_3$ antagonists may be repeated every 6 hours. Repeating the medication given for PONV prophylaxis within 6 hours postoperatively does not provide any additional benefit. Readministration of dexamethasone or scopolamine is not recommended because it is not

effective. Propofol, in small doses, is a powerful antiemetic. It may be used as a rescue antiemetic when all other therapies have failed, but because of potential complications must only be administered by trained anesthesia personnel in a monitored setting (ie, PACU).[59]

OPTIONS FOR POSTOPERATIVE PAIN MANAGEMENT

Uncontrolled pain and opioid-related side effects are major contributors to delayed recovery and discharge after surgery. A multimodal analgesia

Table 7
Antiemetics

Drug Class	Dose	Timing	Side Effects
5-HT₃ Antagonists			
Ondansetron	4 mg IV	End of surgery	Increased LFTs
Granisetron	0.35–1.5 mg IV		Headache
Dolasetron	12.5 mg IV		Constipation
Tropisetron	2 mg IV		
Antihistamine			
Dimenhydrinate	1 mg/kg IV	Unknown	Sedation
Butyrophenones			
Droperidol	0.625–1.25 mg IV	End of surgery	Drowsiness
Halopridol	0.5–2 mg IV		Agitation
			Extrapyramidal side effects
			QT prolongation
Phenothiazines			
Promethazine	6.25–25 mg IV	End of surgery	Agitation
Prochlorperazine	5–10 mg IV		Extrapyramidal side effects
			Drowsiness
Steroid			
Dexamethasone	4–5 mg IV	At induction Unknown	No adverse events with single administration
Other			
Propofol	20 mg IV	In PACU by anesthesiologist	Respiratory
Other			
Scopolamine	Transdermal Patch	4 h before end of anesthesia	Sedation
			Confusion
			Dry mouth

Abbreviations: IV, intravenous; LFTs, liver function tests; PACU, postanesthesia care unit.
Adapted from Galway U. Ambulatory anesthesia. In: Urman RD, Ehrenfeld JM, editors. Pocket anesthesia. 2nd edition. Philadelphia: Lippincott Williams & Wilkins; 2009; with permission.

Table 8
Intravenous analgesics

Drug Class	IV Dose and Interval	Side Effects
NSAIDs		
Ketorolac	Ketorolac 30 mg q 4–6 h	Renal failure
		Peptic ulcer
		Platelet dysfunction
Opioids		
Fentanyl	Fentanyl 25–100 µg q 30–60 min	Sedation
Morphine	Morphine 1–5 mg q 2–4 h	Respiratory depression
Hydromorphone	Hydromorphone 0.2–0.6 mg q 2–3 h	Pruritus
Meperidine	Meperidine 25–100 mg q 1–2 h	PONV
		Constipation
		Dysphoria
Acetaminophen	1000 mg IV q 6 h	Hepatic failure with overdose
Mixed Agonists/Antagonists		
Butorphanol	Butorphanol 20 µg/kg q 3–4 h	Sedation with no significant respiratory depression
Nalbuphine	Nalbuphine 0.25 µg/kg q 3–6 h	

Adapted from Galway U. Ambulatory anesthesia. In: Urman RD, Ehrenfeld JM, editors. Pocket anesthesia. 2nd edition. Philadelphia: Lippincott Williams & Wilkins; 2009; with permission.

Table 9
Oral analgesics

Drug Class	Dose and Interval	Side Effects
NSAIDs		
Ibuprofen	Ibuprofen 400–800 mg q 6–8 h	Renal failure
Naproxen	Naproxen 500 mg q 8 h	Peptic ulcer
Ketorolac	Ketorolac 10–20 mg q 4–6 h	Platelet dysfunction
Diclofenac	Diclofenac 50 mg q 8 h	
Cyclooxygenase-2 Inhibitors		
Celecoxib (Celebrex)	200–400 mg q 12 h	Hypertension
		Edema
		Heart failure
Opioids		
Oxycodone	Oxycodone 5–10 mg q 4–6 h	Sedation
Morphine	Morphine 10–30 mg q 3–4 h	Respiratory depression
Hydrocodone	Hydrocodone 5–10 mg q 4–6 h	Pruritus
Codeine	Codeine 15–60 mg q 4–6 h	Nausea
Meperidine	Meperidine 50–150 mg q 3–4 h	Constipation
Hydromorphone	Hydromorphone 2–4 mg q 4–6 h	Dysphoria
Tramadol	Tramadol 50–100 mg q 4–6 h	
Opioid/Nonopioid Combinations		
Acetaminophen/propoxyphene napsylate (Darvocet)	1–2 tablets q 4–6 h	Sedation
Acetaminophen/oxycodone (Percocet)		Respiratory depression
		Pruritus
Acetaminophen/codeine (Tylenol) with codeine		Nausea
		Constipation
Acetaminophen/hydrocodone (Vicodin)		Dysphoria
Aspirin/oxycodone (Percodan)		Hepatic failure with overdose
Acetaminophen	Acetaminophen 650–1000 mg q 4–6 h	Hepatic failure with overdose

Adapted from Galway U. Ambulatory anesthesia. In: Urman RD, Ehrenfeld JM, editors. Pocket anesthesia. 2nd edition. Philadelphia: Lippincott Williams & Wilkins; 2009; with permission.

Table 10
Alternative analgesics

Local anesthetics	Neuraxial anesthesia
	Regional nerve block
	Local infiltration
	Subcutaneous catheter placement with continuous infusions of dilute local anesthetic
Intranasal	Fentanyl
	Meperidine
	Butorphanol
Intramuscular	Meperidine
	Morphine
	Hydromorphone
Transdermal	Fentanyl patch
Others	Transcutaneous electrical nerve stimulation
	Acupuncture
	Acupressure

Adapted from Galway U. Ambulatory anesthesia. In: Urman RD, Ehrenfeld JM, editors. Pocket anesthesia. 2nd edition. Philadelphia: Lippincott Williams & Wilkins; 2009; with permission.

or balanced technique refers to the use of more than 1 medication or class of analgesic medication combined with regional anesthesia to produce adequate analgesia. This technique should be used whenever possible to limit the potential side effects associated with opioid use. Adjunct medications such as nonsteroidal anti-inflammatories and cyclooxygenase-2 inhibitors have been shown to reduce opioid requirements and improve pain control after surgery. Options for intravenous, oral, or alternative pain medications are listed in **Tables 8–10**.[61]

DISCHARGE CRITERIA AND FAST-TRACKING

Recovery from anesthesia is generally divided into 2 phases. Phase 1 lasts from discontinuation of anesthetic until patients awaken and regain their vital protective airway reflexes. Phase 1 generally begins in the operating room and continues in a PACU.

The authors use a postanesthesia recovery score, such as the Aldrete score (**Table 11**), to evaluate initial patient recovery.[63] The patient

Table 11 The modified Aldrete scoring system for determining patient readiness for discharge from the postanesthesia care unit	
Discharge Criteria from PACU	**Score**
Activity: able to move voluntarily or on command	
Four extremities	2
Two extremities	1
Zero extremities	0
Respiration	
Able to deep breathe and cough freely	2
Dyspnea, shallow or limited breathing	1
Apneic	0
Circulation	
Blood pressure ±20 mm of preanesthetic level	2
Blood pressure ±20–50 mm preanesthesia level	1
Blood pressure ±50 mm of preanesthesia level	0
Consciousness	
Fully awake	2
Arousable on calling	1
Not responding	0
O_2 saturation	
Able to maintain O_2 saturation >92% on room air	2
Needs O_2 inhalation to maintain O_2 saturation >90%	1
O_2 saturation <90% even with O_2 supplementation	0

A score ≥9 is required for discharge.
Adapted from Aldrete JA. The post-anesthesia recovery score revisited. J Clin Anesth 1995;7(1):89; with permission.

Table 12 Modified postanesthetic discharge scoring system	
Discharge Criteria	**Score**
Vital Signs	
Within 20% of preoperative value	2
20%–40% of preoperative value	1
40% of preoperative value	0
Ambulation	
Steady gait/no dizziness	2
With assistance	1
None/dizziness	0
Nausea/vomiting	
Minimal	2
Moderate	1
Severe	0
Pain	
Minimal	2
Moderate	1
Severe	0
Surgical bleeding	
Minimal	2
Moderate	1
Severe	0

A score ≥9 is required for discharge.
Adapted from Chung F, Chan VW, Ong D. A postanesthetic discharge scoring system for home readiness after ambulatory surgery. J Clin Anesth 1995;7(6):501; with permission.

must reach a score of 9 before being considered as being in phase 2. Phase 2 is the intensive observation and stabilization of the patient until fit for discharge home. This phase generally occurs in the day-surgery step-down unit, which is not likely to be present in an OBS facility.

Home-readiness can be evaluated by a modified postanesthetic discharge scoring system, with a score of 9 required for discharge (**Table 12**).[64] Oral intake is not necessary before discharge. Voiding is also unnecessary unless the patient received neuraxial anesthesia or has undergone gynecologic, hernia, anorectal, or genital surgery.[64,65]

For patients who have received spinal/epidural anesthesia, resolution of the sensory and motor block must occur and be documented before discharge. Patients who have received an extremity peripheral nerve block may be discharged before full regression of motor and sensory block, with instructions to protect the limb.[66]

Fast-tracking refers to bypassing the PACU or phase 1 and going straight to phase 2 from the operating room (Aldrete score of 10 in the operating room; see **Table 11**). These patients can be discharged home earlier without any increase in complications or side effects. White and Song[67] proposed fast-tracking criteria that take into consideration pain and emetic symptoms (**Table 13**).

The office-based practice depends on a rapid transition from the initial stages of recovery to formal discharge in a short period of time, with as little postanesthetic cognitive and psychomotor impairment as possible. In general, fast-tracking applies to most patients who undergo OBA, owing

Table 13
White's scoring system to determine whether outpatients can be transferred directly from the operating room to the step-down (phase II) unit (fast-tracked)

Discharge Criteria	Score
Level of consciousness	
Awake and oriented	2
Arousable with minimal stimulation	1
Responsive only to tactile stimulation	0
Physical activity	
Able to move all extremities on command	2
Some weakness in movement of extremities	1
Unable to voluntarily move extremities	0
Hemodynamic stability	
Blood pressure <15% of baseline mean arterial pressure (MAP) value	2
Blood pressure 15%–30% of baseline MAP value	1
Blood pressure >30% below baseline MAP value	0
Respiratory stability	
Able to breathe deeply	2
Tachypnea with good cough	1
Dyspneic with weak cough	0
Oxygen saturation status	
Maintains value >90% on room air	2
Requires supplemental oxygen (nasal prongs)	1
Saturation <90% with supplemental oxygen	0
Postoperative pain assessment	
None, or mild discomfort	2
Moderate to severe pain controlled with IV analgesics	1
Persistent severe pain	0
Postoperative emetic symptoms	
None, or mild nausea with no active vomiting	2
Transient vomiting or retching	1
Persistent moderate to severe nausea and vomiting	0

Total possible score is 14. A minimal score of 12 (with no score <1 in any individual category) would be required for a patient to be fast-tracked (ie, bypass the postanesthesia care unit) after general anesthesia.

Adapted from White PF, Song D. New criteria for fast-tracking after outpatient anesthesia: a comparison with the modified Aldrete's scoring system. Anesth Analg 1999;88:1071; with permission.

to the administration of anesthesia with a quick recovery and few side effects.

The same standards for hospital-based or ASC recovery and discharge apply to the OBS setting. A formal recovery area with recovery-room orders and postoperative record should be the standard. A nurse trained in recovery-room procedures should be available to provide care in a properly equipped location until the patient is discharged. The anesthesiologist or equivalent should remain on the premises until the patient meets discharge criteria. The ASA recommend standard monitoring for all patients in the recovery room regardless of the type of anesthesia.[68] The patient should receive written instructions that include the management of pain, postoperative complications, and routine and emergency follow-up. Other than procedures occurring under LA only, the patient should be discharged into the care of a responsible adult. Personnel trained in basic life support/advanced cardiac life support should be present until the last patient leaves the facility.

SUMMARY

Advances in surgical techniques, coupled with the development of faster-acting, safer anesthetics, allow for more invasive procedures to be performed in an office setting. In addition, economic demands to decrease health costs and patients' preference for a nonhospital setting have contributed to the growth of OBS, and will continue to fuel its growth in the future.

Regulation of OBS is suboptimal at present, and monitoring of safety is questionable. It is imperative that we continue to strive to hold the OBS centers to the same standards as in ambulatory and hospital settings with regard to patient safety. We must continue to inform and train anesthesiologists in this field such that they can be an integral part of the continuing growth and safety of OBS.

Anesthesia for OBS should be such that the patient recovers quickly with few side effects or pain, and has a timely discharge. Options for this include GA with TIVA with consideration of LMA instead of endotracheal tube, MAC sedation, regional anesthesia, neuraxial anesthesia with the use of short-acting agents, local infiltration by the surgeon with light sedation, and minimization of PONV and pain.

REFERENCES

1. Koch ME, Dayan S, Barinholtz D. Office based anesthesia: an overview. Anesthesiol Clin North America 2003;21(2):417–43.

2. American Hospital Association (AHA). Trendwatch chartbook 2007: trends affecting hospitals and health systems, April 2007 Chart 2.5: percentage of outpatient surgeries by facility type, 1981-2005. Available at: http://www.aha.org/research/reports/tw/chartbook/2007chartbook.shtml. Accessed March 1, 2013.

3. Etzioni DA, Liu JH, Maggard MA, et al. The aging population and its impact on the surgery workforce. Ann Surg 2003;238:170–7.

4. Center for Medicare and Medicaid services 2011. Available at: http://www.asaassociatino.org/About Us/WhatisanASC. Accessed March 1, 2013.

5. Byrd HS, Barton FE, Orenstein HH. Safety and efficiency in an accredited outpatient plastic surgery facility: a review of 5316 consecutive cases. Plast Reconstr Surg 2003;112(2):636–41.

6. Woo P. Office based laryngeal procedures. Otolaryngol Clin North Am 2006;39:111–33.

7. Coyle T, Helfrick J, Gonzalez M, et al. Office based ambulatory anesthesia: factors that influence patient satisfaction or dissatisfaction with deep sedation/general anesthesia. J Oral Maxillofac Surg 2005;63:163–72.

8. Kurrek M, Twersky RS. Office based anesthesia. Can J Anaesth 2010;57(3):256–72.

9. Evron S, Ezri T. Organizational prerequisites for anesthesia outside the operating room. Curr Opin Anaesthesiol 2009;22(4):514–8.

10. Twersky RS. Office based anesthesia: challenges and success. Available at: http://www.csaol.cn/img/2007ASA/RCL_src/204_Twersky.pdf. Accessed March 1, 2013.

11. Federation of State Medical Boards. Office based surgery. Available at: http://www.fsmb.org/pdf/grpol_regulation_office_based_surgery.pdf. Accessed March 1, 2013.

12. American Medical Association. Office based surgery core principles. Chicago: American Medical Association; 2003. Available at: http://www.ama-assn.org/ama1/pub/upload/mm/370/obscoreprinciples.pdf. Accessed March 1, 2013.

13. American Society of Anesthesiologists. Guidelines for office-based anesthesia. 2009. Available at: http://www.asahq.org/For-Members/Standards-Guidelines-and-Statements.aspx. Accessed March 1, 2013.

14. Kurrek MM, Twersky RS. Office based anesthesia: how to start an office based practice. Anesthesiol Clin 2010;28(2):353–67.

15. American Society of Anesthesiologists. Statement on nonoperating room anesthetizing locations. 2008. Available at: http://www.asahq.org/For-Members/Standards-Guidelines-and-Statements.aspx. Accessed March 1, 2013.

16. American Society of Anesthesiologists. Standards for basic anesthesia monitoring. 2010. Available at: http://www.asahq.org/For-Members/Standards-Guidelines-and-Statements.aspx. Accessed March 1, 2013.

17. Iverson RE, ASPS Task Force on Patient Safety in Office-Based Surgery Facilities. Patient safety in office-based surgery facilities II. Patient selection. Plast Reconstr Surg 2002;110(5):1337–42 [discussion: 1343–6].

18. Shapiro FE, editor. Manual of office-based anesthesia procedures. Philadelphia: Lippincott Williams & Wilkins; 2007.

19. Coldiron BM, Healy C, Bene NI. Office surgery incidents: what seven years of Florida data show us. Dermatol Surg 2008;34:285–92.

20. Vila H, Soto R, Cantor AB, et al. Comparative outcome analysis of procedures performed in physicians offices and ambulatory surgical center. Arch Surg 2003;138:991–5.

21. Domino KB. Office-based anesthesia: lessons learned from the closed claims project. ASA Newsl 2001;65:427–33.

22. Morello DC, Colon GA, Fredricks S, et al. Patient safety in accredited office surgical facilities. Plast Reconstr Surg 1997;99(6):1496–500.

23. Venkat AP, Coldiron B, Balkrishnan R, et al. Lower adverse event and mortality rates in physician offices compared with ambulatory surgery centers: a reappraisal of Florida adverse event data. Dermatol Surg 2004;30(12 Pt 1):1444–51.

24. Fleisher LA, Pasternak LR, Herbert R, et al. Inpatient hospital admission and death after outpatient surgery in elderly patients: importance of patient and system characteristics and location of care. Arch Surg 2004;139(1):67–72.

25. American Society of Anesthesiologists. ASA physical status classification system. Available at: http://www.asahq.org/Home/For-Members/Clinical-Information/ASA-Physical-Status-Classification-System. Accessed March 1, 2013.

26. Friedman Z, Chung F, Wong DT, et al, Canadian Anesthesiologists' Society. Ambulatory surgery adult patient selection criteria—a survey of Canadian anesthesiologists. Can J Anaesth 2004; 51(5):437–43.

27. Gandhimani P, Jackson JB. UK guidelines for day surgery. Surgery 2006;24:346–9.

28. Segerdahl M, Warren-Stomberg M, Rawal N, et al. Clinical practice and routines for day surgery in Sweden: results from a nation-wide survey. Acta Anaesthesiol Scand 2008;52(1):117–24.

29. Sabate S, Gomar C, Huguet J, et al, ANESCAT Group. Anesthesia for urological surgery in a European region with 6.7 million inhabitants (Catalonia, Spain). J Clin Anesth 2009;21(1):30–7.

30. American Society of Anesthesiology. Office based anesthesia: considerations for anesthesiologists in setting up and maintaining a safe office anesthesia

environment. Available at: http://ftp.asahq.org/
p-319-office-based-anesthesia-considerations-in-
setting-up-and-maintaining-a-safe-office-anesthesia-
environment.aspx. Accessed March 1, 2013.

31. Chung F, Mezei G. Adverse events in ambulatory
anesthesia. Can J Anaesth 1999;46(5 Pt 2):18–34.

32. American Society of Anesthesiologists Task Force
on Preoperative Fasting. Practice guidelines for
preoperative fasting and the use of pharmacolog-
ical agents for the prevention of pulmonary aspiration: application to healthy patients undergoing
elective procedures. Anesthesiology 1999;90:
896–905.

33. Etzioni DA, Liu JH, O'Connell JB, et al. Elderly patients in surgical workloads: a population-based
analysis. Am Surg 2003;69(11):961–5.

34. Bettelli G. High risk patients in day surgery.
Minerva Anestesiol 2009;75(5):259–68.

35. Stierer T, Fleisher LA. Challenging patients in an
ambulatory setting. Anesthesiol Clin North America
2003;21(2):243–61.

36. Canet J, Raeder J, Rasmussen LS, et al. Cognitive
dysfunction after minor surgery in the elderly. Acta
Anaesthesiol Scand 2003;47(10):1204–10.

37. Lean ME. Obesity and cardiovascular disease: the
waisted years. Br J Cardiol 1999;6:269–73.

38. Young T, Palra M, Dempsy J, et al. The occurrence
of sleep-disordered breathing among middle-aged
adults. N Engl J Med 1993;328:1230–5.

39. Gross JB, Bachenberg KL, Benumof JL, et al. Practice guidelines for the perioperative management
of patients with obstructive sleep apnea. A report
by the American Society of Anesthesiologists task
force on perioperative management of patients
with obstructive sleep apnea. Anesthesiology
2006;104:1081–93.

40. Galway U, Kominsky A. Anesthesia for obstructive sleep apnea surgery. In: Abdelmalak B,
Doyle DJ, editors. Anesthesia for otolaryngologic
surgery. 1st edition. Cambridge University Press;
2013. p. 175–85.

41. Kheterpal S, Han R, Tremper KK, et al. Incidence
and predictors of difficult and impossible mask
ventilation. Anesthesiology 2006;105(5):885–91.

42. Siyam MA, Benhamou D. Difficult endotracheal
intubation in patients with sleep apnea syndrome.
Anesth Analg 2002;95(4):1098–102.

43. Bryson GL, Chung F, Cox RG, et al, Canadian
Ambulatory Anesthesia Research Education
group. Patient selection in ambulatory anesthesia—an evidence-based review: part II. Can J
Anaesth 2004;51(8):782–94.

44. Fleisher LA, Pasternak LR, Lyles A. A novel index of
elevated risk of inpatient hospital admission immediately following outpatient surgery. Arch Surg
2007;142(3):263–8.

45. Joshi GP, Chung F, Vann MA, et al, Society for
Ambulatory Anesthesia. Society for Ambulatory
Anesthesia consensus statement on perioperative
blood glucose management in diabetic patients
undergoing ambulatory surgery. Anesth Analg
2010;111(6):1378–87.

46. Fleisher LA, Beckman JA, Brown KA, et al. ACC/
AHA 2007 guidelines on perioperative cardiovas-
cular evaluation and care for noncardiac surgery.
Circulation 2007;116(17):e418–99.

47. Grines CL, Bonow RO, Casey DE Jr, et al. Prevention of premature discontinuation of dual antiplatelet therapy in patients with coronary artery stents.
Circulation 2007;115(6):813–8.

48. Mukerji G, Munasinghe I, Raza A. A survey of the
peri-operative management of urological patients
on clopidogrel. Ann R Coll Surg Engl 2009;91(4):
313–20.

49. Uptodateonline.com. Perioperative medication
management. Available at: http://www.uptodate.
com/contents/perioperative-medication-manage
ment. Accessed March 1, 2013.

50. American Society of Anesthesiologists Task Force
for Preanesthesia Evaluation. Practice advisory for
preanesthesia evaluation: a report by the American
Society of Anesthesiologists Task Force on preanesthesia Evaluation. Anesthesiology 2002;96:485–96.

51. Liu LL, Dzankic S, Leung JM. Preoperative electrocardiogram abnormalities do not predict postoperative complications in geriatric surgical patients.
J Am Geriatr Soc 2002;96:1186–91.

52. McDonald HP Jr. Office ambulatory surgery in urology. Urol Clin North Am 1987;14(1):27–30.

53. American Society of Anesthesiology. Continuum of
depth of sedation: definition of general anesthesia
and levels of sedation/analgesia. 2009. Available
at: http://www.asahq.org/For-Members/Standards-
Guidelines-and-Statements.aspx. Accessed March
1, 2013.

54. American Society of Anesthesiology. Distinguishing
monitored anesthesia care (MAC) from moderate
sedation/analgesia (conscious sedation). 2009.
Available at: http://www.asahq.org/For-Members/
Standards-Guidelines-and-Statements.aspx. Accessed March 1, 2013.

55. Bhananker SM, Posner KL, Cheney FW, et al. Injury
and liability associated with monitored anesthesia
care: a closed claims analysis. Anesthesiology
2006;104(2):228–34.

56. Gupta A, Stierer T, Zuckerman R, et al. Comparison
of recovery profile after ambulatory anesthesia with
propofol, isoflurane, sevoflurane and desflurane.
Anesth Analg 2004;98(3):632–41.

57. Higgins PP, Chung F, Mezei G. Postoperative sore
throat after ambulatory surgery. Br J Anaesth
2002;88(4):582–4.

58. Rosenblatt MA, Abel M, Fischer GW, et al. Successful use of a 20% lipid emulsion to resuscitate a patient after presumed bupivacaine-related cardiac arrest. Anesthesiology 2006;105:217–8.

59. Gan TJ, Meyer TA, Apfel CC, et al. Society for ambulatory anesthesia guidelines for the management of postoperative nausea and vomiting. Anesth Analg 2007;105(6):1615–28.

60. Apfel CC, Laara E, Koivuranta M, et al. A simplified risk score for predicting postoperative nausea and vomiting: conclusions from cross-validations between two centers. Anesthesiology 1999;91(3):693–700.

61. Galway U. Ambulatory anesthesia. In: Urman RD, Ehrenfeld JM, editors. Pocket anesthesia. 2nd edition. Lippincott Williams & Wilkins; 2012.

62. Bailey PL, Streisand JB, Pace NL, et al. Transdermal scopolamine reduces nausea and vomiting after outpatient laparoscopy. Anesthesiology 1990;72(6):977–80.

63. Aldrete JA. The post-anesthesia recovery score revisited. J Clin Anesth 1995;7(1):89–91.

64. Chung F, Chan VW, Ong D. A post-anesthetic discharge scoring system for home readiness after ambulatory surgery. J Clin Anesth 1995;7(6):500–6.

65. Awad IT, Chung F. Factors affecting recovery and discharge following ambulatory surgery. Can J Anaesth 2006;53(9):858–72.

66. Moemen ME. Recovery characteristics after ambulatory anesthesia and surgery. Eg J Anaesth 2004;20:449–57.

67. White PF, Song D. New criteria for fast-tracking after outpatient anesthesia: a comparison with the modified Aldrete's scoring system. Anesth Analg 1999;88:1069–72.

68. American Society of Anesthesiologists. Standards for postanesthetic care. 2009. Available at: http://www.asahq.org/For-Members/Standards-Guidelines-and-Statements.aspx. Accessed March 1, 2013.

Office-Based Management of Impotence and Peyronie's Disease

Ashley H. Tapscott, DO, Lawrence S. Hakim, MD*

KEYWORDS

- Erectile dysfunction • Impotence • Peyronie's disease • Office-based

KEY POINTS

- Even though increased basic science research into the pathophysiology of Peyronie's disease has brought about new insights into the potential cause and treatment options, a reliable and effective nonsurgical therapy still eludes practicing urologists.
- A key to elucidating the beneficial effects of various medical therapies lies in the standardized evaluation of patients with Peyronie's disease across various studies, allowing these proposed benefits to be confirmed and applied to all populations.
- Some combination of intralesional injection with traction therapy may provide a synergy between the chemical effects of the drugs and the mechanical effects of traction.
- Currently available nonsurgical treatments can be used safely and may result in some reduction of deformity with improved sexual function.

INTRODUCTION

In the expanding field of men's health, much recent attention has been directed toward sexual health, an integral part of overall male wellness. Erectile dysfunction (ED) or impotence is a multifactorial disorder that continues to be an evolving public health concern. With the introduction of readily accessible, effective, and generally safe oral medications, men are now turning to primary care physicians and midlevel providers to manage conditions of sexual dysfunction and are often offered therapy with inadequate or no evaluation. Typically, the failure or poor efficacy of first-line treatments often leads to urology referral. Other reasons for specialty referral may be trauma, uncertainty of diagnoses, or simply the wish of patients or providers to better understand the cause of the ED. This article focuses on the office-based work-up, diagnosis, and management of 2 important and variable conditions in male sexual dysfunction, ED and Peyronie's disease (PD).

BACKGROUND

ED is the consistent or recurrent inability to attain or maintain penile erection adequate for sexual intercourse.[1] ED is a common male disability associated with aging that significantly impacts quality of life and interpersonal well-being.[2–7] A 3-month minimum duration is generally accepted for establishment of the diagnosis, although in certain cases of trauma or surgically induced ED, a 3-month minimum may not be necessary. Although objective testing or partner reports help support a diagnosis of ED, these cannot replace patients' self-reports in classifying the dysfunction or establishing the diagnosis.[8]

Early landmark studies, such as the Massachusetts Male Aging Study (MMAS) and the National Health and Social Life Survey, used single-item scales, which assessed erection difficulties over several months or in the past year.[9,10] In the MMAS, a community-based survey of men between 40 and 70 years of age, 52% of all

Department of Urology, Cleveland Clinic Florida, 2950 Cleveland Clinic Boulevard, Weston, FL 33331, USA
* Corresponding author.
E-mail address: hakiml@ccf.org

Urol Clin N Am 40 (2013) 521–543
http://dx.doi.org/10.1016/j.ucl.2013.07.003
0094-0143/13/$ – see front matter © 2013 Elsevier Inc. All rights reserved.

respondents reported some degree of ED: 17% mild, 25% moderate, and 10% complete.[11] The MMAS showed that the incidence increased with patient age, with an incidence of 12.4 for men aged 40 to 49 years, 29.8 for men aged 50 to 59 years, and 46.4 for men aged 60 to 69 years. Other studies from the 1990s estimated that half of men older than 40 years had ED.[2] The degree of bother associated with ED has been shown to be inversely related to aging. Men older than 70 years typically report a lesser degree of bother as compared with their younger counterparts. Distress and treatment seeking related to ED is found to be higher in younger and middle-aged men.[12–14] Recent investigation of the causes and risk factors for ED has revealed an association between ED, benign prostatic hyperplasia, and lower urinary tract symptoms.[15–18]

The prevalence and incidence of ED are highly correlated with the presence of specific risk factors and comorbidities, suggesting that ED may be an early marker for cardiovascular and other disease states.[19–24] In fact, the symptoms of ED can predate the clinical diagnosis of associated vascular disease by up to 3 years. Cardiovascular comorbidities (such as hypertension and hypercholesterolemia), diabetes mellitus, and metabolic syndrome have been associated with ED in multiple cross-sectional and longitudinal studies.[13,19,25,26] Recent studies in hypogonadal men with testosterone deficiency syndrome (TDS) have demonstrated the positive benefits of normalizing testosterone in men with sexual problems. The development of new treatment options has provided men with TDS with improved and effective methods for hormone replacement, including topical gels and time-released pellets. In addition, the introduction of oral phosphodiesterase-5 (PDE-5) inhibitors resulted in patients presenting to their physicians in increasing numbers for evaluation and treatment earlier.[27] It is estimated that 25 to 30 million men worldwide are taking PDE-5 inhibitors and that an additional 50 million or more are potential candidates for treatment.[12,23,28]

IDENTIFICATION OF RISK FACTORS/ COMORBIDITIES

The Second International Consultation on Sexual Dysfunction identified specific risk factors for ED.[1] The factors have been well studied and include cigarette smoking; diabetes mellitus; hormonal disorders; cardiovascular disease; hypertension; chronic renal failure; lower urinary tract symptoms; poor overall health; chronic neurologic diseases; spinal cord injury; surgery and radiotherapy for prostate cancer; psychiatric

conditions, including anxiety disorders and depression; medications; and recreational drugs. Recognition of screening for these important risk factors is vital in the proper clinical evaluation of ED. The International Society of Sexual Medicine (ISSM) categorizes ED into 3 main groups: (1) psychogenic; (2) organic; and (3) mixed (organic and psychogenic), the most common type.[4] The first goal of the in-office evaluation is the identification of risk factors and classification of patients with ED into one of these 3 groups.

PSYCHOGENIC ED

Identifying the proper psychogenic component to ED helps in guiding the treatment plan. According to the ISSM's classification, psychogenic ED may be generalized or situational. Generalized psychogenic ED usually relates to a primary lack of sexual arousability, aging-related decline in arousability, personality characteristics, or a chronic disorder of sexual intimacy. It is usually not associated with a particular sexual partner, situation, or performance concern.[8,29] The situational type of psychogenic ED is associated with a specific partner, performance concerns, or adjustment-related issues. Partner-related issues may include lack of arousability in a specific relationship, sexual object preference, and partner conflict or threat.[30] Performance-related issues can be associated with situational performance anxiety or with other sexual dysfunctions, such as premature ejaculation or disorders of orgasm.[31,32] Adjustment-related issues include major life stress, such as significant illness and death of a partner.[32] Concomitant depressive and anxiety disorders have been associated with ED. The treatment of these disorders often reduces the severity and may treat the ED, although it is important to recognize the potential sexual side effects of the various antidepressant agents.[33–36] In certain patients, psychological counseling and behavioral therapy may be helpful in addition to medical treatments for ED.[32,36–39]

ORGANIC ED

If the clinical evaluation suggests an organic cause, the ISSM's classification system identifies the following major subgroups: neurogenic, hormonal, arterial, cavernosal (venogenic), and drug induced.[1] In addition, various disease states are identified as potential causes of ED through unclear mechanisms.

Lifestyle factors, including smoking, obesity, and lack of exercise, have been shown to be significant predictors of organic ED.[25,40,41] In a randomized, prospective, controlled trial, intensive lifestyle modification improved erectile function and associated cardiovascular and inflammatory markers.[26]

NEUROLOGIC

There are many neurologic conditions that can affect ED. In theory, any neurologic condition involving autonomic innervation of the corpora cavernosa may impact the ability to produce a normal erection. Polyneuropathy, which commonly involves autonomic dysfunction, has been shown to be a source of ED.[42] A study by Vardi and colleagues[43] reported a 38% coincidence of polyneuropathy and ED in patients with diabetes and a 10% coincidence of the two in patients without diabetes. Male sexual dysfunction is also seen in other neurologic conditions, such as Parkinson disease, dementia, multiple sclerosis, and other neurodegenerative diseases.[39,44–48] In these disorders, the cause of ED is thought to result from a complex relationship of altered erectile nerve function, generalized sensorimotor impairment, cognitive decline, illness-related stress, and decreased interpersonal interaction.[44–46] Epilepsy has also been linked to neurologic ED as well as reduced sexual interest/libido and desire.[44] Multiple sclerosis has been found to have an incidence of ED in the range of 40% to 80%. In these cases, ED typically presents 5 to 10 years after the onset of progressive neurologic symptoms.[47] Stroke, one of the most common neurologic conditions worldwide, is associated with ED in 50% to 65% of patients. Patients who have had a stroke also report a loss of sexual interest and desire and ejaculatory dysfunction.[48–50] Patients with various spinal cord injuries may have significant problems with ED and other related sexual dysfunction. These problems tend to be most bothersome in regard to future quality of life.[39,44]

ENDOCRINE

Erections, sexual behavior, desire, and interest can be affected by abnormalities of endocrine function.[51,52] Gonadal function in men may deteriorate in a progressive way as part of the normal aging process.[53,54] A low testosterone level is the most widely recognized and investigated hormonal alteration associated with the aging process, and hypogonadotropic hypogonadism may be an associated finding in ED. There is increasing evidence that androgens are fundamental, not just for sexual behavior and desire but also for various physiologic and signaling pathways regulating erection as well as for preserving bone density and muscle mass.[55] Although hypogonadism is the most common endocrine cause of ED, thyroid disease, other pituitary disorders, adrenal disease, and hyperprolactinemia may all be associated with ED. The production of several hormones, including dehydroepiandrosterone, thyroxine, melatonin, prolactin, and growth hormone, is also affected by age and may have implications in erectile function.[52,56] In significantly hypogonadal men, androgen-replacement therapy has been shown to improve nocturnal penile tumescence testing as well as erotic stimulus-evoked erections.[57–59] The exact role of androgens in normal and abnormal erectile function remains an area of investigation.

VASCULAR

Vascular disease is the most common cause of organic ED.[60] Vasculogenic ED accounts for approximately 60% to 80% of all cases and can be classified into 3 subtypes: arterial, venoocclusive, or mixed vascular insufficiency.[60] ED shares a common pathophysiology with other vascular disease states, such as heart disease, stroke, and peripheral vascular disease. The accepted pathophysiologic mechanism is thought to be a reduction of inflow into the cavernosal arteries and venoocclusive dysfunction secondary to atherosclerotic occlusive disease.[60] The concept of ED as a marker of other underlying vascular disease is, in part, based on the finding that penile vascular disease shares a causal pathway with other vascular disease states, such as cerebrovascular disease, myocardial infarction, coronary artery disease, hypertension, hyperlipidemia, and peripheral vascular disease.[61] In studies, the quality of penile inflow has been related directly to common vascular comorbidities, including age, diabetes mellitus, hypertension, atherosclerotic vascular diseases, hyperlipidemia, and cigarette smoking.[35] Another study, surveying men during hospitalization for myocardial infarction, showed 64% reported some degree of ED.[62] There have also been reports showing an 18% prevalence of ED in men before experiencing a myocardial infarction, compared with 45% after the event.[63]

Other conditions are commonly revealed during the clinical evaluation of patients with ED, including cigarette smoking, diabetes mellitus, chronic renal failure, and history of prostate cancer. Cigarette smoking deleteriously affects the arterial endothelium on a microvascular level and is a risk factor for other vascular disease states.[64,65] A meta-analysis of the available literature over the last 20 years revealed that 40% of men with ED were smokers compared with 28% of men in the general population.[66]

ED is present in at least 50% of men with diabetes mellitus, with the onset of symptoms occurring at an earlier age than in those without diabetes.[67] Several studies suggest that 26% to 35% of men with diabetes will develop ED.[2] In the MMAS, the age-adjusted probability of complete ED was 3 times higher in men who had treated diabetes mellitus than in men without diabetes.[2] There are several proposed mechanisms by which diabetes mellitus is thought to cause ED. Among these, diabetes-induced microvascular and atherosclerotic disease and diabetes-induced autonomic and somatic peripheral neuropathies seem to be the most important.[60] Chronic renal failure (CRF) is a risk factor for ED and should be revealed during a basic urologic evaluation. Effective treatment of CRF with renal transplantation reduces the severity of ED in these patients.[68]

A common ED patient population encountered by the urologist includes those treated for prostate cancer by radical prostatectomy (open and laparoscopic/robotic), radiotherapy (external beam radiation therapy [XRT], intensity-modulated radiation therapy [IMRT], brachytherapy), hormonal therapy, and cryosurgery. A recent report indicates that there is more than a 50% incidence of ED after radical prostatectomy, regardless of whether a nerve-sparing procedure had been performed.[69] Other reports have shown that in younger men, bilateral nerve-sparing radical prostatectomy results in higher retention of baseline erectile function compared with the non–nerve sparing procedure.[70,71] External-beam prostate radiotherapy and interstitial prostate brachytherapy also result in posttreatment ED, although typically less immediate in onset.[72] Interstitial prostate cryosurgery is an emerging treatment modality for prostate cancer, but recent reports indicate a high likelihood of posttreatment ED.[73] Although the medical and surgical treatment of symptomatic benign prostate hyperplasia (BPH) is generally not harmful to the cavernosal nerves, reports show that sexual function may be adversely impacted, especially after the surgical treatment of BPH.[74]

THE FIRST OFFICE VISIT

Patients may present independently to the urologist's office with a complaint of ED, may have been referred from a primary care provider, or may already have an established relationship for other urologic conditions (BPH/LUTS [lower urinary tract symptoms], calculi, and so forth). Studies have suggested, however, that the average man with ED waits up to 3 years before seeking medical evaluation (reinforcing the importance of the clinician initiating the discussion

regarding ED at each elective visit). In any case, a thorough, systematic evaluation of ED should start with a complete history and physical, including the identification of any risk factors for sexual dysfunction. Remember, ED is a couple's disease, affecting both the patients and their partners; therefore, their partners should be encouraged to be present during the office visit. Of primary importance is the building of a clinician-patient partnership established within an atmosphere of trust.[75]

The visit should flow in a sequential manner, with each component generating and contributing information: (1) identify the chief complaint and sexual history; (2) a detailed medical and surgical history, including all comorbidities, medications and lifestyle factors; (3) a physical examination; (4) basic laboratory testing; (5) identification of the need for specialized evaluation and testing or referrals; and (6) treatment and reassessment (Box 1).

PATIENTS' HISTORY OF ED: THE CLINICAL ASSESSMENT

The first step in the evaluation of ED is a complete medical, social, and sexual history, recognizing

---

Box 1
Office-based ED work-up

- Always evaluate couple, together if possible
- Obtain a complete sexual history to define the ED
- Complete medical history
  - Comorbidities: cardiovascular disease, diabetes, hypertension, LUTS
  - Medications (especially antidepressants, antihypertensive agents)
  - Cigarette use/alcohol abuse/illicit drug use
- Complete surgical history (especially prior prostate surgery)
- Directed physical examination (gynecomastia, penile stretch, presence of Peyronie's plaques, testes consistency and size, digital rectal examination)
- Diagnostic tests
  - Blood tests include prostate-specific antigen, fasting glucose, testosterone, lipid panel
  - Assess hormonal status
  - Vascular assessment (intracavernous injection testing, possible penile duplex Doppler study)
  - Neurologic assessment (if indicated)

that ED may be a presenting symptom or marker of an associated disease state, such as cardiovascular disease. Any specific existing medical comorbidities, especially vascular and/or neurogenic, should be noted. A brief history of cardiovascular symptoms, including exercise tolerance, presence of angina, dyspnea, claudication, transient ischemic attacks, smoking history, and family history of cardiovascular disease, may identify patients with cardiac and vascular risk factors.[76] A detailed urologic history should be taken, with special attention to lower urinary tract symptoms, urologic trauma, urologic malignancies, urinary tract infections, and sexually transmitted infections. Prior urologic procedures (prostatectomy, BPH-related procedures, vasectomy) should be recorded as well as ED symptoms before, surrounding, and after those surgeries. An accurate medication list should be obtained, including herbal medicines, nutritional supplements, and other alternative therapies. Attention should be given to the documentation of any allergies and confirmation of any current nitrate usage. This time is also the point to inquire about any other drug use, illicit or supplemental, especially because numerous medications can cause ED.

The foundation to confirming the diagnosis and in evaluating patients' sexual function is a comprehensive sexual history. A validated pre-evaluation questionnaire can elucidate specific patient concerns and the need for further investigation. Assessing patients' sexual history should encompass any concerns regarding arousal, libido, performance, ejaculation and orgasm, and overall satisfaction. Levels of desire and libido should be addressed because these can also be important in identifying some symptoms of hypogonadism. A detailed inquiry should be made into the quality of the erections themselves. Patients should be asked about their ability to attain and maintain their erection, specifically about the inconsistencies in their erections (spontaneity, ability to maintain) and the progression of their problem. The clinician's goal in the process should be to differentiate between potential organic and psychogenic causes in a patient's sexual problem. The practitioner should also recognize any potential overlap between organic and psychogenic etiologies.

SYMPTOMS AND QUANTIFICATION

It is often difficult to quantify the symptoms of sexual dysfunction because of its variable nature and complex issues involving its cause. The practitioner should incorporate the use of ED symptom scales and questionnaires for patient self-assessment whenever possible. There are many types of validated sexual questionnaires available for use.[77] Multidimensional questionnaires, such as the International Index of Erectile Function (IIEF) or the Sexual Health Inventory for Men, are very helpful in the identification of risk factors and potential causes of male sexual dysfunction. The IIEF may be used as a 5- or 15-item version to assess male sexual function over a 4-week period.[28] Single-item instruments have the advantage of high completion rates and low patient burden. On the other hand, multidimensional scales provide a broader and more complete assessment of disease severity. Despite such differences, similar results have been obtained across studies using these different measures. Symptom scales offer cost-efficient, validated measures for the identification of problems and also provide an assessment of past and current sexual function.[75]

PHYSICAL EXAMINATION

On the first visit for ED, routine office vital signs should be taken and recorded, in addition to height and weight. The physical examination should include a broad screening for medical comorbid conditions relevant to ED, such as body habitus and blood pressure measurements. The medical history should help direct the examination of the organ systems, including a focused cardiovascular and neurologic examination. The urologic examination should include an assessment of proper development of secondary sexual characteristics; an abdominal and inguinal examination; and scrotal examination with assessment of testicular size, consistency, and any abnormal palpable or visual scrotal findings. The examination of the penis should include an assessment of cutaneous sensation as well as screening for any cutaneous lesions, congenital anomalies, traumatic lesions, or plaques. The penis should also be examined for stretched penile length, presence of a suprapubic or pelvic fat pad affecting such length, and any evidence of phimosis or penile adhesions and scarring. A proper digital rectal examination (DRE) should document prostate size, consistency, and the presence or absence of masses. The evaluation of cutaneous sensation in the perineum is useful in identifying potential neurogenic causes of ED.[78]

BASIC LABORATORY EVALUATION

The goal of basic laboratory testing for ED is to perform cost-efficient screening for common systemic disorders. The Second International

Consultation on Sexual Dysfunction (2004) Committee on Sexual Dysfunction Assessment in Men has recommended that fasting blood glucose, fasting cholesterol and lipid panel, and testosterone levels be obtained routinely as part of a basic ED evaluation.[75] Other diagnostic laboratory values should be obtained when indicated specifically by the medical history and physical examination. These values include levels of prolactin, luteinizing hormone, follicle-stimulating hormone, prostate-specific antigen (PSA), complete blood count, and a thyroid function panel.

VASCULAR ASSESSMENT AND ADVANCED (SPECIALIZED) EVALUATION

Specialized evaluation of ED is often necessary to formally define its cause so that the practitioner may offer the most effective treatments. For many patients with ED, a detailed medical and sexual history, general medical examination with a focused genitourinary component, and a thorough review of all comorbidities and medications and laboratory evaluation can recognize the likely cause and allow the design of a treatment plan. Advanced or specialized evaluation is indicated if the initial treatments fail; if there is a diagnosis of PD; primary ED; history of pelvic or perineal trauma; in cases involving vascular or neurosurgical intervention; complicated endocrinopathy; complicated psychiatric disorder; complex relationship problems; when patients desire a better understanding of the underlying cause of the disease, especially as a marker of cardiovascular disease; and for medicolegal concerns.[75]

Considerable research for the vascular assessment of ED over the past few decades has produced methods allowing for the quantitative and qualitative assessment of penile arterial and venoocclusive function. There are many tests available to evaluate penile vascular integrity, erectile function and anatomy, and venoocclusive function, including intracavernous injection (ICI) pharmacotesting, penile duplex Doppler ultrasonography (PDDU), dynamic infusion cavernosometry, and selective penile angiography, although the last two tests are typically not office based and are mentioned here for the sake of completeness.[75]

The first-line in-office diagnostic test for vasculogenic ED has historically been the combination of ICI and visual sexual stimulation with direct assessment by an observer. This test bypasses both neurologic and hormonal influences and enables the direct evaluation of the vascular and physical status of the penis (ie, curvature). The ICI pharmacotest is simple to perform, minimally invasive, and can be done relatively quickly in the office. The most common intracavernosal vasoactive agent used for this test is prostaglandin-E1 (PGE1). The initial dose should be 10 to 20 mcg for injection. Once the intracavernosal injection is administered, a subjective assessment of response should be documented: patients should give a visual rating of their erection, comparing it with their best erection at home. This rating allows a subjective assessment to be made between an inadequate versus adequate in-office erection. Redosing of vasoactive agents may be necessary to achieve the best (or bedroom) quality erection (BQE) because patient anxiety during testing situations may prevent achieving their BQE.

A normal result produced from an ICI pharmacotest in neurologically intact patients may suggest the diagnosis of psychogenic ED. According to Rosen and colleagues,[75] "comparison to other hemodynamic tests suggests a normal ICI pharmacotest is associated with normal venoocclusive function (flow to maintain rigidity values of 0.5–3 mL/min)." If the response from ICI pharmacotesting is insufficient, it may be difficult to distinguish pure arterial insufficiency from venoocclusive dysfunction. An abnormal ICI pharmacotest raises several diagnostic questions that may require further study. The clinician should be aware that an ICI pharmacotest alone might be a misleading diagnostic test to exclude vascular ED unless performed in combination with PDDU.[79] False-negative results can be found in almost 20% of patients with intermediate arterial inflow. False-positive results are also commonly known to occur. If the results are not thoroughly conclusive, or operative intervention is being considered, a second-line study is warranted.

PDDU

PDDU with vasoactive agents is the gold standard office-based diagnostic modality for determining the subtype of vasculogenic ED and in assessing the degree of its severity. The PDDU uses ICI and the assessment of penile vascular flow by color duplex Doppler ultrasound. It is the most informative and least invasive means of evaluating vasculogenic ED.[75] This test can be performed easily in the office setting, allowing for a direct and a quantifiable evaluation of ED and a useful baseline before therapy. The test provides an objective measurement of penile hemodynamics, especially arterial inflow. Ultrasonography may reveal other penile problems or anatomic genital abnormalities, such as PD. Another indication for PDDU is in preoperative planning to provide critical data for operations involving plaque grafts, excisions, and even penile prostheses. It is also an effective test for demonstrating the classic arterial-lacunar fistula associated with high-flow arterial priapism.

To perform the study, one should have an understanding of the relevant penile anatomy and physiology of erection as well as their clinical correlations to ED. As with any procedure, a proper informed consent should be undertaken with patients outlining the purpose, alternatives, risks, and benefits of the testing process. The examination room should be comfortable and safe from intrusion and distraction. False-positive test results, displayed as a partial erection when there is no underlying vascular abnormality, may be secondary to patient anxiety, needle phobia, and/or inadequate medication dosage. Although PDDU is a noninvasive testing modality, ICIs do have potential morbidity that the examiner and patients should be aware of. Up to 20% of neurologically intact men report aching in the penis after PGE1 injections. Prolonged erection is another well-known risk and should be pharmacologically reversed with dilute intracorporeal phenylephrine injections to avoid priapism and its subsequent morbidity.

To perform the study in the office, a high-resolution ultrasonographic probe (7–10 MHz) is required for real-time ultrasonography and color pulsed Doppler, which allows the examiner to evaluate penile blood flow changes throughout the various phases of erection. With color-coded duplex sonography, the direction of blood flow is designated with red (toward the probe) or blue (away from the probe), making identification of the small cavernous vessels and recording of blood flow easier.[80,81] Following intracorporeal injection of the vasoactive medication, baseline penile blood flow measurements are taken and subsequently measured at approximately 5-minute intervals until BQE is achieved, with redosing as necessary; resolution of the erection is then documented. Dosing information during the study is also useful as a basis for intracavernosal therapy.[82] Studies have demonstrated the combination of injection plus manual self-stimulation leads to higher rates of rigid erections compared with injection alone.[83] For recording purposes, a recent validated scale, the Erection Hardness Score (scale 1–4), can be used to standardize responses.[84] If necessary, patients should be reexamined after self-stimulation.[85,86]

The combination of oral sildenafil citrate and a visual erotic stimulation has also been studied as an effective noninvasive pharmacologic induction of erection.[87] Studies are mixed regarding a comparable increase in the peak flow velocities as is

achieved with ICI; the time frame is considerably longer, up to 90 minutes after an oral medication is given. This method may be useful in predicting treatment success with phosphodiesterase inhibitors (PDE5Is).[88–90]

The important vascular parameters assessed by PDDU include cavernous artery diameters, peak systolic velocity (PSV), and end-diastolic arterial velocity. Normal cavernous arterial flow is defined as a PSV greater than 30 cm/s. A PSV measurement of less than 25 cm/s following ICI pharmaco-testing and erotic stimuli has 100% sensitivity and 95% specificity in selecting patients with abnormal penile arteriography.[75] Cavernous venous occlusive disease (CVOD) is defined as the inability to achieve and maintain adequate erections despite appropriate arterial inflow.[83–85,91,92] Many investigators include another value that takes PSV into account. This value is the resistive index (RI). The formula for RI is as follows: $RI = (PSV-EDV)/PSV$, where EDV is the end-diastolic velocity. As the penile pressure equals or exceeds the diastolic pressure, the diastolic flow in the corpora (EDV) approaches zero and the value for RI approaches 1. During the initial tumescence phase, as well as in partial erections, the diastolic flow remains and the RI value is less than 1.0. Naroda and colleagues[93,94] concluded that an RI of less than 0.75 predicts CVOD in nearly 95% of patients and that an RI greater than 0.9 to 1 is normal.

Doppler evaluations should include measurements for the evaluation of blood flow as well as any physical deformity noted (such as plaques and penile curvature). Once patients reach full tumescence (or BQE), gray-scale imaging for the presence of nonvascular abnormalities, such as plaques, curvature, and fibrosis, should be performed. At the conclusion of the testing period, it is important to ensure complete detumescence. Occasionally, this will require an intracorporeal injection of a diluted phenylephrine solution, which may be repeated at approximately 5-minute intervals as needed, until detumescence is achieved. Alternate agents, including epinephrine, have also been used, although some providers use cardiac monitoring during this process because of their potent and possibly systemic effects. These patients should be monitored for symptoms of acute hypertension, tachycardia, arrhythmias, and palpitations.

NEUROLOGIC EVALUATION

A patient's medical history and physical examination develops the foundation for further neurologic evaluation of ED. Generally, many studies have shown that specialized testing for neurogenic ED is only indicated in cases of underlying neurogenic disease or when normal vascular studies and history suggest a neurologic cause. Neurogenic ED usually involves the following: known neurologic risk factors, younger age at presentation, acute onset of ED, and a normal or excellent response following ICI or oral PDE5 inhibitor pharmacotesting. Although specific neurologic tests are available, evidence suggests that they lack adequate sensitivity and reliability for routine clinical diagnosis.[75] Various testing measures include nerve conduction velocity studies, biothesiometry, bulbocavernosus electromyography (EMG), and corpus cavernosa EMG. One study by Lefaucheur and colleagues[95] did show a strong correlation between abnormal penile thermal sensory testing with the clinical diagnosis of neurogenic ED. However, further evaluations are necessary before this test may be brought into routine clinical practice.

PSYCHOLOGICAL EVALUATION

Most screening evaluations for ED can identify psychological risk factors, both independently and in coexistence with other organic risk factors. Patients (often times with their partners) with a psychogenic component or primary psychogenic sexual dysfunction should be referred to those practitioners with specific expertise (psychiatrists, clinical psychologists, and sex therapists) as part of their management.

OFFICE TREATMENT OF ED

Once a diagnosis of ED has been made, the next step in management is to choose the appropriate treatment plan. There is no single treatment that is appropriate for every patient, and an individual treatment plan should be discussed with patients and their partners to assure the best level of satisfaction. Treatment can be considered in terms of first-, second-, and third-line therapies (**Box 2**). First-line therapies include addressing reversible lifestyle issues (smoking cessation, healthy diet, alcohol moderation, and exercise), correcting hormonal abnormalities, and simple noninvasive therapies, such as oral medications and vacuum devices. Second-line therapies involve more invasive options, including intracorporeal injection therapy and intraurethral medication. Third-line treatments are not considered as office-based therapies, including surgical implantation of penile prosthesis and penile revascularization, and are typically reserved for those patients who cannot achieve satisfaction with less-invasive therapies (and are not discussed here).

Box 2
Therapeutic options for ED

- First-line therapeutic options
  - Address reversible lifestyle issues
  - Psychosexual therapy, when indicated
  - Oral therapy: PDE5 inhibitors (daily or on demand)
  - Vacuum erection devices
- Second-line therapeutic options
  - ICI therapy
  - Intraurethral therapy
  - Combination therapy
- Third-line therapeutic options
  - Surgery
    - Implantation of penile prosthesis
    - Penile revascularization

HORMONAL REPLACEMENT THERAPY

Testosterone replacement therapy should only be used in the treatment of sexual dysfunction in the presence of symptomatic hypogonadism and is based on repeat values from early morning specimens of low serum testosterone levels (**Box 3**). In these cases, testosterone replacement is used to maintain normal serum levels of testosterone in an attempt to restore potency and libido. In addition, maintenance of muscle mass and bone density may be achieved. Because of the potential side effects and relatively unpredictable serum levels obtained by oral administration of testosterone preparations, parenteral administration is preferred.

Currently, there are multiple testosterone formulations available for the treatment of hypogonadism. These formulations include intramuscular testosterone, buccal testosterone, topical gels and patches, and time-released testosterone pellets. Intramuscular testosterone is typically administered in dosages of 200 to 300 mg every 2 to 3 weeks. The amount and frequency of administration will vary with the individual and can be titrated. Topical and buccal administration must be used on a daily basis and may offer more stable hormone levels as compared with intramuscular therapy. Considerations of drug transference (ie, to spouse or children) and local skin reactions are issues of concern associated with topical agents. Testosterone pellets can also be placed under the skin (typically in the hip or buttocks), and their effectiveness lasts an average of 3 to 6 months,

Box 3
Office-based management of low testosterone

- Clinical presenting symptoms often seen in patients with low testosterone
  - Decreased sexual function
  - Poor libido, lack of interest
  - Decreased energy levels, fatigue, depression
- Other possible effects of decreased testosterone levels
  - Medical ED treatments (PDE5Is) may be less effective
  - Decreased muscle mass and bone density
  - Potential adverse effects on memory and cardiovascular function
- Therapeutic measures include
  - Assure low morning testosterone; normal PSA and DRE
  - Testosterone enanthate intramuscular every 1 to 3 weeks (in office or home use)
  - Topical therapy, including gels or patches (used daily)
  - Testosterone pellets (in office, every 4–6 months)
  - Monitor testosterone, PSA, lipids, complete blood count (CBC) on regular basis; adjust dose or change regimen as indicated

This form of treatment eliminates the need for daily treatment (improving convenience for some men) and eliminates the risk of transference.

Of note, all forms of testosterone replacement therapy may have some risks of increasing BPH symptoms, a rising PSA, and potentially increasing stroke risk. Regular close monitoring of hormone levels, PSA, CBC, and lipids is recommended. Finally, hormone replacement therapy is relatively contraindicated in men with untreated adenocarcinoma of the prostate or breast because administration may increase the rate of growth of their cancer. It would, therefore, seem prudent that before beginning testosterone replacement therapy in men older than 40 years, serum PSA levels, a DRE, and possibly transrectal ultrasound studies should be performed.

Hyperprolactinemia, another hormonal abnormality effecting sexual function, is treated by (1) cessation of medication causing hyperprolactinemia (eg, estrogens, alpha methyldopa), (2) administration of bromocriptine, or (3) surgical ablation or extirpation of a pituitary prolactin secreting tumor. Treatment with exogenous testosterone to restore the diminished levels of serum testosterone usually seen with this disorder has not been demonstrated to reverse the ED.

ORAL AGENTS: PDE5IS

In order for a normal erection to occur, an interrelated sequence of events that leads to vascular smooth muscle relaxation is necessary. Nitric oxide (NO), produced by vascular endothelial cells and nonadrenergic/noncholinergic neurons, is released and taken up by vascular smooth muscle cells. The level and activity of NO synthase is under the partial influence of testosterone. NO activates the enzyme guanylate cyclase, catalyzing the conversion of guanosine triphosphate into cyclic guanosine monophosphate (cGMP), which then acts as a second messenger with multiple intracellular effects; the most important effect with regard to erectile function is a decrease in intracellular calcium ion concentration, which facilitates smooth muscle relaxation. Unfortunately, the activity of cGMP is limited by its reconversion into GMP PDE5. PDE5Is suppress this pathway, resulting in higher intracellular levels of the second messenger, cGMP, and increased smooth muscle relaxation.

This important discovery has led to the development of specific PDE5I agents that are effective in the treatment of ED. These oral agents include sildenafil, vardenafil, tadalafil, and avanafil and are highly specific for PDE5, with efficacies approaching 60%. The pharmacokinetic properties of these agents differ, resulting in changes in their half-life (T1/2), which effects their period of efficacy. In addition, because there are differences in the degree of selectivity for the various agents, there is the possibility of cross-reactivity with different phosphodiesterases in other parts of the body, such as muscle and retina. As compared with other ED treatments, the PDE5I agents offer certain advantages: they are oral medications, and patients and partners place a high priority on this; they are well tolerated; they require stimulation; and daily agents improve spontaneity. The disadvantages include decreased efficacy in severe ED cases, as compared with other therapies; the need for systemic administration; an absolute contraindication with nitrates; delayed time of onset of action; high cost; and class-specific side effects (SEs), including headache, flushing, rhinitis, dyspepsia, occasional visual changes, and muscle pain.

VACUUM ERECTION DEVICES

Vacuum erection devices (VEDs) are a noninvasive and viable therapeutic option and may be offered as a first-line of treatment of patients with ED. Most VEDs have 3 common components: a vacuum cylinder, a vacuum pump that creates negative pressure within the chamber, and a constrictor or tension band that is applied to the base of the penis after the erection is achieved. The erection resulting from the vacuum device differs from the physiologically induced erection. The latter type is achieved by the initial relaxation of the corporal smooth musculature, thus allowing for engorgement of blood into the lacunar spaces. In the case of a vacuum-induced erection, corporal smooth muscle relaxation does not occur initially and blood is simply trapped in both the intracorporeal and extracorporeal compartments of the penis.

Complications associated with the use of a VED may include difficulty with ejaculation, penile pain, ecchymosis, hematomas, and petechiae (especially if the device is used for more than 30 minutes). Patients taking aspirin or warfarin sodium are more likely to develop vascular complications. Finally, only physician-prescribed, pressure-regulated VEDs should be used in the treatment of ED. Severe morbidities, including the development of PD and worsening of ED, are more likely to occur with the use of commercial, nonprescription, magazine-ad–type devices that lack the pop-off pressure mechanism that is incorporated in the prescription devices.

INTRACAVERNOSAL INJECTION OF VASOACTIVE AGENTS

An effective therapeutic option for men with ED is intracavernosal pharmacotherapy. These self-administered intracavernosal injections of vasoactive agents serve either to directly relax the corporal smooth musculature or block adrenergic tone of the corporal smooth muscle and involve the use of papaverine hydrochloride, phentolamine mesylate, and the prostanoid prostaglandin El. The mechanism of action of papaverine hydrochloride and prostaglandin El is via direct smooth muscle relaxation. Therefore, when injected intracavernosally, they maximize arterial inflow as well as corporal venoocclusion via the relaxation of both arterial and trabecular smooth musculature, respectively. Phentolamine, on the other hand, blocks adrenergically induced muscle tone and, therefore, does not, alone, initiate erections but is effective in prolonging the erectile response. A variety of solutions containing the aforementioned agents are presently being used in clinical practice: papaverine alone, papaverine and phentolamine, prostaglandin El alone, phentolamine and prostaglandin El, or a mixture of all 3 (papaverine, prostaglandin E1, phentolamine).

In general, intracavernosal pharmacotherapy, like vacuum constrictor therapy, may be offered to most patients with organic ED, although patients with poor manual dexterity, poor visual acuity, morbid obesity, or those in whom a transient hypotensive episode may have a deleterious effect (eg, unstable cardiovascular disease and transient ischemic attacks) should be carefully screened before being offered this therapeutic option. Successful treatment of impotence with this therapy has been achieved in patients with diabetes concomitantly taking aspirin or warfarin sodium. Patients with significant psychiatric disease or potential for misuse or abuse of this therapy should be excluded from treatment. The usual therapeutic goal is to be able to create a rigid enough erection satisfactory for vaginal penetration that lasts between 30 minutes and 1 hour.

The initial objective of the dosage determination phase is to define the lowest dose required for achieving an appropriate erectile response. Patients are injected at first in the office with low doses, which are then increased incrementally. After an appropriate dose has been determined and detumescence observed, patients are instructed in proper injection techniques by reviewing printed material showing them the site and sterile technique of injection. An insulin syringe with a 27- to 30-gauge needle is usually used, which minimizes pain and bleeding. Patients are also taught to compress the site of injection for 3 minutes following therapy. Patients are told not to inject more frequently than 3 times per week. Those patients who enter a pharmacologic erection program should first understand a detailed informed consent, which states the known complications of this treatment and discusses the possibility of significant side effects, including nodules, plaques, curvature, and priapism. Patients must be cautioned to seek immediate medical care if an erection persists for 4 hours or longer.

MEDICAL URETHRAL SYSTEM FOR ERECTION

The medical urethral system for erection (MUSE) is a safe and effective formulation of PGE1, which causes erection by inducing the formation of cAMP in the erectile tissue. MUSE is formulated into a pellet, which the man places into the tip of the penis, via the meatus, into the distal urethra, before sexual activity. After manipulation of the penis, the medication is absorbed into the erectile tissue and leads to penile engorgement. The main advantages of the MUSE system are that it involves no needles or injections, it is safe and effective, and the erection typically occurs within 10 to 15 minutes. There are, however, significant disadvantages for some men, including penile pain and burning (caused, in part, by the high doses of PGE1 required for absorption); occasional hypotension; often inadequate penile rigidity, sometimes necessitating the use of a constriction band; the high cost; the fact that it should be refrigerated before use; and the actual procedure of administration may be difficult for some men.

THIRD-LINE TREATMENT OPTIONS

Despite excellent office-based first- and second-line management options for ED, some patients require a third-line treatment to restore their sexual function and quality of life: implantation of a penile prosthesis. The safety, longevity, and success of these devices have currently reached an all-time high. There are fewer mechanical malfunctions and a lower incidence of infection rates (leading to and maintaining the highest patient and partner satisfaction measures of all ED therapies) and should be considered for any patient with ED that does not achieve a satisfactory response to first- or second-line treatment alternatives.

PENILE REHABILITATION

Penile rehabilitation refers to the management of ED in men following radical prostatectomy. Although many of these men may have had normal erectile function before surgery, despite bilateral nerve-sparing procedures and robotic surgery, a significant percentage of these men will notice a decrease in their erectile function and penile length postoperatively. The goal of penile rehabilitation in theory is to minimize these detrimental effects of surgery, maximize sexual function, and improve quality of life. Although there is no accepted universal algorithm for penile rehabilitation, it is generally accepted that by starting early in the postoperative phase (weeks, not months), using a combination of oral agents (daily when possible) or ICI (when oral agents fail), in addition to the application daily of the VED, patients may be able to maximize their restoration of function. Further studies are necessary to determine the ideal therapeutic regimen.

SUMMARY

The introduction of PDE5Is has broadened the scope of ED evaluations to include primary care providers, urologists, cardiovascular specialists, endocrinologists, neurologists, psychiatrists, psychologists, and other specialties. A multidisciplinary approach is vital to patients with ED seeking evaluation and treatment. A systematic approach in the clinical evaluation of ED should

identify sexual problems through the appropriate use of questionnaires and symptom scales, a detailed medical and sexual history, directed physical examination, and basic laboratory testing. For proper diagnosis, the practitioner must be aware of all medical comorbidities associated with ED. Along with in-office diagnostic testing, patients will be able to understand the cause and nature of their ED, and physicians will be able to offer the most appropriate and successful treatments.

OFFICE-BASED MANAGEMENT OF PD

PD is a male sexual disorder that may be associated with ED, pain with erections, and penile curvature. It is a condition involving the tunica albuginea of the corporal bodies. It is characterized by the formation of plaques of fibrous tissue that results in various severities of penile curvature. In some men, there is significant ED or severe curvature that precludes sexual intercourse. This section reviews the potential mechanisms of PD as well as the current office-based evaluation and treatment options for PD.

BACKGROUND AND CAUSE

Francois de la Peyronie[96] first described "induration penis plastic" in 1743 and was the first to offer the treatment of what is now known as PD. PD is now generally thought to be a fibrotic wound-healing disorder of the tunica albuginea. The true pathophysiology of PD and the mechanism of plaque formation are unknown. What is known is that this plaque formation results in penile deformity, curvature, hinging, narrowing, shortening, and painful erections. PD is not only a physically but also a psychologically devastating disorder for these men and is essentially a disease of fibrosis. One model of disease is centered on repeated microtrauma in genetically susceptible individuals. The localized response to injury releases endogenous factors (such as transforming growth factor beta [TGF-b]). This response can lead to the biologic transformation of cells within the tunica albuginea; cell-cycle dysregulation; genotypic changes; and increased expression of cytokines and free radicals that can lead to unregulated extracellular matrix deposition, including fibronectin and collagen, and ultimately plaque formation. This plaque, which does not seem to undergo proper scar remodeling, results in an inelastic segment in the involved tunica albuginea.[97–105] Some other theories included infection, such as sexually transmitted diseases (gonorrhea and syphilis).[106,107] The most common theory among researchers is that PD is a disorder of wound healing, with repetitive microtrauma as a causative origin.[108] From this paradigm, much research has been performed into the immunologic, biochemical, and cytogenetic factors that may play a role in plaque formation.[109,110] As initially reported by Abernathy[107] in 1828, Dupuytren contracture may be associated with PD, and the pathophysiologic pathways in both seem similar. In both conditions, collagen synthesis is abnormally increased with respect to collagen breakdown. It is through this mechanism that the cells responsible for the collagen synthesis and wound contraction (myofibroblasts) seem to occur in excessive amounts. This excess activates an abnormal response to local injury in a man with genetic predisposition to abnormal scar formation and healing. As part of the routine examination in patients with PD, patients' hands should be evaluated for evidence of contracture.

The process of wound healing is divided into 3 phases. The acute phase is described to involve enzymatic cleanup of dead, damaged, or infected tissue with concurrent release of cytokines. Fibrin then is generated and deposited into tissues, including the tunica albuginea in men with PD, and has been proposed to result in the persistent stimulation of scar formation. Overexpression of other cytokines, such as TGF-b, may also play a role. The second phase encompasses strengthening or repairing the wound through scar formation. With normal individuals, cytokines activate the migration of fibroblasts and macrophages. In PD, these fibroblasts may differentiate to become myofibroblasts, which can respond differently to injury. In the final (contractile) phase of wound healing, the scar undergoes remodeling. At this time, metalloproteinases are released (collagenases and gelatinases), remodeling the tissue. This action results in a smaller, more organized scar. Patients with PD may have atypical amounts or dysfunctional types of these collagenases, causing the abnormal plaque or scar.[111]

EPIDEMIOLOGY

Accurate epidemiologic information regarding PD is limited. Polkey[112] first published data in 1928, with 550 case reports. In 1968, Ludvik and Wasserburger[113] described experience within a private clinic, with a prevalence rate of 0.3% to 0.7%. Thirty years later, Devine[114] reported a prevalence of symptomatic PD in 2 populations of male physicians of approximately 1%. The first cross-sectional study was provided in a report by Lindsay and colleagues[115] in 1991, showing the proposed incidence and prevalence rates of PD of

0.38%. Recent studies suggest that the actual prevalence rate may be closer to 9% or even higher. In a study by Mulhall and colleagues[116] in 2004, of the 534 men presenting to a group of geographically diffuse urologists in the United States for prostate cancer screening, 8.9% were found to have objective evidence of PD. The impact of PD is probably not accurately represented in common urologic practice because the true prevalence rate may be even higher and easily underestimated because patients are likely to underreport such a condition that causes embarrassment. Disparity also exists regarding the natural history of PD, which was initially thought to be a disease of spontaneous resolution; however, recent studies have dispelled this myth.[117–119] Another popular misconception is that PD is mainly a disease of older men. PD has been reported to occur over a wide range of ages, with reports in patients as young as 18 years.[120,121]

EVALUATION AND TREATMENT

The first step in the evaluation of men with PD should include a complete medical and sexual history, including duration of onset, history of trauma, degree of curvature, loss of penile length, penile pain (and resolution), degree of erectile function, and the ability to have comfortable intercourse. A detailed physical examination should describe the presence of any palpable plaque, tenderness, numbness, and decreased penile stretch. PDDU is helpful to objectively document the degree of penile curvature, narrowing, or other anatomic abnormality, as well as to objectively define the degree of erectile function. This information is critical to document before any intervention. Several nonsurgical options are currently being used in the treatment of PD, which may reduce or stabilize objective measures, such as penile curvature and erectile function, and also improve subjective measures, such sexual satisfaction, pain, and partner satisfaction. In addition, oral PDE5I agents are often used as a component of the treatment regimen in these patients.[117,122–124]

MEDICAL THERAPY OF PD

Many medical therapies have been described in the search for a successful treatment regimen for PD. Certain medical treatments are based on anecdotal experiences because existing studies are characterized by small numbers of patients with limited follow-up; the absence of placebo or control groups; and few, if any, objective measures of improvement. Another confounding issue is the reporting of spontaneous remission rates, ranging from 7% to 29%.[117,125,126]

VITAMIN E

Vitamin E was one of the first oral therapies to be described in the treatment of PD. Initially studied by Scott and Scardino[127] in 1948, vitamin E was suspected to be of clinical value because of its mechanism of limiting oxidative stress of reactive oxygen species, which increase during the acute and proliferative phases of wound healing.[127,128] The antioxidant properties of vitamin E were thought to be helpful against the prolonged inflammatory phase of wound healing, previously demonstrated in PD.[99,128] Despite multiple studies looking at the use of vitamin E in these patients, a review of the literature reveals no large placebo-controlled trials with vitamin E demonstrating any true benefit in the treatment of PD. That knowledge, paired with the evidence that high doses of vitamin E may increase the risk of cerebrovascular events, does not support its continued empiric use in PD.[129–131]

COLCHICINE

Colchicine, first proposed by in 1994 for the treatment of PD, was thought to hinder fibrosis and collagen deposition primarily by inhibiting neutrophil microtubules.[132] Several small studies, including the only randomized trial examining the effects of colchicine as a monotherapy, revealed that colchicine was no better than placebo in improving pain, curvature, or plaque size.[133–135] With its lack of demonstrable efficacy and a significant side effect profile (gastrointestinal distress, diarrhea, aplastic anemia), the authors do not recommend colchicine as a therapy for PD.

POTASSIUM AMINOBENZOATE

Another oral agent used in the therapy for PD is potassium aminobenzoate, which is thought to increase the activity of monoamine oxidase in tissues, thereby decreasing local levels of serotonin, which may contribute to fibrogenesis and scar formation. A review of the literature did not reveal any large, placebo-controlled studies demonstrating its efficacy in the treatment of PD.[136–140] In addition, this drug is costly, can require taking up to 24 tablets daily, and is known for its low tolerability caused by the gastrointestinal side effects. With its limited evidence of benefit, increased side effect profile, and inconvenient administration regimen, most experts do not support the use of potassium aminobenzoate as a treatment of PD.

TAMOXIFEN CITRATE AND CARNITINE

Tamoxifen is a selective estrogen receptor modulator that has both agonist and antagonist effects on target tissues depending on tissue-specific estrogen receptor expression. Tamoxifen is also reported to affect the release of TGF from fibroblasts, blocking TGF receptors, thus potentially reducing fibrogenesis.[141–144] Carnitine, a naturally occurring metabolic intermediate, works via the inhibition of acetyl coenzyme A, may help in the repair of damaged cells, and has been proposed as a treatment of PD. A review of the literature did not reveal any large, placebo-controlled studies demonstrating improvement in pain, curvature, or plaque size in the treatment of PD for either agent; they are not currently recommended for the treatment of PD.

PENTOXIFYLLINE

Pentoxifylline (PTX) is a nonspecific phosphodiesterase inhibitor, with combined antiinflammatory and antifibrogenic properties by downregulating TGF-b and increasing fibrinolytic activity. Its use has been suggested in the management in PD, after studies have shown its effects in vitro to attenuate both collagen fiber deposition and elastogenesis.[145,146] Although small, uncontrolled studies suggested some improvement in penile curvature, this has not been demonstrated in large, placebo-controlled trials. In addition, patients taking PTX may experience significant side effects, including nausea, vomiting, dyspepsia, and diarrhea.[147,148] Further randomized, placebo-controlled trials are necessary before recommending this as an effective treatment option for PD.

In summary, no oral therapy to date has been shown to reliably reduce penile deformity in a clinically meaningful way. The 2010 published guidelines on PD by Ralph and colleagues[149] state: "There is evidence that there is no benefit with respect to deformity reduction with any oral therapy, including vitamin E, potassium aminobenzoate, colchicine, Tamoxifen, and Carnitine."

TOPICAL THERAPY

Verapamil as a treatment of PD has been suggested, in part, based on studies demonstrating that exocytosis of extracellular matrix molecules, including collagen, fibronectin, and glycosaminoglycan, is a calcium ion–dependent process.[150] Aggeler and colleagues[151] noted changes in cell shape when fibroblasts were exposed to calcium antagonists in vitro, associated with increased extracellular matrix collagenase secretion, and decreased collagen and fibronectin synthesis and secretion.[152] In 2002, Martin and colleagues[153] initiated a study to confirm that topically applied verapamil gel could penetrate into the tissues of the tunica albuginea. This research investigated tissue concentrations in men who were exposed to topical verapamil gel before penile prosthesis implantation surgery. At the time of prosthetic implantation, a sample of tunica albuginea was excised and analyzed. No verapamil was detected in the tunica albuginea specimens, leading the investigators to conclude that transdermal application of topical verapamil has no scientific basis.[153] In addition, no controlled trial has been performed demonstrating the benefit of topical verapamil.

INTRALESIONAL THERAPY
Steroids

Teasley[154] described the first use of intralesional steroids for PD in 1954. However, despite multiple studies, objective efficacy in the treatment of PD has not been demonstrated.[154–157] Currently, the treatment of PD with intralesional steroid injections is discouraged. There are no consistent beneficial effects of this treatment, and local tissue may atrophy. Of note, steroid use can distort tissue planes between Buck fascia and the tunica albuginea, making subsequent surgical correction more difficult.

Collagenase

Collagen, specifically type I and III collagen, has been established as the primary component of the dense, fibrotic PD plaque and collagenase is the enzyme that catalyzes the breakdown of collagen. Gelbard and colleagues[158,159] were the first to study clostridial collagenase in vitro for the treatment of PD in 1982. Their early results reported objective improvement in 20 (64%) of 31 patients within 4 weeks of treatment with collagenase injections.[160] A double-blind, placebo-controlled trial demonstrated a statistically significant improvement in curvature in the collagenase-treated group, documenting the efficacy and safety of intralesional clostridial collagenase injection therapy. The most common adverse events (edema, penile pain, and ecchymosis) occurred in 20 (80%) patients.[161] Collagenase clostridium histolyticum is currently in large-scale, multicenter, randomized, placebo-controlled trials and is awaiting US Food and Drug Administration approval for the treatment of PD.

Verapamil

Levine[162] first reported the use of intralesional verapamil, a calcium channel blocker in 1994. In their initial nonrandomized study, 14 men received biweekly injections of verapamil into their Peyronie's plaques for 6 months. Subjectively, there was significant improvement in plaque-associated penile narrowing in all patients (100%) and improvement in curvature in 6 (42%). Objectively, a decreased plaque volume of more than 50% was noted in 4 (30%) of the patients. Plaque softening was noted in all patients; 12 patients (83%) noticed that plaque-related changes in erectile function had improved. No adverse effects were noted.[162] A second trial of men with early stage disease, (PD <1 year) demonstrated a rapid reduction of pain after a mean of 2.5 injections in 97% of men, with improvement in sexual function, reduction in deformity, and a mean reduction of curvature in 65% of patients. In late-stage disease, (PD >1 year) Levine reported that intralesional verapamil decreased curvature in 8 men (44%).[108] The third trial was the largest published single-center trial using intralesional verapamil. This trial was a prospective nonrandomized study of 140 men (mean duration of disease of 17.7 months), with 77.5% of the patients documented as receiving previous therapy with vitamin E, potassium aminobenzoate, or colchicine. In this study, a local penile block using 0.5% bupivacaine (10–20 mL) was administered at the base of the penis. Next, using a short (five-eighths in) needle (25-gauge to prevent needle breakage), 1 to 5 punctures were made through the skin. However, multiple passes were made through the plaque as verapamil was delivered, with the goal of leaving the drug in the tracks. A standardized dose of 10 mg verapamil (5 mg/2 mL), diluted to 10 mL total volume with injectable saline, was used for injection. Each set of injections was administered at a prescribed interval of 2 weeks for a total of 12 treatment sessions. Of the 121 men tested, penile curvature decreased in 73 (60%), increased in 10 (8%), and remained unchanged in 38 (31%).[163] In these studies, the patients received 12 biweekly injections over 6 months. The rationale by Levine and colleagues is that scar remodeling occurs at glacial speed, suggesting that repeated treatment over time would produce better results. Bennett and colleagues[164] evaluated intralesional verapamil biweekly and reported curve improvement in 22%; they stated that 60% showed no disease progression, suggesting a stabilizing effect. Rehman and colleagues[165] published the first randomized single-blind trial of intralesional injection of verapamil versus saline, in 14 patients and reported significant differences in subjective improvement in quality of erections and objective measurements of plaque volume. A nonsignificant improvement trend was also noted in degree of curvature in the verapamil group.

Recently nicardipine, also a calcium channel blocker, was compared with saline injection as a potential treatment of PD. Although significant improvement in penile curvature was seen in both the nicardipine and saline groups, a significant reduction in the IIEF-5 score and in plaque size was seen only in the nicardipine group.[166] In 2009, a randomized, single-blind, placebo-controlled trial comparing intralesional verapamil with saline did not demonstrate any significant improvements in penile deformity, pain, plaque softening, or sexual function in either groups.[167] Although there are limited controlled data showing clear benefit with intralesional verapamil, the larger-scale trials suggest a curvature improvement rate in up to 60% of men completing 12 injections. Currently, the recommended regimen in experts that use verapamil is a trial of 6 injections, with each injection occurring every 2 weeks. If no improvement is noted, they suggest the injection therapy may be terminated, the dose of verapamil increased to 20 mg (in men with no cardiovascular disease), or interferon (IFN) injections may be offered.

IFN

The potential for the use of intralesional IFN as a therapy for PD was first demonstrated by Duncan and colleagues[168] in 1991. These investigators reported that IFN a, b, and g decreased the rate of proliferation of fibroblasts in Peyronie's plaques in vitro as well as reduced the production of extracellular collagen and increased the activity of collagenase. Initial clinical trials published by Wegner and colleagues[169,170] in 1995 and 1997 demonstrated a significant incidence of side effects, specifically myalgia and fever. In 1997, Judge and Wisniewski[171] published the results of their study in which the dose of IFN was modified, resulting in improvements in the side effects. Ahuja and colleagues[172] performed a nonrandomized study of 20 men who received 1 million units biweekly for 6 months. In this trial, 100% of the men had softening of the plaque, 90% of those presenting with pain had improvement, and 55% had a subjective reduction in plaque size. In 2004, Dang and colleagues[173] administered a reduced dosage of IFN (2×10^6 U) biweekly for 6 weeks. Objective improvements in curvature, using pharmacologic stimulation and a protractor, of greater than 20% were noted in 67% of men. Of those presenting with pain, 80% claimed

improvement, and 71% with presenting complaints of ED also noted improvement in function. In 2006, Hellstrom and colleagues[174] reported their multicenter, single-blind, placebo-controlled trial of 117 men with PD, with a duration of disease for more than 12 months. This trial was the first placebo-controlled trial of intralesional injection therapy for PD to offer evidence of treatment benefit. These men underwent 6 biweekly injections of either IFN-a2b or saline, for a total of 12 weeks.[148] Average curvature in the treatment group improved 13° versus 4° in the placebo arm. Pain resolution was noted in 67% of the treatment patients versus 28% for the placebo. Pretreatment nonsteroidal antiinflammatory drugs (NSAIDS) and assuring excellent hydration during therapy significantly reduced the degree of flulike SEs. Further investigation is clearly needed regarding IFN therapy as well as the possible effects of plaque injection in general because it seems that saline injection itself may offer some benefit to certain patients.[175]

External Energy Therapy

Local penile electro-shockwave therapy (ESWT) has been suggested as a treatment option for PD. The proposed mechanism of action involves direct damage to the plaque resulting in an inflammatory reaction. This reaction is thought to increase macrophage activity leading to lysis of the plaque. ESWT is also hypothesized to improve vascularity, resulting in plaque resorption and to create contralateral scarring, resulting in false straightening.[176] In most studies, the efficacy of ESWT is limited to only subjective reports of improvement of deformity, plaque size, or pain.[177–180] At this time, published studies have not shown reliable clinical benefit in terms of curvature, plaque size, or objective improvement in sexual function or rigidity. The International Consultation on Sexual Medicine's (ICSM's) guidelines state: "There is evidence that ESWT does not improve PD related deformity."[148]

Iontophoresis

Iontophoresis is the use of electric current to transport ions through tissue. This current has been studied and used in dermatology to induce wound healing.[181] Levine and colleagues[182] verified the efficacy of this mode of transmission of verapamil in 2002 using surgically retrieved tunica albuginea specimens after a single intraoperative exposure before partial plaque excision and grafting surgery. In 2009, Stancik and colleagues[183] compared excised-treated Peyronie's plaques to therapy naive plaques. They demonstrated a decreased expression of basic fibroblast growth factor (bFGF), mRNA, and bFGF protein expression in excised Peyronie's plaques after having undergone electromotive drug therapy with dexamethasone, verapamil, and lidocaine. Greenfield and colleagues[184] performed a randomized, double-blind, placebo-controlled trial in 42 men with PD, comparing iontophoresis with verapamil to saline. Their results demonstrated similar measured curve reduction in both groups. In 2005, a prospective, randomized, placebo-controlled study compared the results of patients receiving iontophoresis with verapamil and dexamethasone versus 2% lidocaine. In the verapamil treatment group, the plaque volume decreased and mean measured erect penile curvature was reduced by up to 50%, as compared with no changes in the lidocaine group. The only side effect reported was temporary erythema at the electrode site.[185] The ICSM's guidelines state: "Several controlled trials had evidence of reduced deformity following iontophoresis treatment using verapamil and dexamethasone." Although larger trials remain to be done, current studies suggest that iontophoresis is nontoxic and noninvasive, potentially lending its most beneficial use to those with mild to moderate curvature or those with plaque-related pain.[148,186–189]

Penile Traction Devices

The mechanisms through which mechanical strain can yield a biologic response have been studied in several nonpenile models, including bone, muscle, and Dupuytren scar. Research has shown that mechanical stress modulates cell function in a process called mechano-transduction by activating multiple signal transduction pathways via the internal cytoskeleton and extracellular matrix.[190] Histologically, tension has been demonstrated to reorient collagen fibrils parallel to the axis of stress.[191,192] Genetically, mechanical shear stress has been shown to cause an upregulation of antifibrotic genes.[193] Levine[194] published the first pilot study on traction therapy in men with PD. Penile traction therapy was initiated with the Fast Size Penile Extender (Alison, Viejo, California) for a period of 6 months, 2 to 8 hours per day. Curvature was reduced in all men with a mean reduction of 22°, and the mean IIEF increased from 44.6 to 55.0 for the treatment group. Stretched penile length improved in all patients (100%), with an increase in length up to 2.5 cm. There was no change in penile sensation or new ED.[194] Gontero and colleagues[195] performed a study on traction therapy, evaluating its efficacy in change in curvature. Traction was performed using the Andropenis

(Andromedical, Madrid, Spain) penile extender for 6 months, 5 to 9 hours per day. After 6 months, penile curvature decreased in 6 patients from a mean baseline value of 31° to 27°. Curvature worsened in 1 patient and remained unchanged in 8 patients. Greenfield[196] performed a critical review of these 2 studies and suggested factors that may account for the different results, including the duration of disease, plaque calcification, and methodology of measuring curvature.[196] The ICSM's guidelines state: "Early evidence from two small non-controlled prospective trials have reported a reduction of deformity and increased penile length with traction therapy."[148] Although further large-scale trials are necessary, in regard to this relatively noninvasive, safe treatment option, the primary limitation of traction is that prolonged daily use is necessary to obtain a clinical benefit.

SUMMARY

Even though increased basic science research into the pathophysiology of PD has brought about new insights into the potential cause and treatment options for PD, an ideal, reliable, and effective nonsurgical therapy still eludes the practicing urologist. It is apparent from the review of the literature regarding medical options for the treatment of PD that we still lack controlled clinical trials with uniform standardized assessments and objective measures of deformity, including curvature and circumference. A key to elucidating the beneficial effects of various medical therapies lies in the standardized evaluation of patients with PD across various studies, allowing these proposed benefits to be confirmed and applied to all populations.[197] At this time, it seems that some combination of intralesional injection with traction therapy may provide a synergy between the chemical effects of the drugs and the mechanical effects of traction. Until a reliable medical treatment emerges, it does seem that currently available nonsurgical treatments can be used safely and may result in some reduction of deformity with improved sexual function. Because this is both a physically and psychologically devastating disorder for some patients, any degree of improvement in curvature and pliability of the erection, or even stabilization of the disease, with the goal of allowing comfortable intercourse for patients and their partners may be better than no treatment at all or surgery.

REFERENCES

1. Lizza EF, Rosen RC. Definition and classification of erectile dysfunction: report of the nomenclature

committee of the International Society of Impotence Research. Int J Impot Res 1999;11:141–3.

2. Feldman HA, Goldstein I, Hatzichristou DG, et al. Impotence and its medical and psychosocial correlates: results of the Massachusetts Male Aging Study. J Urol 1994;151(1):54–61.

3. Fugl-Meyer AR, Lodnert G, Branholm IB, et al. On life satisfaction in male erectile dysfunction. Int J Impot Res 1997;9:141–8.

4. Guest JF, Das Gupta R. Health-related quality of life in a UK-based population of men with erectile dysfunction. Pharmacoeconomics 2002;20:109–17.

5. Laumann EO, Paik A, Rosen RC. The epidemiology of erectile dysfunction: results from the National Health and Social Life Survey. Int J Impot Res 1999;11(Suppl 1):S60–4.

6. Litwin MS, Nied RJ, Dhanani N. Health-related quality of life in men with erectile dysfunction. J Gen Intern Med 1998;13:159–66.

7. Lue TF. Erectile dysfunction. N Engl J Med 2000; 342(24):1802–13.

8. Lewis RW, Fugl-Meyer KL, Bosch R, et al. Definitions, classification, and epidemiology of sexual dysfunction. In: Lue TF, Basson R, Rosen R, et al, editors. Sexual medicine: sexual dysfunctions in men and women. 2004 edition. Paris: Health Publications; 2004. p. 39–72.

9. Derby CA, Araujo AB, Johannes CB, et al. Measurement of erectile dysfunction in population-based studies: the use of a single question self-assessment in the Massachusetts Male Aging Study. Int J Impot Res 2000;12(4):197–204.

10. Feldman HA, Goldstein I, Hatzichristou DG, et al. Construction of a surrogate variable for impotence in the Massachusetts Male Aging Study. J Clin Epidemiol 1994;47(5):457–67.

11. Johannes CB, Araujo AB, Feldman HA, et al. Incidence of erectile dysfunction in men 40–69 years old: longitudinal results from the Massachusetts Male Aging Study. J Urol 2000;163:460–3.

12. Fisher W, Rosen RC, Eardley I, et al. The multinational men's attitudes to life events and sexuality (MALES) study phase II: understanding PDE5 inhibitor treatment seeking patterns among men with erectile dysfunction. J Sex Med 2004;1:150–60.

13. Braun M, Wassmer G, Klotz T, et al. Epidemiology of erectile dysfunction: results of the Cologne Male Survey. Int J Impot Res 2000;12(6):305–11.

14. Holden CA, McLachlan RI, Pitts M, et al. Men in Australia, Telephone Survey (MATeS) I: a national survey of the reproductive health and concerns of middle aged and older Australian men. Lancet 2005;366:218–24.

15. Blanker MH, Bohnen AM, Groeneveld FP, et al. Correlates for erectile and ejaculatory dysfunction in older Dutch men: a community-based study. J Am Geriatr Soc 2001;49(4):436–42.

16. Rosen R, Altwein J, Boyle P, et al. Lower urinary tract systems and male sexual dysfunction: the multinational survey of the aging male (MSAM-7). Eur Urol 2003;44(6):637–49.

17. Rosen RC, Giuliano F, Carson CC. Sexual dysfunction and lower urinary tract symptoms (LUTS) associated with benign prostatic hyperplasia (BPH). Eur Urol 2005;47:824–37.

18. Rosen R, Seidman S, Menza M, et al. Quality of life, mood, and sexual function: a path analytic model of treatment effects in men with erectile dysfunction and depressive symptoms. Int J Impot Res 2004; 16:334–40.

19. Feldman HA, Johannes CB, Derby CA, et al. Erectile dysfunction and coronary risk factors: prospective results from the Massachusetts Male Aging Study. Prev Med 2000;30(4):328–38.

20. Fung MM, Bettencourt R, Barrett-Connor E. Heart disease risk factors predict erectile dysfunction 25 years later. The Rancho Bernardo Study. J Am Coll Cardiol 2004;43:1405–11.

21. Jackson G. Erectile dysfunction and cardiovascular disease. Int J Clin Pract 1999;53:363–8.

22. Martin-Morales A, Sanchez-Cruz JJ, Saenz deTejada I, et al. Prevalence and independent risk factors for erectile dysfunction in Spain: results of the Epidemiologia de la Disfuncion ErectilMasculina Study. J Urol 2001;166(2):569–74.

23. McKinlay JB. The worldwide prevalence and epidemiology of erectile dysfunction. Int J Impot Res 2000;12(Suppl 4):S6–11.

24. Shabsigh R, Klein LT, Seidman S, et al. Increased incidence of depressive symptoms in men with erectile dysfunction. Urology 1998;52:848–52.

25. Bacon CG, Mittleman MA, Kawachi I, et al. Sexual function in men older than 50 years of age: results from the Health Professionals Follow-Up Study. Ann Intern Med 2003;139:161–8.

26. Esposito K, Giugliano D. Obesity, the metabolic syndrome and sexual dysfunction. Int J Impot Res 2005;17:391–8.

27. Gopalakrishnan M, Buckner SA, Wyllie MG. Directions in urological research and drug therapies. Drug News Perspect 2001;4(9):544–50.

28. Rosen RC, Riley A, Wagner G, et al. The International Index of Erectile Function (IIEF): a multidimensional scale for assessment of erectile dysfunction. Urology 1997;49:822–30.

29. Mas M. The influence of personality traits on the erectile response to intracavernosal PGE-1 injections. Int J Impot Res 2002;14(Suppl 4):S3.

30. Wiederman MW. The state of theory in sex therapy. J Sex Res 1998;35:88–99.

31. Feil MG, Richter-Appelt H. Control beliefs and anxiety in heterosexual men with erectile disorder: an empirical study. Zeitschrift für Sexualforschung 2002;15:1–20.

32. Levine S. Sexual life, a clinicians guide. New York: Plenum; 1992.

33. Araujo AB, Durante R, Feldman HA. The relationship between depressive symptoms and male erectile dysfunction: cross-sectional results from the Massachusetts Male Aging Study. Psychosom Med 1998;60:458–65.

34. Barlow DH. Causes of sexual dysfunction: the role of anxiety and cognitive interference. J Consult Clin Psychol 1986;54:140–8.

35. Althof S. When an erection alone is not enough: biopsychosocial obstacles to lovemaking. Int J Impot Res 2002;14(Suppl 1):99–104.

36. Wincze JP, Carey MP. Sexual dysfunction: a guide for assessment and treatment. 2nd edition. New York: Guilford Press; 2001.

37. Wylie KR. Treatment outcome of brief couple therapy in psychogenic male erectile disorder. Arch Sex Behav 1997;26(5):527–45.

38. Perelman MA. The impact of the new sexual pharmaceuticals on sex therapy. Curr Psychiatry Rep 2001;3:195–201.

39. Nehra A, Moreland RB. Neurologic erectile dysfunction. Urol Clin North Am 2001;28(2): 289–308.

40. Derby CA, Mohr BA, Goldstein I, et al. Modifiable risk factors and erectile dysfunction: can lifestyle changes modify risk? Urology 2000;56:302–6.

41. Nicolosi A, Glasser DB, Moreira ED, et al. Prevalence of erectile dysfunction and associated factors among men without concomitant diseases: a population study. Int J Impot Res 2003;15:253–7.

42. Low PA. Autonomic neuropathies. Curr Opin Neurol 2002;15(5):605–9.

43. Vardi Y, Sprecher EK, Kanter Y, et al. Polyneuropathy in impotence. Int J Impot Res 1996;8:65–8.

44. Lundberg PO, Brackett NL, Denys P, et al. Neurological disorders: erectile and ejaculatory dysfunction. In: Jardin A, Wagner G, Khoury S, et al, editors. Erectile dysfunction. London: Health Publication; 1999. p. 591–649.

45. Kaufman JM, Hatzichristou DG, Mulhall JP, et al. Sexual function in Parkinson's disease. Clin Neuropharmacol 1990;13:461–3.

46. Brown RG, Jahanshahi WT, Quinn N, et al. Sexual dysfunction in patients with Parkinson's disease and their partners. J Neurol Neurosurg Psychiatry 1990;53(6):480–6.

47. Litwiller SE, Frohman EM, Zimmern PE. Multiple sclerosis and the urologist. J Urol 1999;161: 743–57.

48. Monga TN, Lawson JS, Inglis J. Sexual dysfunction in stroke patients. Arch Phys Med Rehabil 1986;67: 19–22.

49. Sjogren K, Damber JE, Liliequist B. Sexuality after stroke. Aspects of sexual function. Scand J Rehabil Med 1983;15:55–61.

50. Hawton K. Sexual adjustment of men who have had strokes. J Psychosom Res 1984;28:243–9.

51. Morales A. Androgens, sexual endocrinopathies and their treatment. In: Morales A, editor. Erectile dysfunction: issues in current pharmacotherapy. London: Martin-Dunitz; 1998. p. 141–55.

52. Morales A, Buvat J, Gooren LJ, et al. Endocrine aspects of male sexual dysfunction. In: Lue TF, Basson R, Rosen R, et al, editors. Sexual medicine: sexual dysfunctions in men and women. 2004 edition. Paris: Health Publications; 2004. p. 345–83.

53. Vermeulen A. Andropause. Maturitas 2000;35: 5–15.

54. Feldman HA, Longcope C, Derby CA. Age trends in the levels of serum testosterone and other hormones in middle-aged men: longitudinal results of the Massachusetts Male Aging Study. J Clin Endocrinol Metab 2002;87:589.

55. Wespes E. The ageing penis. World J Urol 2002; 20(1):36–9.

56. Gray A, Feldman HA, McKinley JB, et al. Age, disease and changing sex hormone levels in middle-aged men: results of the Massachusetts Male Aging Study. J Clin Endocrinol Metab 1991;73: 1016–105.

57. Nehra A. Treatment of endocrinologic male sexual dysfunction. Mayo Clin Proc 2000;75(Suppl): S40–5.

58. Bancroft J, Wu FW. Changes in erectile responsiveness during androgen replacement therapy. Arch Sex Behav 1983;12:59–66.

59. Carani G, Granata AR, Bancroft J, et al. The effects of testosterone replacement on nocturnal penile tumescence testing, rigidity and erectile response to visual erotic stimuli in hypogonadal men. Psychoneuroendocrinology 1995;20:743–53.

60. Russell S, Nehra A. The physiology of erectile dysfunction. Herz 2003;28(4):277–83.

61. Sullivan ME, Thompson CS, Dashwood MR, et al. Nitric oxide and penile erection: is erectile dysfunction another manifestation of vascular disease? Cardiovasc Res 1999;43:658–65.

62. Wabrek AJ, Burchell RC. Male sexual dysfunction associated with coronary artery disease. Arch Sex Behav 1990;9:69–75.

63. Sjogren K, Fugl-Meyer AR. Some factors influencing quality of sexual life after myocardial infarction. Int Rehabil Med 1983;5(4):197–201.

64. Puranik R, Celermajer DS. Smoking and endothelial function. Prog Cardiovasc Dis 2003;45(6):443–58.

65. Bazzano LA, He J, Muntner P, et al. Relationship between cigarette smoking and novel risk factors for cardiovascular disease in the United States. Ann Intern Med 2003;138(11):891–7.

66. Tengs TO, Osgood ND. The link between smoking and impotence: two decades of evidence. Prev Med 2001;32:447–52.

67. Benet AE, Melman A. The epidemiology of erectile dysfunction. Urol Clin North Am 1995;22(4): 699–709.

68. Abdel-Hamid I. Mechanisms of vasculogenic erectile dysfunction after kidney transplantation. BJU Int 2004;94(4):497–500.

69. Stanford JL, Feng Z, Hamilton AS, et al. Urinary and sexual function after radical prostatectomy for clinically localized prostate cancer: the Prostate Cancer Outcomes Study. JAMA 2000;283:354–60.

70. Rabbani F, Stapleton AM, Kattan W, et al. Factors predicting recovery of erections after radical prostatectomy. J Urol 2000;164:1929–34.

71. Nehra A. Medical and surgical advances in the radical prostatectomy patient. Int J Impot Res 2000;12(Suppl 4):S47–52.

72. Goldstein I, Feldman MI, Deckers PJ, et al. Radiation associated impotence: a clinical study of its mechanism. JAMA 1984;251:903–10.

73. Robinson JW, Donnelly BJ, Saliken JC, et al. Quality of life and sexuality of men with prostate cancer 3 years after cryosurgery. Urology 2002; 60(2 Suppl 1):12–8.

74. Leliefeld HH, Stovelaar HJ, McDonnell JM. Sexual function after various treatments for symptomatic benign prostatic hyperplasia. BJU Int 2002;89: 208–13.

75. Rosen R, Hatzichristou D, Broderick G, et al. Clinical evaluation and symptom scales: sexual dysfunction assessment in men. In: Lue TF, Basson R, Rosen R, et al, editors. Sexual medicine: sexual dysfunctions in men and women. 2004 edition. Paris: Health Publications; 2004. p. 175–206.

76. Russell ST, Khandheria BK, Nehra A. Erectile dysfunction and cardiovascular disease. Mayo Clin Proc 2004;79(6):782–94.

77. Rosen R, Hatzichristou D, Broderick G, et al. Clinical evaluation and symptom scales: sexual dysfunction assessment in men [annex I]. In: Lue TF, Basson R, Rosen R, et al, editors. Sexual medicine: sexual dysfunctions in men and women. 2004 edition. Paris: Health Publications; 2004. p. 207–20.

78. Klausner AP, Batra AK. Pudendal nerve somatosensory evoked potentials in patients with voiding and/or erectile dysfunction: correlating test results with clinical findings. J Urol 1996;156(4):1425–7.

79. Aversa A, Isidori AM, Caprio M, et al. Penile pharmacotesting in diagnosing male erectile dysfunction: evidence for lack of accuracy and specificity. Int J Androl 2002;25(1):6–10.

80. Broderick GA, Arger P. Duplex Doppler ultrasonography: noninvasive assessment of penile anatomy and function. Semin Roentgenol 1993;28:43–56.

81. Landwehr P. Penile vessels: erectile dysfunction. In: Wolf KJ, Fobbe F, editors. Color duplex sonography: principles and clinical application. Stuttgart (Germany): Thieme Medical; 1995. p. 204–15.

82. Seyam R, Mohamed K, Akhras AA, et al. A prospective randomized study to optimize the dosage of trimix ingredients and compare its efficacy and safety with prostaglandin E1. Int J Impot Res 2005;17:346–53.

83. Donatucci CF, Lue TF. The combined intracavernous injection and stimulation test: diagnostic accuracy. J Urol 1992;148:61–2.

84. Cappelleri JC, Bushmakin AG, Symods T, et al. Scoring correspondence in outcomes related to erectile dysfunction treatment on a 4-point scale (SCORE-4). J Sex Med 2009;6(3):809–19.

85. Halls J, Bydawell G, Patel U. Erectile dysfunction: the role of penile Doppler ultrasound in diagnosis. Abdom Imaging 2009;34:712–25.

86. Lewis RW, King BF. Dynamic color Doppler sonography in the evaluation of penile erectile disorders [abstract]. Int J Impot Res 1994;6:A30.

87. Speel TG, Bleumer I, Diemont WL, et al. The value of sildenafil as a mode of stimulation in pharmaco-penile duplex ultrasonography. Int J Impot Res 2001;13(4):189–91.

88. Arslan D, Esen AA, Secil M, et al. A new method for the evaluation of erectile dysfunction: sildenafil plus Doppler ultrasonography. J Urol 2001;66(1):181–4.

89. Copel L, Katz R, Blachar A, et al. Clinical and duplex US assessment of effects of sildenafil on cavernosal arteries of the penis: comparison with intracavernosal injection of vasoactive agent- initial experience. Radiology 2005;237(3):986–91.

90. Erdogru T, Usta MF, Ceken K, et al. Is sildenafil citrate an alternative agent in the evaluation of penile vascular system with color Doppler ultrasound. Urol Int 2002;68(4):255–60.

91. Teh HS, Lin MB, Tsou IY, et al. Color duplex ultrasonography as a screening tool for venogenic erectile dysfunction. Ann Acad Med Singapore 2002;31(2): 165–9.

92. Wilkins CJ, Sriprasad S, Sidhu PS. Color Doppler ultrasound of the penis. Clin Radiol 2003;58(7): 514–23.

93. Naroda T, Yamanaka M, Matsushita K, et al. Clinical studies for venogenic impotence with color Doppler ultrasonography- evaluation of resistance index of the cavernous artery. Nippon Hinyokika Gakkai Zasshi 1996;87(11):1231–5 [in Japanese].

94. Bellorofonte C, Dellacqua S, Mastromarino G, et al. Penile nuclear magnetic resonance. Arch Ital Urol Androl 1994;66(4):187–93.

95. Lefaucheur KP, Yiou R, Colombel M, et al. Relationship between penile thermal sensory threshold-measurement and electrophysiologic tests to assess neurogenic impotence. Urology 2001; 57(2):306–9.

96. de la Peyronie F. Sur quelques obstacles qui s'opposent a l'ejaculation naturelle de la semence. Mem Acad Royale Chir 1743;1:337–42.

97. El-Sakka AI, Hassoba HM, Chui RM, et al. An animal model of Peyronie's like condition associated with an increase of transforming growth factor beta mRNA and protein expression. J Urol 1997; 158:2284–90.

98. El-Sakka AI, Hassoba HM, Pillarisetty RJ, et al. Peyronie's disease is associated with an increase in transforming growth factor-beta protein expression. J Urol 1997;158:1391–4.

99. Mulhall JP, Anderson MS, Lubrano T, et al. Peyronie's disease cell culture models: phenotypic, genotypic and functional analyses. Int J Impot Res 2002;14:397–405.

100. Nachtsheim DA, Rearden A. Peyronie's disease is associated with an HLA class II antigen, HLA-DQ5, implying an autoimmune etiology. J Urol 1996;156:1330–4.

101. Schiavino D, Sasso F, Nucera E, et al. Immunologic findings in Peyronie's disease: a controlled study. Urology 1997;50:764–8.

102. Cantini LP, Ferrini MG, Vernet D, et al. Profibrotic role of myostatin in Peyronie's disease. J Sex Med 2008;5:1607–22.

103. Ryu JK, Piao S, Shin HY, et al. IN-1130, a novel transforming growth factor-beta type I receptor kinase (activin receptor-like kinase 5) inhibitor, promotes regression of fibrotic plaque and corrects penile curvature in a rat model of Peyronie's disease. J Sex Med 2009;6:1284–96.

104. Murphy LJ. Miscellanea: Peyronie's disease (fibrous cavernositis). In: The history of urology. 1st edition. Springfield (IL): Charles C. Thomas; 1972. p. 485–6.

105. Wesson MB. Peyronie's disease (plastic induration) cause and treatment. J Urol 1943;49:350–6.

106. Hunter J. Of the treatment of occasional symptoms of the gonorrhea. In: Nicol G, Johnson J, editors. A treatise on the venereal disease. 2nd edition. Philadelphia: J. Webster; 1818. p. 88–9.

107. Abernethy J. The consequences of gonorrhea. Lecture on anatomy, surgery, and pathology: including observations on the nature and treatment of local diseases, delivered at St. Bartholomew's and Christ's Hospitals. 1st edition. London: James Balcock; 1828. p. 205.

108. Levine LA. Treatment of Peyronie's disease with intralesional verapamil injection. J Urol 1997;158(4): 1395–9.

109. Devine CJ Jr, Somers KD, Jordan SG, et al. Proposal: trauma as the cause of the Peyronie's lesion. J Urol 1997;157(1):285–90.

110. Zargooshi J. Trauma as the cause of Peyronie's disease: penile fracture as a model of trauma. J Urol 2004;172(1):186–8.

111. Cole A. Increased endogenous inhibitors of collagenases within Peyronie's plaques may represent a scar remodeling disorder [abstract 944]. Annual Meeting of the American Urological Association. San Antonio, May 21–26, 2005.

112. Polkey HJ. ID induratio penis plastica. Urol Cut Rev 1928;32:287–308.

113. Ludvik W, Wasserburger K. Die Radiumbehandlung der induratio penis plastica. Z Urol Nephrol 1968;61:319–25.

114. Devine CJ. Introduction to Peyronie's disease. J Urol 1997;157:272–5.

115. Lindsay MB, Schain DM, Grambsch P, et al. The incidence of Peyronie's disease in Rochester, Minnesota, 1950 through 1984. J Urol 1991;146(4):1007–9.

116. Mulhall JP, Creech SD, Boorjian SA, et al. Subjective and objective analysis of the prevalence of Peyronie's disease in a population of men presenting for prostate cancer screening. J Urol 2004; 171(6 Pt 1):2350–3.

117. Gelbard MK, Dorey F, James K. The natural history of Peyronie's disease. J Urol 1990;144(6):1376–9.

118. Kadioglu A, Tefekli A, Erol H, et al. A retrospective review of 307 men with Peyronie's disease. J Urol 2002;168(3):1075–9.

119. Mulhall JP, Guhring P, Depierro C. Intralesional verapamil prevents progression of Peyronie's disease [abstract 936]. Annual Meeting of the American Urological Association. San Antonio, May 21–26, 2005.

120. Levine LA, Estrada CR, Storm DW, et al. Peyronie's disease in younger men: characteristics and treatment results. J Androl 2003;24(1):27–32.

121. Tefekli A, Kandirali E, Erol H, et al. Peyronie's disease in men under 40: characteristics and outcome. Int J Impot Res 2001;13(1):18–23.

122. Deveci S, Hopps CV, O'Brien K, et al. Defining the clinical characteristics of Peyronie's disease in young men. J Sex Med 2007;4:485–90.

123. Furlow WL, Swenson HE Jr, Lee RE. Peyronie's disease: a study of its natural history and treatment with orthovoltage radiotherapy. J Urol 1975; 114(1):69–71.

124. Deveci S, Hopps CV, O'Brien K, et al. A retrospective review of 307 men with Peyronie's disease. J Urol 2002;168:1075–9.

125. Williams JL, Thomas GG. The natural history of Peyronie's disease. J Urol 1970;103(1):75–6.

126. Kadioglu A, Tefekli A, Sanly O, et al. Lessons learned from 307 men with Peyronie's disease. J Urol 2001;165(Suppl 5):202–3 [abstract 838].

127. Scott WW, Scardino PL. A new concept in the treatment of Peyronie's disease. South Med J 1948;41: 173–7.

128. Sikka SC, Hellstrom WJ. Role of oxidative stress and antioxidants in Peyronie's disease. Int J Impot Res 2002;14:353–60.

129. Pryor JP, Farell CF. Controlled clinical trial of vitamin E in Peyronie's disease. Progress in Reproductive Biology and Medicine 1983;9:41–5.

130. Safarinejad MR, Hosseini SY, Kolahi AA. Comparison of vitamin E and propionyl-L-carnitine, separately or in combination, in patients with early chronic Peyronie's disease: a double-blind, placebo controlled, randomized study. J Urol 2007; 178(4 Pt 1):1398–403.

131. Brown BG, Zhao XQ, Chait A, et al. Simvastatin and niacin, antioxidant vitamins, or the combination for the prevention of coronary disease. N Engl J Med 2001;345(22):1583–92.

132. Furst DE, Munster T. Nonsteroidal anti-inflammatory drugs, disease-modifying antirheumatic drugs, nonopioid analgesics & drugs used in gout. In: Bertram G, editor. Basic and clinical pharmacology. New York: Katzung Lange; 2001. p. 596.

133. Akkus E, Carrier S, Rehman J, et al. Is colchicine effective in Peyronie's disease? A pilot study. Urology 1994;44(2):291–5.

134. Kadioglu A, Tefekli A, Koksal T, et al. Treatment of Peyronie's disease with oral colchicine: long-term results and predictive parameters of successful outcome. Int J Impot Res 2000;12(3):169–75.

135. Safarinejad MR. Therapeutic effects of colchicine in the management of Peyronie's disease: a randomized double-blind, placebo-controlled study. Int J Impot Res 2004;16:238–43.

136. Zarafonetis CJ, Horrax TM. Treatment of Peyronie's disease with potassium para-aminobenzoate (potaba). J Urol 1959;81(6):770–2.

137. Griffiths MR, Priestley GC. A comparison of morphoea and lichen sclerosus et atrophicus in vitro: the effects of para-aminobenzoate on skin fibroblasts. Acta Derm Venereol 1992;72(1):15–8.

138. Hasche-Klunder R. Treatment of Peyronie's disease with para-aminobenzoacidic potassium (POTOBA) (author's transl). Urologe A 1978;17(4):224–7 [in German].

139. Weidner W, Schroeder-Printzen I, Rudnick J, et al. Randomized prospective placebo-controlled therapy of Peyronie's disease (IPP) with Potaba* (aminobenzoate potassium). J Urol 1999;6(Suppl 4): 205 [abstract 785].

140. Weidner W, Hauck EW, Schnitker J, et al. Potassium paraaminobenzoate (Potaba) in the treatment of Peyronie's disease: a prospective, placebo controlled, randomized study. Eur Urol 2005;47: 530–6.

141. Ralph DJ, Brooks MD, Bottazzo GF, et al. The treatment of Peyronie's disease with tamoxifen. Br J Urol 1992;70(6):648–51.

142. Colletta AA, Wakefield LM, Howell FV, et al. Anti-oestrogens induce the secretion of active transforming growth factor beta from human fetal fibroblasts. Br J Cancer 1990;62(3):405–9.

143. Teloken C, Rhoden EL, Grazziotin TM, et al. Tamoxifen versus placebo in the treatment of Peyronie's disease. J Urol 1999;162(6):2003–5.

144. Biagiotti G, Cavallini G. Acetyl-L-carnitine vs tamoxifen in the oral therapy of Peyronie's disease: a preliminary report. BJU Int 2001;88(1):63–7.

145. Shindel AW, Lin G, Ning H, et al. Pentoxifylline attenuates transforming growth factor-b1-stimulated collagen deposition and elastogenesis in human tunica albuginea-derived fibroblasts part 1: impact on extracellular matrix. J Sex Med 2010; 7(6):2077–85.

146. Lin G, Shindel AW, Banie L, et al. Pentoxifylline attenuates transforming growth factor-beta1-stimulated elastogenesis in human tunica albuginea-derived fibroblasts part 2: interference in a TGF-beta1/Smad-dependent mechanism and downregulation of AAT1. J Sex Med 2010;7(5): 1787–97.

147. Safarinejad MR, Asgari MA, Hosseini SY, et al. A double-blind placebo-controlled study of the efficacy and safety of pentoxifylline in early chronic Peyronie's disease. BJU Int 2010;106(2):240–8.

148. Althof SE, Corty EW, Levine SB. EDITS: development of questionnaires for evaluating satisfaction with treatments for erectile dysfunction. Urology 1999;53:793–9.

149. Ralph D, Gonzalez-Cadavid N, Mirone V, et al. The management of Peyronie's disease: evidence based 2010 guidelines. J Sex Med 2010;7(7): 2359–74.

150. Kelly RB. Pathways of protein secretion in eukaryotes. Science 1985;230(4721):25–32.

151. Aggeler J, Frisch SM, Werb Z. Changes in cell shape correlate with collagenase gene expression in rabbit synovial fibroblasts. J Cell Biol 1984;98(5): 1662–71.

152. Lee RC, Ping JA. Calcium antagonists retard extracellular matrix production in connective tissue equivalent. J Surg Res 1990;49(5):463–6.

153. Martin DJ, Badwan K, Parker M, et al. Transdermal application of verapamil gel to the penile shaft fails to infiltrate the tunica albuginea. J Urol 2002; 168(6):2483–5.

154. Teasley GH. Peyronie's disease a new approach. J Urol 1954;71(5):611–4.

155. Bodner H, Howard AH, Kaplan JH. Peyronie's disease: cortisone-hyaluronidase-hydrocortisone therapy. J Urol 1954;72:400–31.

156. Winter CC, Khanna R. Peyronie's disease: results with dermo-jet injection of dexamethasone. J Urol 1975;14:898–900.

157. Williams G, Green NA. The non-surgical treatment of Peyronie's disease. Br J Urol 1980;52:392–5.

158. Gelbard MK, Walsh R, Kaufman JJ. Collagenase for Peyronie's disease: experimental studies. Urol Res 1982;10:135–40.

159. Gelbard MK, Linkner A, Kaufman JJ. The use of collagenase in the treatment of Peyronie's disease. J Urol 1985;134:280–3.

160. Gelbard MK, James K, Riach P, et al. Collagenase versus placebo in the treatment of Peyronie's disease: a double-blind study. J Urol 1993;149(1): 56–8.

161. Jordan GH. The use of intralesional clostridial collagenase injection therapy for Peyronie's disease: a prospective, single-center, non-placebo-controlled study. J Sex Med 2008;5(1):180–7.

162. Levine LA, Merrick PF, Lee RC. Intralesional verapamil injection for the treatment of Peyronie's disease. J Urol 1994;151(6):1522–4.

163. Levine LA, Goldman KE, Greenfield JM. Experience with intraplaque injection of verapamil for Peyronie's disease. J Urol 2002;168(2):621–5.

164. Bennett NE, Guhring P, Mulhall JP. Intralesional verapamil prevents the progression of Peyronie's disease. Urology 2007;69(6):1181–4.

165. Rehman J, Benet A, Melman A. Use of intralesional verapamil to dissolve Peyronie's disease plaque: a longterm single-blind study. Urology 1998;51(4): 620–6.

166. Soh J, Kawauchi A, Kanemitsu N, et al. Nicardipine vs. saline injection as treatment for Peyronie's disease: a prospective, randomized, single-blind trial. J Sex Med 2010;7(11):3743–9.

167. Shirazi M, Haghpanah AR, Badiee M, et al. Effect of intralesional verapamil for treatment of Peyronie's disease: a randomized single-blind, placebo controlled study. Int Urol Nephrol 2009;41(3):467–71.

168. Duncan MR, Berman B, Nseyo UO. Regulation of the proliferation and biosynthetic activities of cultured human Peyronie's disease fibroblasts by interferons-alpha, -beta and -gamma. Scand J Urol Nephrol 1991;25(2):89–94.

169. Wegner HE, Andresen R, Knispel HH, et al. Treatment of Peyronie's disease with local interferon alpha 2b. Eur Urol 1995;28(3):236–40.

170. Wegner HE, Andresen R, Knispel HH, et al. Local interferon-alpha 2b is not an effective treatment in early-stage Peyronie's disease. Eur Urol 1997; 32(2):190–3.

171. Judge IS, Wisniewski ZS. Intralesional interferon in the treatment of Peyronie's disease: a pilot study. Br J Urol 1997;79(1):40–2.

172. Ahuja S, Bivalacqua TJ, Case J, et al. A pilot study demonstrating clinical benefit from intralesional interferon alpha 2B in the treatment of Peyronie's disease. J Androl 1999;20(4):444–8.

173. Dang G, Matern R, Bivalacqua TJ, et al. Intralesional interferon-alpha-2B injections for the treatment of Peyronie's disease. South Med J 2004; 97(1):42–6.

174. Hellstrom WJ, Kendirci M, Matern R, et al. Single-blind, multicenter placebo controlled parallel study to assess the safety and efficacy of intralesional interferon alpha-2B for minimally invasive

treatment for Peyronie's disease. J Urol 2006; 176:394–8.

175. Inal T, Tokatli Z, Akand M, et al. Effect of intralesional interferon-alpha 2b combined with oral vitamin E for treatment of early stage Peyronie's disease: a randomized and prospective study. Urology 2006;67:1038.

176. Levine LA. Review of current nonsurgical management of Peyronie's disease. Int J Impot Res 2003; 15:S113–20.

177. Manikandan R, Islam W, Srinivasan V, et al. Evaluation of extracorporeal shock wave therapy in Peyronie's disease. Urology 2002;60(5):795–9.

178. Lebret T, Loison G, Herve JM, et al. Extracorporeal shock wave therapy in the treatment of Peyronie's disease: experience with standard lithotriptor (siemens-multiline). Urology 2002;59(5):657–61.

179. Palmieri A, Imbimbo C, Longo N, et al. A first prospective, randomized, double-blind, placebo-controlled clinical trial evaluating extracorporeal shock wave therapy for the treatment of Peyronie's disease. Eur Urol 2009;56(2):363–9.

180. Hauck EW, Altinkilic BM, Ludwig M, et al. Extracorporeal shock wave therapy in the treatment of Peyronie's disease. First results of a case-controlled approach. Eur Urol 2000;38(6):663–9.

181. Weiss DS, Kirsner R, Eaglestein WH. Electrical stimulation and wound healing. Arch Dermatol 1990;126(2):222–5.

182. Levine LA, Estrada CR, Shou W, et al. Tunica albuginea tissue analysis after electromotive drug administration. J Urol 2003;169(5):1775–8.

183. Stancik I, Schäfer R, Andrukhova O, et al. Effect of transdermal electromotive drug therapy on fibrogenic cytokine expression in Peyronie's disease. Urology 2009;74(3):566–70.

184. Greenfield JM, Shah SJ, Levine LA. Verapamil versus saline in electromotive drug administration (EDMA) for Peyronie's disease: a double blind, placebo controlled trial. J Urol 2007;177:972–5.

185. Di Stasi SM, Giannantoni A, Capelli G, et al. Transdermal electromotive administration of verapamil and dexamethasone for Peyronie's disease. BJU Int 2003;91(9):825–9.

186. Prieto Castro RM, Leva Vallejo ME, Regueiro Lopez JC, et al. Combined treatment with vitamin E and colchicine in the early stages of Peyronie's disease. BJU Int 2003;91(6):522–4.

187. Mirone V, Palmieri A, Granata AM, et al. Ultrasound- guided ESWT in Peyronie's disease plaques. Arch Ital Urol Androl 2000;72(4):384–7.

188. Mirone V, Imbimbo C, Palmieri A, et al. Our experience on the association of a new physical and medical therapy in patients suffering from induratio penis plastica. Eur Urol 1999;36(4):327–30.

189. Cavallini G, Biagiotti G, Koverech A, et al. Oral propionyl-l-carnitine and intraplaque verapamil in

the therapy of advanced and resistant Peyronie's disease. BJU Int 2002;89(9):895–900.

190. Alenghat FJ, Ingber DE. Mechanotransduction: all signals point to cytoskeleton, matrix, and integrins. Sci STKE 2002;2002(119):PE6.

191. Molea G, Schonauer F, Blasi F. Progressive skin extension: clinical and histological evaluation of a modified procedure using Kirschner wires. Br J Plast Surg 1999;52(3):205–8.

192. Shapiro F. Bone development and its relation to fracture repair. The role of mesenchymal osteoblasts and surface osteoblasts. Eur Cell Mater 2008;15:53–76.

193. Fong KD, Trindade MC, Wang Z, et al. Microarray analysis of mechanical shear effects on flexor tendon cells. Plast Reconstr Surg 2005;116(5): 1393–404.

194. Levine LA, Newell MM. FastSize Medical Extender for the treatment of Peyronie's disease. Expert Rev Med Devices 2008;5(3):305–10.

195. Gontero P, Di Marco M, Giubilei G, et al. Use of penile extender device in the treatment of penile curvature as a result of Peyronie's disease. Results of a phase II prospective study. J Sex Med 2009; 6(2):558–66.

196. Greenfield JM. Penile traction therapy in Peyronie's disease. F1000 Med Rep 2009;1(pii):37.

197. Levine LA, Greenfield JM. Establishing a standardized evaluation of the man with Peyronie's disease. Int J Impot Res 2003;15(Suppl 5):S103–12.

Urodynamics
With a Focus on Appropriate Indications

Sara M. Lenherr, MD*, J. Quentin Clemens, MD, MSCI

KEYWORDS

- Urodynamic • Uroflowmetry • Incontinence • Sphincter electromyography • Pressure-flow study
- Detrusor-sphincter dyssynergia

KEY POINTS

- Optimal use of urodynamic testing requires the formulation of urodynamic questions.
- The purpose of urodynamic testing is to supplement a patient's clinical history and physical examination with a series of tests that are designed to assess the storage and voiding phases of micturition using noninvasive and invasive methods.
- Appropriate ancillary staff training and patient preparation are essential to a successful urodynamic examination.

INTRODUCTION

Urodynamic testing has become a standard part of the available diagnostic armamentarium for the evaluation of patients with lower urinary tract dysfunction.[1] Optimal use of an urodynamic test requires the formulation of urodynamic questions, namely, "What is the information I need to obtain from the test?" and "What is the most appropriate urodynamic technique to obtain these results?"[2] An understanding of when to use certain urodynamic tests can be derived from the literature, from clinical practice guidelines, and from clinical experience.

URODYNAMIC TESTING IN CONTEXT

The purpose of urodynamic testing is to supplement a patient's clinical history and physical examination with a series of tests that are designed to assess the storage and voiding phases of micturition, using noninvasive and invasive methods. Observations seen during these tests and the clinician's interpretation can help identify potential bladder safety issues (eg, elevated bladder storage pressures), help to guide treatment, predict outcomes, and correlate with patient quality of life.

Before performing a urodynamic test, a clinical evaluation should be completed to identify the relevant urodynamic questions. A thorough history is necessary to obtain a clear understanding of the patient's complaints, including type of symptoms (ie, urgency, frequency, urge incontinence, stress incontinence, pain, other voiding and storage symptoms), severity and duration of symptoms, bother associated with the symptoms, previous therapies, and relevant medical comorbidities. A physical examination can identify specific findings (pelvic prolapse, urethral diverticulum, pelvic mass), which may contribute to or cause the symptoms of interest. Patients can also be asked to complete a voiding diary to assess objectively fluid intake, voided volumes, episodes of incontinence, and voiding frequency. Pad-weight testing helps quantify the amount of urine lost during incontinence episodes.[3] Data from validated questionnaires help to quantify symptoms and their affect on quality of life.[4–8] To be most useful, data obtained from a urodynamic test must be considered as supplemental to clinical data. For instance,

Disclosures: The authors have nothing to disclose.
Department of Urology, University of Michigan, 1500 East Medical Center Drive, 3875 Taubman Center, SPC 5330, Ann Arbor, MI 48109-5330, USA
* Corresponding author.
E-mail address: slenherr@med.umich.edu

identification of stress incontinence on a urodynamic test is of limited importance if the patient reports severe urge incontinence as the primary complaint.

OVERVIEW OF URODYNAMIC TESTING

Both noninvasive and invasive urodynamic techniques can be used to help qualify and quantify lower urinary tract activity during the micturition cycle. Noninvasive tests include uroflowmetry and postvoid residual (PVR). Invasive tests include cystometry, sphincter electromyography (EMG), videourodynamics (VUDs), pressure-flow study (PFS), and urethral function tests. An appropriately formulated urodynamic question might warrant one or more of these individual procedures to answer the question. We will begin with an overview of noninvasive urodynamic tests. We will then discuss invasive urodynamic tests, with separate sections devoted to the storage and voiding components of the micturition cycle.

Preparing the patient for invasive urodynamic testing can greatly affect usefulness and efficacy of the test. Patients generally tolerate urodynamic testing well, but feelings of anxiety, discomfort, and embarrassment are not rare.[9] Studies of patient experiences with urodynamic testing indicate that more than 70% of patients would be willing to repeat invasive urodynamic testing if medically indicated[9,10] and most thought the testing was the same or better than they expected it would be.[11,12] As with all invasive procedures, informed consent should be obtained and all questions addressed.

It is the authors' practice to distribute standard patient instructions about urodynamics before the testing. These explain the testing procedures using nonmedical terminology, as well as the rationale for the testing. Patients are instructed to maintain their regular diet and to take their scheduled home medications. They are asked to arrive to the clinic with a full bladder to provide a urine specimen and possibly perform an initial noninvasive uroflow study. Poststudy instructions explain that they can resume routine activities and that they may experience mild dysuria, hematuria, and/or increased bladder sensitivity for 24 to 48 hours after the test.

All patients should undergo urinalysis to screen for signs a urinary tract infection at the time of procedure. Patients with a symptomatic infection should have the urodynamic test deferred until the infection has been treated. Limited data exist regarding the usefulness of preprocedural antibiotic administration.[11,12] The American Urological Association (AUA) *Best Practice Statement on*

Urologic Surgery Antimicrobial Prophylaxis states that antibiotic prophylaxis before urodynamic testing is indicated only in patients with risk factors, specified as advanced age, anatomic anomalies of the urinary tract, poor nutrition status, smoking, chronic corticosteroid use, immunodeficiency, externalized catheters, colonized material, coexistent infection, and recent prolonged hospitalization.[11] Recommended antibiotics include oral fluoroquinolones or trimethoprim-sulfamethoxazole; however, patient allergies, prior urine cultures, and local antibiogram patterns should be considered.

Patients with spinal cord injuries above T6 are at risk for experiencing autonomic dysreflexia (AD) during bladder filling, characterized by an acute increase in blood pressure and bradycardia, accompanied by symptoms such as headache, piloerection, skin pallor, profuse sweating, or skin flushing.[13] Untreated AD can result in intracranial hemorrhage, retinal detachment, seizures, and death. A prior history or the risk for AD should be noted and appropriate preparations and/or precautions followed. Many patients know their typical triggers and these most often involve simulation of the bowel or bladder.[14] Preparations in the urodynamic test suite include monitoring blood pressure and heart rate throughout the study. If symptoms of AD are identified during urodynamic testing, the trigger (usually filling of the bladder or catheter placement) should be removed by draining the bladder and then removing catheters if needed. Additionally, the patient should be placed in reverse Trendelenburg (head up) to take advantage of any gravitational reduction in blood pressure and loosen any tight clothing or restrictive devices. If blood pressure elevation does not resolve, 1 to 2 inches of nitropaste can be applied to the chest and wiped off after blood pressure values normalize.[13]

As with all invasive procedures, certain patients may also experience vasovagal syncope during urodynamic testing. For this reason, some centers have a policy that all patients, male and female, perform the voiding phase of the study in the seated position. In contrast to treatment of AD, vasovagal syncope requires the patient be placed in the Trendelenburg position to increase blood flow to the head and/or chest.

Noninvasive Emptying Assessment

Uroflowmetry (uroflow) is a noninvasive method to measure the flow of urine during micturition. Patients are instructed to void with a comfortably full bladder. Measurements obtained during uroflow are peak flow rate (Qmax), average flow rate, voiding time, voided volume, and flow pattern (eg, flat, bell-shaped curve, saw-tooth, intermittent). Voided volume must be equal to or greater than 150 mL for uroflowmetry results to be valid.[15,16] A reduced flow rate suggests the presence of bladder outlet obstruction, reduced bladder contractility, or both. Because patients are not always able to complete the voiding phase of multichannel urodynamic testing, noninvasive uroflow can be a useful adjunct after the filling portion of a PFS has been completed.

PVR can be measured directly by draining the bladder with a catheter, or indirectly with bladder ultrasound or fluoroscopy (if radiopaque contrast has been instilled into the bladder before voiding). Bladder outlet obstruction can be due to many causes that can be suggested by clinical history, but cannot be diagnosed with just PVR testing.

Assessment of Bladder Storage Function

Simple cystometry is an inexpensive evaluation that can assess bladder sensation and detrusor behavior during filling. It can be performed in a regular examination suite in either the standing or supine position. The study requires a small sterile catheter (usually 12–14F) and a 60 mL catheter-tip syringe with the plunger removed. Room temperature sterile saline or water is used as the filling fluid. The catheter is inserted per urethra with sterile technique and PVR volume measured. The syringe is attached to the end of the catheter as a funnel. Using gravity, the fluid is gradually poured (approximately 50 mL/min increments) into the funnel to fill the bladder. As filling proceeds, the patient is asked to report their first sensation of bladder filling, normal desire to void, strong desire to void, and maximum bladder capacity.[17] In the authors' practice, the scripted questions we ask our patients are (1) first sensation, "Tell me when you first feel any fluid or a coolness in your bladder;" (2) first desire to void, "If you're watching TV, tell me when you would go to the bathroom at the next commercial;" (3) strong desire to void, "Tell me when you can't wait for the next commercial;" and (4) maximum capacity, "Let me know when you can't hold any more in your bladder." Involuntary detrusor contractions can be seen by watching the meniscus in the syringe as a back-pressure against gravity. Care should be taken to correlate these observations with any patient movement. If indicated, a full bladder cough stress test can be performed after the catheter is removed.

Complex filling cystometrogram (CMG) allows for measurement of bladder pressure during filling. Single-channel recording of bladder pressure can offer information about bladder sensation, capacity, compliance, and involuntary detrusor contractions.[1] The urodynamic catheter (6–10F) is placed into the bladder and room temperature fluid is instilled at 30 to 50 mL per minute. Bladder sensation (first sensation, normal desire, strong desire, and maximum capacity) is assessed. Studies in healthy volunteers indicate that these sensations are reproducible.[17] Extremes in sensation likely represent a pathologic abnormality.

Commonly, disposable air-charged or water-filled urodynamic pressure-measurement catheters are used to perform cystometry. Air-charged catheters are newer in design; therefore, most prior research was based on water-filled systems. There are notable differences in how each catheter responds to changes transient and sustained pressures and they do not give interchangeable results.[18] However, both catheter types are widely accepted for clinical use, and most observed differences are outside the range of what is generally relevant to urodynamic studies. Standard double- and triple-lumen catheters are available. Double-lumen catheters have one port for fluid inflow and a second port to measure vesical pressure (Pves). Triple-lumen catheters provide a third, more proximal, sensor port, which can be positioned at the level of the external urethral sphincter to measure bladder and urethral pressure simultaneously.

Multichannel urodynamic testing is the stepwise addition of a rectal catheter to a filling CMG, to measure abdominal pressure (Pabd). This allows the testing clinician to incorporate information about the relative contribution of Pabd changes (ie, with cough or Valsalva) to bladder behavior. Rectal catheters come in multiple styles, including fluid-filled rectal balloon and air-charged catheters. Both types of catheters are placed in the rectal vault, proximal to the anal sphincters. Presence of stool in the rectum can affect Pabd readings. In patients without a rectum, the catheter can be placed either in the vaginal vault or in a fecal stoma to allow measurement of the Pabd. Regardless of catheter system, the International Continence Society (ICS) recommends that all urodynamic catheters be zeroed to atmospheric pressure and reference height is set to the level of the upper edge of the pubic symphysis.[16]

In urodynamic terminology, Pves is the measure of the bladder pressure and Pabd is the abdominal pressure measured by the catheter in the rectum. Detrusor pressure (Pdet) is the difference of Pves minus Pabd. Calculation of Pdet is often important as a measure of detrusor muscle function in patients who are able to generate Pabd. Whereas the calculated Pdet represents the viscoelastic properties and tone of the bladder wall, all three tracings (Pves, Pabd, and Pdet) should be evaluated when looking at a urodynamic study to monitor for artifacts and other factors contributing to the Pdet tracing.

Sphincter EMG is an indirect measure of pelvic floor and urethral sphincter muscle contractility.[19] This is a measurement of depolarization of the sphincter muscle membrane. Urodynamic questions that can be answered include information about outlet contraction and relaxation in relation to the timing of other components of the urodynamic study. EMG is typically performed with surface patch electrodes, placed on the perineum. Needle electrodes EMG can be used but are more invasive and uncomfortable.

In a normal urodynamic study, the sphincter EMG has a baseline resting activity that may increase slightly as the bladder fills (guarding reflex). EMG activity will also increase with stress or Valsalva maneuvers. During the first phase of voiding, there should be cessation of activity as the urethral sphincter relaxes. If EMG activity increases with voiding, this may represent detrusor-sphincter dyssynergia (DSD), dysfunctional voiding, or normal attempts to prevent voiding in the presence of an involuntary detrusor contraction.[20] DSD is found in patients with suprasacral spinal cord lesions. As an example, a 58-year-old man with an incomplete C2/3 spinal cord injury demonstrates a strong involuntary detrusor contraction, with DSD based on both increased intraluminal urethral pressure and increased sphincter EMG activity (**Fig. 1**).

VUDs, or fluorourodynamics, involve synchronous radiographic imaging of the bladder with multichannel urodynamic testing. It was originally (1970) called this because the information was recorded to videotape.[21] Ultrasonography is an alternative imaging modality but not used widely. Fluoroscopy is used to offer dynamic images of the anatomy with maneuvers. Other pathologic findings can be visualized with these images, including vesicoureteral reflux, urinary tract stones, and bladder diverticula.

The use of fluoroscopy offers useful information in complex patients. For example, a 75-year-old man presented for evaluation of stress urinary incontinence, urinary frequency, and recurrent urinary tract infections (**Fig. 2**). He had a urologic history notable for a robotic-assisted laparoscopic radical prostatectomy for prostate cancer with concomitant bladder diverticulectomy 1 year before presentation. Postoperatively, he developed a bladder neck contracture that was dilated and he now performs obturation daily. Urodynamic evaluation showed first desire to void at 90 mL, strong urge at 121 mL, and capacity of 144 mL. Pdet rose from a baseline of 0 cm H_2O to 9 cm H_2O at a volume of 144 mL. Pves, on the

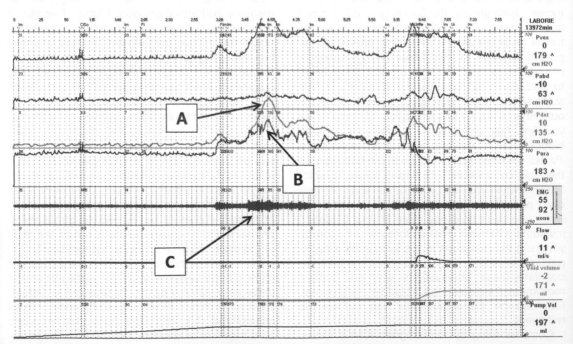

Fig. 1. (A) Strong voluntary detrusor contraction (Pdet) with (B) simultaneous increased external urethral sphincter contraction (Pura) and (C) increased EMG activity.

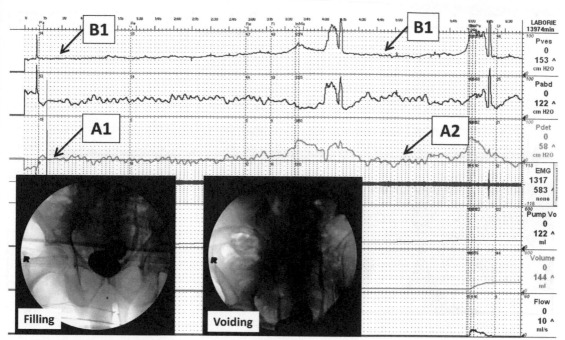

Fig. 2. Pabd has significant baseline variability. When trying to determine compliance, the baseline variability affects Pdet; therefore, there is not a notable change in compliance (*A1* vs *A2*). However, Pves baseline is about 34 cm H_2O (*B1*) and increases to 48 cm H_2O (*B2*), for a change of 14 cm H_2O. Although this is not a clinically significant compliance change, the addition of fluoroscopy shows a diverticulum and bilateral vesicoureteral reflux (*right* grade II–V, *left* grade III–V). The diverticulum filled more and reflux increased bilaterally with voiding.

other hand, rose from a baseline of 34 cm H_2O to 48 cm H_2O at a volume of 144 mL. He had involuntary detrusor contractions at 90 mL and 122 mL, with incontinence. Overall, these findings suggest normal detrusor compliance, reduced bladder capacity, detrusor overactivity, and intrinsic sphincter deficiency. However, fluoroscopy demonstrated a bladder diverticulum and bilateral vesicoureteral reflux (grade II–V on the left side and grade III–V on the right side occurred at 33 mL with 0 cm H_2O and 70 mL with 3 cm H_2O, respectively). The diverticulum filled more and the reflux increased bilaterally with voiding. Because of the vesicoureteral reflux, comment cannot be made about the patient's true bladder compliance because there is no longer a closed pressure reservoir and the bladder pressure may appear falsely safe.[22] Addition of fluoroscopy alters both interpretation and recommended treatment of this patient.

Although fluoroscopy is often useful, providers should limit the number of images that do not contribute to the diagnostic value of the study.[23,24] For many urodynamic studies, the essential static images include one for each of the following stages of the urodynamic study: scout, filling phase low volume, Valsalva maneuver (dynamic) at approximately 200 mL (or lower in patients with decreased capacity), dynamic images during incontinence, cystometric capacity, during voiding, and postvoid. Additional images without the catheter may be needed during voiding if the patient is unable to void with catheter in place.[23]

Assessment of Urethral Function

Abdominal leak point pressure (ALPP) is defined by the ICS as the "intravesical pressure at which urine leakage occurs due to increased abdominal pressure in the absence of a detrusor contraction."[1] Lower ALPP values correspond to more severe stress urinary incontinence. The ALPP can be induced either by cough (cough leak point pressure) or by Valsalva maneuver (Valsalva leak point pressure). ALPP values can be used to quantify the severity of stress urinary incontinence, and this information can be used to guide treatment selection. The usefulness of urodynamics to evaluate incontinence is demonstrated with a case of a 36-year-old woman referred for evaluation of incontinence after repair of a urethral diverticulum. Office cystoscopy showed no evidence of persistent urethral diverticulum. The 24-hour pad weight testing was 248 g. Urodynamic testing showed severe intrinsic sphincter deficiency with urethral hypermobility (**Fig. 3**).

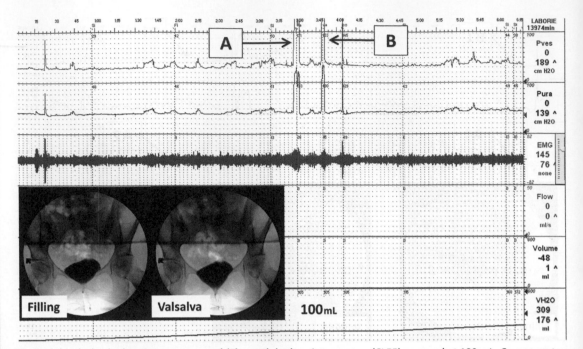

Fig. 3. (*A*) Valsalva leak point pressure and (*B*) cough leak point pressure (CLPP) assessed at 100 mL. Compensatory urethral pressure and EMG activity noted. Bladder neck was open with rest on fluoroscopy and urethral hypermobility with leakage was seen with Valsalva and cough.

Bladder volume can affect ALPP measurements. The testing was first performed at a bladder volume of 150 mL[25] and has since been performed at volumes of 200 to 300 mL.[26] Catheter size is another important consideration in the measurement of ALPP. A transurethral catheter can partially occlude the urethral lumen, potentially distorting the value of the ALPP.[27,28] Although there is no standard catheter size recommended for urodynamic testing, it is generally agreed that smaller catheters have less occlusive potential and are usually preferred.

Urethral pressure measurements are used to assess urethral competence and incontinence severity. Although it is fully accepted that urethral pressure is an important and integral component to urinary continence, it remains challenging to measure and characterize this pressure in a reliable manner.[29] The urethral pressure profile (UPP), maximum urethral pressure, and maximum urethral closure pressure (MUCP) may be used as part of the urodynamic evaluation for stress urinary incontinence. UPP is the graph of intraluminal pressure that is produced when urethral pressure is measured by a catheter along the entire length of the urethra. The maximum urethral pressure is recorded on this graph and the maximum difference between the urethral pressure and the Pves is the MUCP,[1] which is the most commonly used measurement of the urethra in current practice. MUCP has been assessed in multiple studies to determine whether it can be used to predict success among women undergoing anti-incontinence procedures, with mixed results.[30,31]

Invasive Assessment of Bladder Emptying Function

A PFS involves the simultaneous measurement of Pves, Pabd, and voiding flow. Flow is recorded as a milliliter per second and Qmax is the highest flow rate recorded in the study. Urodynamic questions that can be answered include information about detrusor contractility and evidence of bladder outlet obstruction. Detrusor contractility and coordination with the external urethral sphincter and pelvic floor is assessed during the PFS by correlating Pdet increase with urethral pressure or EMG relaxation. As an example, a 46-year-old man with multiple sclerosis was evaluated for straining and double voiding. Office cystoscopy showed prostatic hypertrophy with concentric bladder neck narrowing. Multichannel urodynamic testing with fluoroscopy confirmed the presence of bladder outlet obstruction without any evidence of DSD (**Fig. 4**). The patient was offered a transurethral resection of the prostate rather than interventions to manage DSD.

There are several nomograms developed to help characterize the PFS in men. Perhaps the most

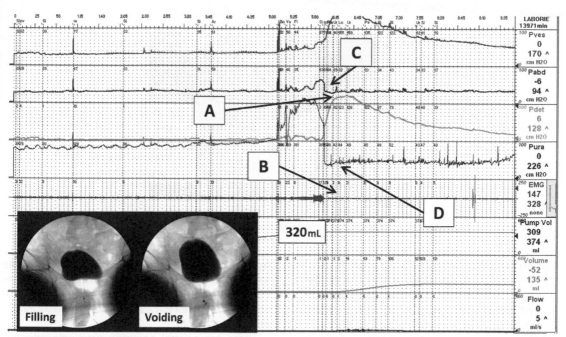

Fig. 4. (*A*) Voluntary detrusor contraction (Pdet) at 320 mL coincided with (*B*) decreased EMG activity and (*C*) no evidence of Valsalva voiding. Fluoroscopy showed the bladder neck did not open with voiding but (*D*) external urethral sphincter pressure (urethral pressure) did decrease. There was urine flow but with high voiding pressure (92 cm H_2O) and Qmax of 4 mL/sec.

widely used is the ICS nomogram for pressure flow analysis.[32] This analysis represents a plot of Pdet versus urethral flow to provide characterization of the flow as obstructed, unobstructed, or equivocal. Several other nomograms have been developed such as CHESS (in chessboard format)[33] and linPURR (linearized passive urethral resistance relation),[34] which can be used in a similar manner to quantify the degree of obstruction.

PITFALLS AND TROUBLE SHOOTING

Avoiding technical complications during urodynamic testing begins with an appropriately planned study and quality control measures. Once urodynamic questions and the appropriate tests have been chosen, the equipment must be set up and calibrated. In most urodynamic testing suites, there is a specially trained registered nurse, nurse practitioner, physician assistant, or medical assistant to facilitate the procedure. Although there are many team members needed to perform the study, it is the responsibility of the physician to ensure quality. An experienced provider with a good team is able to interpret the mechanical, physical, and psychosocial factors that affect urodynamic testing.

One of the first challenges encountered with urodynamic testing is placing the urodynamic catheter, which is small and malleable. If unable to pass the urodynamic catheter into the bladder, the urodynamic catheter can be piggybacked off a stiffer catheter, usually a coudé tip. Once the urodynamic catheter is in the bladder, the larger catheter is pulled out.

If that technique proves unsuccessful, urodynamic information can be obtained from a larger or more rigid catheter such as a red-rubber, Foley, or Mentor catheter. Pves can be transduced via one of these single-channel catheters with some modifications. First, after placement of the catheter, a Christmas-tree adaptor is placed into the catheter for attachment of a Y-connector (**Fig. 5**). The water-charged pressure system is in a direct line with the catheter and the infusion line must go in the side-port.

Because of significant flow turbulence that will be detected with the infusion line and pressure system in direct communication, Pves measurements can only be made when infusion is stopped (**Fig. 6**). It is the authors' practice to fill with a maximum of 30 mL per minute and stop infusion to check Pves every 50 mL volume. Pves measurements and calculation of compliance can be made along the tracing.

Routine cough and Valsalva maneuvers can also be tested (**Fig. 7**). Involuntary detrusor contraction will result in a rise in the vibratory tracing and

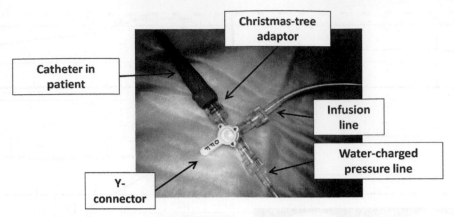

Fig. 5. Set-up for single-channel water-charged pressure monitoring.

infusion should stop to monitor contraction, as with any urodynamic study. Fluoroscopy can be used to augment anatomic evaluation. A PFS cannot be performed with this system but the catheter could be removed and uroflow performed.

ICS criteria for quality control include the following parameters: (1) ensuring that resting values for abdominal, vesical, and Pdet are all in a typical range, indicating they are not influenced by artifact; (2) confirming that abdominal and vesical pressures reflect live signal changes with talking or breathing, but that these variations do not appear in the Pdet tracing; and (3) checking that there is an equal response of abdominal and vesical pressures with a cough every 1 minute (or 50 mL) and before voiding.[16] It is the authors' practice to check coordination of Pabd and Pves with a cough approximately every 200 mL if patient has a

normal to large capacity bladder (**Fig. 8**). This routine measurement allows accurate differentiation of detrusor forces acting on the bladder versus abdominal forces, as well as timely identification of artifacts.

There are several common problems encountered with urodynamic testing. These can be categorized as mechanical versus patient-related events (**Table 1**). Rapid identification and correction should be taken at the time of the study to maximize the usefulness of the study and to prevent incorrect data interpretation.

Mechanical events include a displaced catheter, expelled catheter, and EMG signal artifacts. Displaced tubes do not provide correct values if the sensor tip is against the rectal or bladder wall. Generally, the displaced catheter will not respond to quality control measures with the same

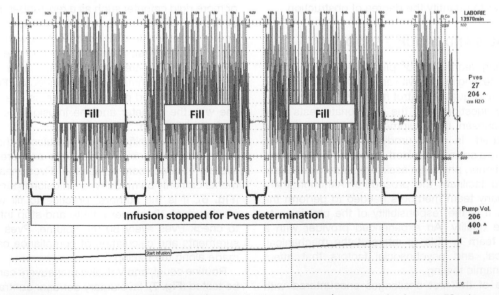

Fig. 6. Example of Pves tracing during single-channel fluid infusion and pressure check every 50 mL.

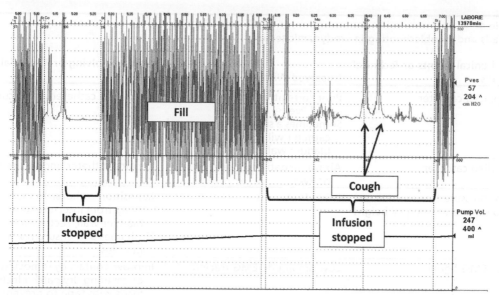

Fig. 7. Example of Pves tracing with cough and Valsalva during single-channel fluid infusion. Compliance can be determined from the Pves when not filling.

amplitude and, therefore, it should be repositioned. Prolonged rise or decrease in Pabd or Pves that does not respond symmetrically to a quality control measure (eg, coughing) can also be assumed to be a displaced tube. Expelled tubes will result in a negative reading for that tracing.

EMG signals are susceptible to artifacts created by electrical potentials that are not generated by those muscles targeted for assessment. Electrical equipment in the room might produce artifacts. A more contemporary source of tracing artifacts is

an implantable sacral neuromodulation device that will give constant background amplitude tracing (**Fig. 9**). To avoid interference, the device can be turned off during testing. Lead placement in a poor location, over-thick hair, or wet skin will also interfere with EMG readings.

There are also technology-related artifacts that are dependent on the type of equipment used. For example, microtransducer sensors will detect urethral pressure differently according to orientation. Staff should be familiar with such equipment

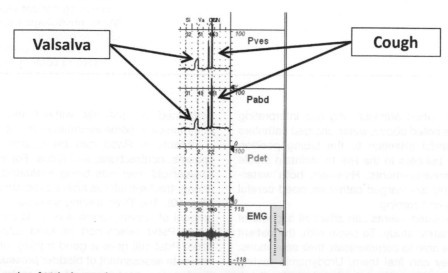

Fig. 8. Example of Valsalva and cough maneuvers to assess appropriate tracing response. Both Pabd and Pves respond with the same magnitude and timing, indicating an appropriate tracing. The calculated Pdet does not show a change in pressure. There is a compensatory EMG contraction.

Table 1
Pitfalls and troubleshooting in urodynamic testing

Mechanical Events or Technical Pitfalls	Observed With	Problem Solving or Remedial Action
Displaced catheter	Poor correlation between Pabd and Pves Sometimes a slowly moving rectal catheter will suggest low bladder wall compliance	Reposition catheter and secure it
Expelled catheter	Abrupt negative value in Pabd or Pves	Replace catheter and secure it
Poor pressure transmission or spikes are of unequal height	Pabd, Pves	Reposition catheter to move away from interference (eg, bladder wall, rectal wall) Flush lines and ensure no air-bubbles
Poor EMG signal	Low-amplitude EMG tracing	Improve contact by removing hair or covering dry patch electrode leads with tape to prevent interference Reposition closer to sphincter
Neuromodulation device	Abundant persistent EMG signal artifact	Turn-off neuromodulation device or disregard EMG tracing
Fluoroscopy does not show bladder neck, urethra, or other anatomy	Fluoroscopic images	Reposition fluoroscopic arm

Patient-Related Events	Observed With	Problem Solving or Remedial Action
Rectal contractions and passing flatus	Fluctuating Pabd or negative tracing	Observe real-time and note on event log Consider during interpretation
Patient movement	Changing Pabd, Pves, EMG that correlate with patient movement	Observe real-time and note on event log Consider during interpretation
Symptom not reproduced	—	Eliminate barriers to study by reducing patient anxiety Mimic physiologic triggers Change position Remove urethral catheter if assessing voiding phase

parameters when administering and interpreting the test. As noted above, water-charged catheters require careful attention to the tubing position and water bubbles in the line to maintain stable pressure measurements. However, both water-charged and air-charged catheters, need careful calibration and zeroing.

Patient-related events can affect all aspects of the urodynamic study. To begin with, the patient may not be able to communicate their sensations, even if they can feel them. Urodynamic testing is an interactive procedure, in which feedback about sensations and discomfort is solicited from the patient. Although urodynamic testing can be performed on patients without the ability to communicate, some information is lost.

Artifacts in Pabd can be caused by rectal spasms, contractions, and flatus. For example, a 51-year-old man was being evaluated for lower urinary tract symptoms after a prostate procedure (**Fig. 10**). The Pves tracing showed a significant amount of activity, which is only clarified by looking at Pabd, which had mirrored values. In this case, Pdet still gave a good tracing, allowing for accurate assessment of bladder pressure. This indicates the usefulness of the rectal catheter. Conversely, in a 67-year-old woman being evaluated for mixed urinary incontinence, the Pabd

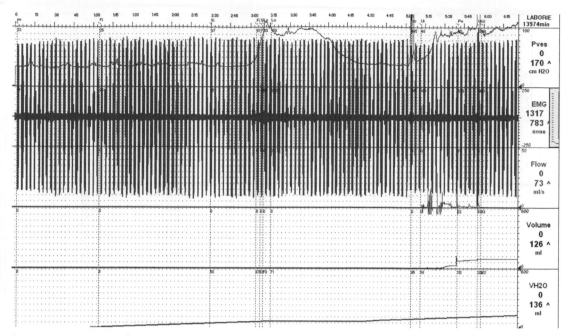

Fig. 9. EMG tracing artifact (*red*) due to sacral neuromodulation device.

was also not stable, but this affected the interpretation of Pdet. In this case, Pves provided a more useful and interpretable tracing to answer whether this patient had detrusor overactivity with filling (**Fig. 11**).

For fluoroscopic imaging, the position of the bladder may look lower and images of the urethra and/or bladder neck may be obstructed if the radiographic angle is straight in the anterior-posterior position. Repositioning the C-arm slightly

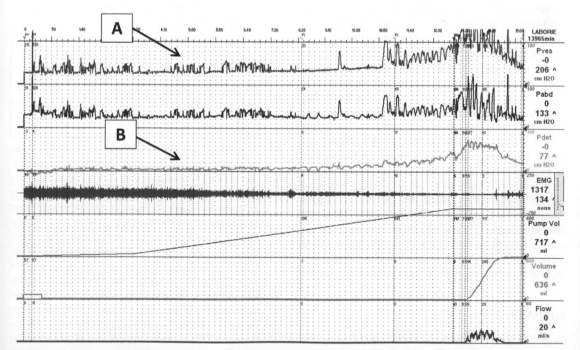

Fig. 10. (A) Pves tracing showed a significant amount of activity, which is only clarified by looking at Pabd, which had mirrored values. (B) Pdet is the accurate assessment of bladder pressure.

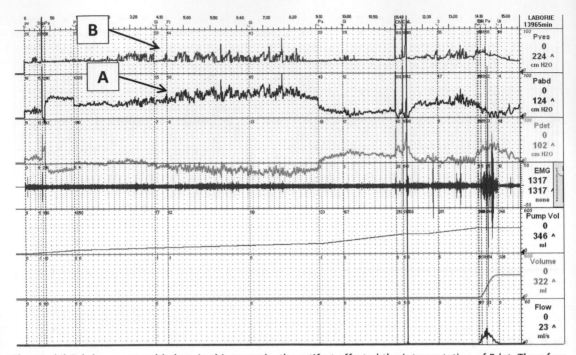

Fig. 11. (*A*) Pabd was not stable but, in this example, the artifact affected the interpretation of Pdet. Therefore, (*B*) Pves provided a more useful and interpretable tracing.

oblique allows these anatomic structures to appear. Similarly, in patients with urinary diversions and other potential pathological conditions, maneuvering the fluoroscopy source or the patient is required to delineate the anatomy.

The final pitfalls of urodynamic testing are that the study may not provide an answer regarding the posed urodynamic question, may give a false answer, or the study may not reproduce the patient's symptoms. If the testing does not reproduce clinical symptoms, some maneuvers can assist in eliciting these symptoms. To help with anxiety-related artifacts when asking the patient to void, leaving the room, or turning on the faucet is useful. Patient-reported triggers for urinary urgency (change in position, turning on the faucet or putting a hand in water) can be performed to illicit detrusor overactivity. Pelvic organ prolapse can be reduced to check for possible bladder function after a prolapse repair. Finally, the study can be repeated, "if the initial test suggests an abnormality, leaves the cause of troublesome lower urinary tract symptoms unresolved, or if there are technical problems preventing proper analysis."[16]

SUMMARY

As widespread access to urodynamic testing increases, appropriate clinical indications must be followed to minimize the possibility of unnecessary testing, which can result in patient morbidity and extra expense. Current urodynamic guidelines[2] provide clinical parameters for some aspects of testing, but the nuances of urodynamic testing are largely in the hands of the practicing urologists to perform tests that will add to diagnosis, prognosis, and surgical planning.

REFERENCES

1. Abrams P, Cardozo L, Fall M, et al. The standardisation of terminology in lower urinary tract function: report from the standardisation sub-committee of the International Continence Society. Urology 2003;61:37–49.
2. Winters JC, Dmochowski RR, Goldman HB, et al. Urodynamic studies in adults: AUA/SUFU guideline. J Urol 2012;188:2464–72.
3. Groutz A, Blaivas JG, Chaikin DC, et al. Noninvasive outcome measures of urinary incontinence and lower urinary tract symptoms: a multicenter study of micturition diary and pad tests. J Urol 2000;164:698–701.
4. Shumaker SA, Wyman JF, Uebersax JS, et al. Health-related quality of life measures for women with urinary incontinence: the incontinence impact questionnaire and the urogenital distress inventory. Continence Program in Women (CPW) Research Group. Qual Life Res 1994;3:291–306.
5. Blaivas JG, Panagopoulos G, Weiss JP, et al. Validation of the overactive bladder symptom score. J Urol 2007;178:543–7 [discussion: 7].

6. Barry MJ, Fowler FJ Jr, O'Leary MP, et al. The American Urological Association symptom index for benign prostatic hyperplasia. The measurement committee of the American Urological Association. J Urol 1992;148:1549–57 [discussion: 64].

7. Barry MJ. Evaluation of symptoms and quality of life in men with benign prostatic hyperplasia. Urology 2001;58:25–32 [discussion: 32].

8. McVary KT, Roehrborn CG, Avins AL, et al. Update on AUA guideline on the management of benign prostatic hyperplasia. J Urol 2011;185:1793–803.

9. Scarpero HM, Padmanabhan P, Xue X, et al. Patient perception of videourodynamic testing: a questionnaire based study. J Urol 2005;173:555–9.

10. Yokoyama T, Nozaki K, Nose H, et al. Tolerability and morbidity of urodynamic testing: a questionnaire-based study. Urology 2005;66:74–6.

11. Wolf JS Jr, Bennett CJ, Dmochowski RR, et al. Best practice policy statement on urologic surgery antimicrobial prophylaxis. J Urol 2008;179:1379–90.

12. Foon R, Toozs-Hobson P, Latthe P. Prophylactic antibiotics to reduce the risk of urinary tract infections after urodynamic studies. Cochrane Database Syst Rev 2012;(10):CD008224.

13. Krassioukov A, Warburton DE, Teasell R, et al. A systematic review of the management of autonomic dysreflexia after spinal cord injury. Arch Phys Med Rehabil 2009;90:682–95.

14. Furusawa K, Tokuhiro A, Sugiyama H, et al. Incidence of symptomatic autonomic dysreflexia varies according to the bowel and bladder management techniques in patients with spinal cord injury. Spinal Cord 2011;49:49–54.

15. Drach GW, Layton TN, Binard WJ. Male peak urinary flow rate: relationships to volume voided and age. J Urol 1979;122:210–4.

16. Schafer W, Abrams P, Liao L, et al. Good urodynamic practices: uroflowmetry, filling cystometry, and pressure-flow studies. Neurourol Urodyn 2002;21:261–74.

17. Wyndaele JJ, De Wachter S. Cystometrical sensory data from a normal population: comparison of two groups of young healthy volunteers examined with 5 years interval. Eur Urol 2002;42:34–8.

18. Cooper MA, Fletter PC, Zaszczurynski PJ, et al. Comparison of air-charged and water-filled urodynamic pressure measurement catheters. Neurourol Urodyn 2011;30:329–34.

19. Mayo ME. The value of sphincter electromyography in urodynamics. J Urol 1979;122:357–60.

20. Castro-Diaz D, Taracena Lafuente JM. Detrusor-sphincter dyssynergia. Int J Clin Pract Suppl 2006;(151):17–21.

21. Bates CP, Whiteside CG, Turner-Warwick R. Synchronous cine-pressure-flow-cysto-urethrography with special reference to stress and urge incontinence. Br J Urol 1970;42:714–23.

22. Wyndaele JJ, Gammie A, Bruschini H, et al. Bladder compliance what does it represent: can we measure it, and is it clinically relevant? Neurourol Urodyn 2011;30:714–22.

23. Lee CL, Wunderle K, Vasavada SP, et al. Reduction of radiation during fluoroscopic urodynamics: analysis of quality assurance protocol limiting fluoroscopic images during fluoroscopic urodynamic studies. Urology 2011;78:540–3.

24. Amis ES Jr, Butler PF, Applegate KE, et al. American College of Radiology white paper on radiation dose in medicine. J Am Coll Radiol 2007;4:272–84.

25. McGuire EJ, Fitzpatrick CC, Wan J, et al. Clinical assessment of urethral sphincter function. J Urol 1993;150:1452–4.

26. Faerber GJ, Vashi AR. Variations in Valsalva leak point pressure with increasing vesical volume. J Urol 1998;159:1909–11.

27. Lane TM, Shah PJ. Leak-point pressures. BJU Int 2000;86:942–9.

28. Turker P, Kilic G, Tarcan T. The presence of transurethral cystometry catheter and type of stress test affect the measurement of abdominal leak point pressure (ALPP) in women with stress urinary incontinence (SUI). Neurourol Urodyn 2010;29:536–9.

29. Lose G, Griffiths D, Hosker G, et al. Standardisation of urethral pressure measurement: report from the Standardisation Sub-Committee of the International Continence Society. Neurourol Urodyn 2002;21:258–60.

30. Harris N, Swithinbank L, Hayek SA, et al. Can maximum urethral closure pressure (MUCP) be used to predict outcome of surgical treatment of stress urinary incontinence? Neurourol Urodyn 2011;30:1609–12.

31. Kawasaki A, Wu JM, Amundsen CL, et al. Do urodynamic parameters predict persistent postoperative stress incontinence after midurethral sling? A systematic review. Int Urogynecol J 2012;23:813–22.

32. Abrams PH, Griffiths DJ. The assessment of prostatic obstruction from urodynamic measurements and from residual urine. Br J Urol 1979;51:129–34.

33. Hofner K, Kramer AF, Tan HK, et al. CHESS classification of bladder-outflow obstruction. A consequence in the discussion of current concepts. World J Urol 1995;13:59–64.

34. Schafer W. Analysis of bladder-outlet function with the linearized passive urethral resistance relation, linPURR, and a disease-specific approach for grading obstruction: from complex to simple. World J Urol 1995;13:47–58.

Vasectomy

Matthew D. Rogers, MD, Peter N. Kolettis, MD*

KEYWORDS

- Vasectomy • Sterilization • No-scalpel vasectomy • Minimally invasive vasectomy • Contraception
- Fascial interposition • Recanalization • Postvasectomy semen analysis

KEY POINTS

- Vasectomy is fast, safe, effective, and underutilized in comparison with tubal ligation.
- The preoperative visit is crucial for educating the patient on the risks and expectations of vasectomy, and especially that vasectomy is considered permanent.
- Minimally invasive vasectomy or no-scalpel vasectomy is preferable to conventional vasectomy.
- Fascial interposition decreases recanalization rates.
- Mucosal cautery appears to have the lowest vasectomy failure rates (<1%), although more high-quality comparative studies are needed.
- Patients must understand that an alternative birth-control method is necessary after the procedure until a postvasectomy semen analysis shows azoospermia.

INTRODUCTION

Vasectomy was first attempted on a canine in the 1800s, and has grown to be the most common operation performed by urologists today in the United States. More than 75% of vasectomies in the United States are performed by urologists. Vasectomy is a safe and effective form of contraception, yet it is underutilized today. Data collected in 2002 revealed that only 5.7% of United States men aged 15 to 44 years used vasectomy as a means of contraception.[1] Couples more commonly used condoms, oral contraceptives, or tubal ligation. Vasectomy is one of the most cost-effective contraceptive methods overall, its cost being is similar to that of the Mirena Intrauterine System ($844), the ParaGard Intrauterine Device ($718), and the Implanon implant ($791). The cost of vasectomy is one-quarter that of tubal ligation ($707 vs $2833).[2,3] Compared with tubal ligation, vasectomy is equally effective in preventing pregnancy; however, vasectomy is less invasive, simpler, safer, faster, and less expensive. The benefits of

vasectomy over tubal ligation include faster recovery and return to work, local rather than general anesthesia, and ability to perform the procedure in the office rather than in the operating suite. Complications are rare for both procedures, but tend to be more serious for tubal ligation because it is more invasive.[4]

Although the advantages of vasectomy over tubal ligation are evident, tubal ligation is 2 to 3 times more prevalent in the United States. This discrepancy is present worldwide, but there are at least 10 countries where the prevalence of vasectomy equals or exceeds tubal ligation: Canada, Bhutan, United Kingdom, New Zealand, Netherlands, Spain, Republic of Korea, Malta, Tajikistan, and Denmark.[5] The patterns of prevalence among the two groups in the United States have been found to be different. Tubal ligation is more prevalent among those with lower income and education levels, and among minority groups, whereas vasectomy use is higher among those with higher education and income and among white men.[6]

Disclosures: None.
Department of Urology, University of Alabama at Birmingham, 1720 2nd Avenue South, Birmingham, AL 35294, USA
* Corresponding author. Department of Urology, University of Alabama at Birmingham, FOT 1105, 1720 2nd Avenue South, Birmingham, AL 35294.
E-mail address: pkolettis@uabmc.edu

Urol Clin N Am 40 (2013) 559–568
http://dx.doi.org/10.1016/j.ucl.2013.07.009

It is clear that vasectomy should be performed equally as or more frequently than tubal ligation, and couples should therefore be counseled about the pros and cons of various contraception options so that an informed decision can be made.

PREOPERATIVE EVALUATION

It is recommended that a face-to-face consult take place with the patient before planning the vasectomy. It is beneficial for the patient's partner to be present, although this is not required. An appropriate medical history should be taken, focusing on his reproductive history. Patients should also be questioned about bleeding tendencies and anticoagulant use as per routine preoperative workup. If there is suspicion of coagulopathy, coagulation tests may be necessary; otherwise, preoperative blood work is not needed. A physical examination of the scrotum should be performed, with emphasis on manually isolating the vas deferens, as well looking for scrotal abnormality such as undescended testis or testis tumors. If the patient is unable to tolerate this examination while isolating the vas deferens, he may not be a good candidate for local anesthesia. The preoperative examination may also alert the physician to patients whose vasa are difficult to locate or isolate; this allows planning of oral sedation or general anesthesia at the time of procedure if necessary.

Preoperative counseling of the patient is extremely important, and may prevent postoperative patient dissatisfaction or even litigation in the case of complications or vasectomy failure. Most patients have decided on vasectomy as their choice of permanent contraception before meeting with the physician, but a discussion of the risks, benefits, alternatives, and expectations should be conducted at the initial consultation. Patients should be counseled that vasectomy is considered irreversible and permanent. If the patient indicates any uncertainty regarding the desire for future fertility (eg, asking about sperm cryopreservation), vasectomy should not be performed and other contraceptive methods should be discussed. Likewise, if the patient seems too young and has not had children, it is reasonable to encourage other contraceptive options that are less permanent. The other benefit of the preoperative consult is to give the patient a "cool-down" period while waiting for the procedure date, thus allowing time for patients to change their mind if an impetuous decision for vasectomy has been made initially.

The following points should be addressed at the preoperative visit, many of which are addressed in more detail in this article.

- Alternatives to vasectomy
- Risk of infection or hematoma (1%–2%)
- Risk of chronic scrotal pain (1%–3%)
- Refrain from ejaculation for 1 week after the procedure
- Vasectomy is considered permanent
- Vasectomy does not produce immediate sterility; another form of contraception is required after the procedure until vasectomy success is confirmed by semen analysis
- Early vasectomy failure: risk of needing repeat vasectomy (<1%)
- Late vasectomy failure: after vasectomy success is confirmed by semen analysis, there is still a small chance of pregnancy (approximately 1 in 2000)

ANESTHETIC TECHNIQUE

Vasectomy can be performed under any type of anesthesia, but most are performed under local anesthesia because it is well tolerated with minimal morbidity. Certain patients may require intravenous sedation or general anesthesia if they cannot tolerate the procedure or if the vas is particularly difficult to isolate. Oral sedation in the form of a benzodiazepine (eg, diazepam) is offered by some clinicians to decrease anxiety and aid in relaxing the patient. Lidocaine or bupivacaine without epinephrine are typically the local anesthetic agent of choice, and are injected using a small needle (eg, 25 gauge or smaller) to reduce patient discomfort. Some clinicians apply an anesthetic cream to the skin before the needle stick, although it is unclear whether this significantly decreases pain.[7,8]

VAS ISOLATION

Vasectomy is performed in 2 distinct steps: delivering and exposing the vas deferens out of the scrotum (vas isolation), and occluding the vas. Before the introduction of the no-scalpel technique, vas isolation was performed using the conventional technique, which used a larger incision and involved more dissection without special instruments. The no-scalpel vasectomy was first described in China in 1974.[9] The no-scalpel technique has been found to have shorter operative times and to decrease the rate of hematomas, infections, and pain during the procedure.[10–12] Today the standard of care is to perform a no-scalpel technique or a variation of such that remains minimally invasive.

In this article the term "minimally invasive vasectomy" is used to describe any vasectomy performed using a variation of the true no-scalpel vasectomy originally described by Li Shunqiang, as long as it maintains a small skin opening and limits the amount of dissection around the vas with specialized vasectomy instruments. **Box 1** lists the exact steps of the original no-scalpel vasectomy.[13] A more detailed description of the no-scalpel technique can be found in EngenderHealth's illustrated guide for surgeons.[14] Note that the no-scalpel technique refers to vas isolation only and does not denote a method of vas occlusion. Two instruments were designed for this procedure: the vas deferens fixation ring clamp (**Fig. 1**), used to grasp the vas, and the vas dissector (**Fig. 2**), which is a sharp, curved mosquito hemostat without serrations. These instruments are widely used today for minimally invasive vasectomies.

Routine preoperative antibiotics are not necessary when performing minimally invasive vasectomy with the sterile technique. Scrotal skin

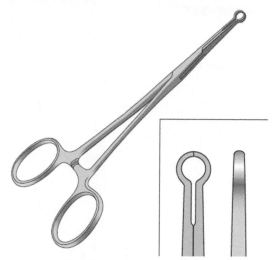

Fig. 1. Vas deferens ring fixation clamp. (© 2003 EngenderHealth. Used with permission.)

should be shaved, and the patient prepped with antimicrobial solution and draped in a standard sterile fashion. The procedure may be noticeably easier if the Dartos smooth muscle is relaxed, so using warm preparation solution and avoiding cold room temperatures may be beneficial.

Begin by isolating the straight portion of the vas with one hand using the 3-finger technique. Separate the vas from the spermatic-cord contents, and trap the vas over the middle finger and under the index finger and thumb (**Fig. 3**). There is no clear advantage of using one midline incision rather than bilateral incisions, and this should be decided upon based on surgeon preference and comfort. The bilateral incision approach may decrease the chance of cutting the same vas

---

Box 1
Dr Li Shunqiang's no-scalpel vasectomy steps

- Isolate the vas manually to a superficial position under the median raphe
- Create skin wheal with local anesthetic and inject into perivasal sheath
- Use vas ring clamp to firmly secure the vas through the skin
- With vas dissector at 45° angle to the vas, puncture the skin, vas sheath, and vas wall with the left tip of the vas dissector, then remove
- Close the vas dissector and puncture the skin and vas sheath. Spread to make small opening in the skin, exposing the bare anterior wall of the vas
- Puncture the vas with one tip of the vas dissector
- Use supination motion to deliver a loop of vas above the skin opening while simultaneously releasing the vas ring clamp with the other hand
- Regrasp the vas with the vas ring clamp. Use vas dissector to gently strip the sheath and vasal vessels away from the vas, yielding a clean segment of vas
- Divide the vas, with or without excision of a vas segment, and occlude the lumen per physician's preference
- Via same puncture hole, fix opposite vas in ring clamp and repeat steps
- Leave puncture hole unsutured except in rare cases requiring closure

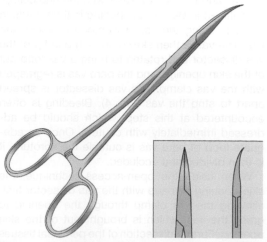

Fig. 2. Vas deferens dissector. (© 2003 EngenderHealth. Used with permission.)

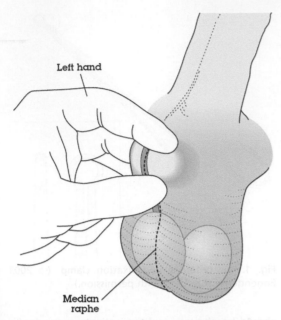

Fig. 3. Three-finger technique of vas deferens isolation. (© 2003 EngenderHealth. Used with permission.)

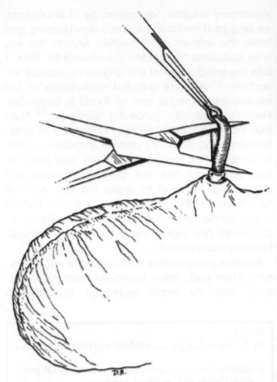

Fig. 4. The vas dissector is spread open, which brings the loop of vas deferens out of the scrotum and strips it of its sheath. (*From* Li SQ, Goldstein M, Zhu J, et al. The no-scalpel vasectomy. J Urol 1991;145:343; with permission.)

twice, although pulling on each vas should raise the testis on that side, which should eliminate this risk. Once the vas is isolated just underneath the skin between the fingers, local anesthetic is injected superficially to create a skin wheal. Injection into the vasal sheath can also facilitate anesthesia for the patient.

The next step of a minimally invasive vasectomy depends on whether an open-access or closed-access technique is performed. The closed-access technique, first described with the no-scalpel vasectomy, is performed by grasping the vas and the skin together with the ring clamp. As outlined in **Box 1**, an opening is then made in the skin using the vas dissector to expose the vas. The vas is then skewered with one tip of the vas dissector and rotated to bring a vas loop out of the skin opening, and the bare vas is regrasped with the vas clamp. The vas dissector is spread apart to strip the vas (**Fig. 4**). Bleeding is often encountered at this step, which should be addressed immediately with cautery. Once an adequate loop of bare vas is outside the scrotum, it is then divided and occluded.

When using the open-access technique, the skin opening is made with the vas dissector first, allowing the vas clamp through the opening to grasp the vas, which is brought out of the skin opening. Further dissection of the perivasal tissues to expose the bare vas is performed with the vas dissector. To facilitate this, a longitudinal incision

with a scalpel can be made through the vasal sheath along the vas, allowing the sheath to be separated from the vas more easily. Once a loop of bare vas is created, the remainder of the procedure is identical. The open-access technique was found in one study have a shorter operative time than the standard no-scalpel vasectomy, with no difference in length of incision.[15]

VAS DIVISION

Once a loop of bare vas deferens is outside of the wound, it is then divided with scissors. With a traditional vasectomy, a segment of vas is then excised. Questions of how much vas to remove and whether excision is even necessary remain unanswered. The optimal length of vas to excise, if any, should be left up to the surgeon. Excising a long (>2 cm) segment of vas may decrease the chance of recanalization,[16] but will also require more dissection along the spermatic cord, increase complications, and make vasectomy reversal more challenging and less successful.[17] The authors believe that if a segment of vas is excised, it should not exceed 1 to 2 cm in length.

As discussed later, the method of occlusion of the vas is more important for vasectomy success than is excision of a long vasal segment.

If a segment of vas is excised, sending the excised segments for histologic examination is not necessary. The measure of vasectomy success is determined by the results of the postvasectomy semen analysis (PVSA) rather than confirming vasal tissue on histologic evaluation. Despite this, some surgeons continue this practice because they find it useful to confirm vasal excision, and also out of fear of litigation in the case of a postvasectomy pregnancy.

VAS OCCLUSION

Vasectomy success can be measured by either azoospermia on PVSA or absence of pregnancy after vasectomy. In terms of achieving vasectomy success, the most important step comes after division of the vas and occlusion of the vas. There are several vas-occlusion techniques, including intraluminal cautery of one or both ends, ligation with suture, occlusion with clips, fascial interposition, and any combination of these. Review of the literature reveals many studies examining each of these techniques, yet it is difficult to conclude which occlusion method is superior, owing to study flaws and lack of uniformity in terms of patient follow-up and measurement of success. Several methods of vas occlusion are presented here, and their efficacy discussed.

Intraluminal cautery, or mucosal cautery, is performed by applying thermal cautery or low-voltage electrical cautery with a needle tip within the lumen of the vas. It is unclear as to what length of cauterized mucosa is required to create occlusion, but most surgeons cauterize between 5 and 15 mm of vas lumen. The goal is to destroy only the mucosal layer, which then scars to create a plug in the lumen. Avoiding thermal injury to the muscular layer prevents complete sloughing of the cauterized vas segment, which could potentially allow recanalization. When mucosal cautery is applied to both the abdominal and testicular ends of the divided vas deferens without using fascial interposition, vasectomy failure rates are less than 1%.[18–20]

Fascial interposition has become a commonly used technique, because when used with other methods of occlusion it decreases vasectomy failure rates.[21] The goal is to separate the two newly divided ends of the vas to reduce the chance of recanalization. To do so, a layer of vas sheath is placed between the two ends of the vas as a tissue barrier with the help of 1 or 2 absorbable sutures (**Fig. 5**). The fascial layer can be placed over the abdominal or the testicular end. When fascial interposition is combined with mucosal cautery of both ends of the divided vas, failure rates are less than 1%.[20,22–26]

Another commonly used method of vas occlusion is suture ligation of the vas. Studies evaluating vasectomy using ligation of the vas without fascial interposition reveal a wide range of failure rates from 0% to 12.7%.[21,27–33] The only randomized study reported a failure rate of 12.7% out of 416 patients who received vasectomy and were followed up postoperatively.[21] A high-quality prospective study revealed a failure rate of 11.5%.[33] Because of the higher rates of failure, ligation of the vas without fascial interposition is not recommended.

Combining fascial interposition with the suture ligation technique improves success rates, as proved in a randomized study in which fascial interposition decreased the failure rate by half, down to 5.8%.[21] Other studies showed better outcomes. A retrospective review of 2150 patients undergoing suture ligation and excision with fascial interposition had no failures.[34] More recently, a large prospective study from Iran reported a 2.1% failure rate.[35] Although fascial interposition increases efficacy when combined with suture ligation, failure rates are often unacceptably high.

In 2002, 29.5% of United States physicians reported using clips as part of their occlusion technique.[36] Similar to ligation with suture, applying clips to the vas without using fascial interposition may result in undesirable rates of vasectomy failure. One study revealed a failure rate of 8.7%,[37] whereas smaller older studies report failure rates

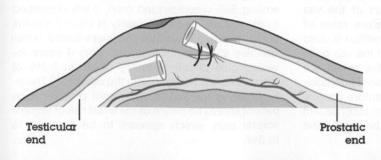

Fig. 5. Fascial interposition is performed by suturing a layer of vas sheath between the two ends of the vas deferens, which separates the ends of the vas and decreases the risk of recanalization. (© 2003 EngenderHealth. Used with permission.)

Testicular end

Prostatic end

of less than 1%.[38,39] There are limited data assessing the efficacy of vasectomy when fascial interposition is used in conjunction with clipping the vas. The only study found reported no failures out of 1073 patients.[40] There is therefore insufficient evidence to determine the exact efficacy of using clips, but fascial interposition is likely to decrease failure rates based on the randomized study of fascial interposition and suture ligation.[21] Some consider that applying too much pressure to the vas with clips or sutures creates ischemia and sloughing of the ligated stump, resulting in recanalization, which could explain some of the higher failure rates seen with these methods.

In an attempt to decrease the risk of postvasectomy chronic pain, some have advocated using a variation of an open-ended vasectomy whereby the testicular end of the vas is left open, the abdominal end is occluded with mucosal cautery, and fascial interposition is then performed. Leaving the testicular end open is proposed to decrease back pressure on the epididymis and decrease the risk of chronic pain, although this has not yet been proved in clinical studies.[12] However, it has been shown to be an effective vasectomy method. Four studies using this technique were found, including one prospective study, with failure rates between 0% and 0.5%.[20,37,41,42] Leaving out the fascial interposition step with this technique results in a higher failure rate (4%) and is not recommended.[43]

One other method of vas occlusion has been found to be effective, although it is rarely, if ever, used in the United States. Known as the Marie Stopes International technique, the vas is not divided. Instead, occlusion of the vas occurs after cauterization of the outside of the vas, creating a full-thickness injury on one side and a partial-thickness injury on the other.[44] The failure rate of this method performed at the Marie Stopes Clinic was reported to be less than 1% after 45,123 vasectomies.

Based on all of this information, no firm conclusion can be drawn as to which occlusion technique is best, but some methods appear to be more effective than others. It is clear that use of fascial interposition reduces rates of vasectomy failure, and mucosal cautery of both ends of the vas seems to consistently result in failure rates of less than 1% whether fascial interposition is used or not. Leaving the testicular end of the vas open has also been consistently effective when the abdominal end is cauterized and fascial interposition is performed. Use of clips or suture ligature with fascial interposition has shown inconsistent results in the literature, and may not be as effective as using mucosal cautery.

The American Urological Association (AUA) released guidelines in 2012 recommending 1 of 4 occlusion techniques should be used, based on available evidence[45]:

- Mucosal cautery of both ends with fascial interposition (without clips or ligatures)
- Mucosal cautery of both ends without fascial interposition (without clips or ligatures)
- Open-ended vasectomy leaving the testicular end of the vas unoccluded, using mucosal cautery on the abdominal end, and performing fascial interposition
- Marie Stopes International technique (nondivisional method of extended electrocautery)

The skin opening can be closed with suture or left open, depending on surgeon preference. Strictly speaking, to be called a no-scalpel vasectomy the skin is not sutured. The authors use one suture to close the wound and apply antibiotic ointment, followed by a sterile gauze and scrotal supporter.

COMPLICATIONS

Complications of infection and hematoma are uncommon using minimally invasive vas isolation, with the rate somewhere on the order of 1% to 2%.[10,46–48] As discussed earlier, the risk of these complications is less with the minimally invasive techniques than with conventional open vasectomy. There are rare reports of Fournier gangrene occurring postoperatively, one case of which resulted in death.[49]

Debilitating chronic scrotal pain may occur in men immediately or years following their vasectomy, and is sometimes referred to as postvasectomy pain syndrome. In some cases, the pain may be severe enough to adversely affect the quality of life. Patients should be warned of this risk before proceeding with surgery. Various studies differ in the reported rate of postvasectomy pain. The only comparative study showed that 6% of a group of 101 vasectomized men had pain severe enough to seek medical attention, compared with 2% of nonvasectomized men.[50] Leslie and colleagues[51] found in a prospective audit that among 593 vasectomized men, 0.9% described a pain that affected their quality of life at 7 months postoperatively. Two questionnaire-based retrospective studies with follow-up over 4 years revealed pain affecting quality of life in 2.2% of men in one study, and 5% in the other.[52,53] Therefore, during the informed consent process each patient should be aware of the small risk of chronic scrotal pain, which appears to be around 1% to 3%.

There has been some discussion about possible association of vasectomy with diseases such as prostate cancer and primary progressive aphasia. Based on available evidence, these claims have not been substantiated. A meta-analysis performed by Dennis and colleagues[54] showed a possible increased risk for prostate cancer only in the pooled hospital-based case-control studies with a relative risk (RR) of 1.92 (95% confidence interval [CI] 1.37–2.67), whereas pooled cohort studies and population-based case-control studies did not show a statistically significant RR. Another group[55] performed a systematic review of the literature and reported an RR of 1.23 (95% CI 1.01–1.49), and concluded that no causal relationship was found between vasectomy and prostate cancer. There was significant unexplained heterogeneity among the studies reviewed, and both groups of investigators were of the opinion that there is high risk of selection bias with these studies, which could explain the statistical differences.

Another independent meta-analysis was more recently performed by the authors of the AUA guidelines for vasectomy,[45] who pooled 10 comparative cohort studies and found an RR of 1.08 (95% CI 0.88–1.32). One group[56] evaluated the possibility of certain subgroups that may have increased risk, and found that there were no associations between prostate cancer and age at vasectomy, years elapsed since vasectomy, or calendar year of vasectomy. Overall, review of the evidence shows no association between vasectomy and prostate cancer. It is not necessary to discuss prostate cancer routinely with patients considering vasectomy, and men who undergo vasectomy should not be screened differently for prostate cancer.

Primary progressive aphasia (PPA) is a dementia syndrome with aphasia as the presenting symptom, and one small study reported vasectomy to be a possible risk factor for PPA.[57] The investigators theorized that the link between the two may be related to vasectomy-induced immune response to the tau protein shared by both sperm and brain. A subsequent study did not find an association between antisperm antibodies and cognitive status or language-function status.[58] Large epidemiologic studies have yet to find an association between vasectomy and dementia, including lack of association with immune-related diseases.[59] It is therefore unlikely that vasectomy poses a risk for dementia, and patients do not need to be counseled regarding this preoperatively. Numerous studies have also examined a possible relationship between vasectomy and cardiovascular disease, atherosclerosis, stroke, and testicular cancer.[60–62] There is no link between these diseases and vasectomy.

POSTOPERATIVE CARE

The authors ask patients to avoid any physical activity for 2 days and to refrain from ejaculation and strenuous activity for 1 week, thus allowing time for luminal occlusion to mature. The procedure does not produce sterility immediately because sperm that could cause pregnancy remain in the reproductive system after vasectomy. Another method of contraception must be used until a favorable PVSA is rendered.

The goal of the PVSA is to rule out vasectomy failure. Vasectomy failure can be due to either technical failure or recanalization. A technical failure can occur by operating on the same vas twice, failing to correctly identify the vas, or, rarely, a duplicated vas deferens. Vasectomy failure is more commonly due to the phenomenon of recanalization. Histologic studies of vasectomy sites after failure reveal 1 or more channels (canaliculi) formed through the scar tissue, which allow passage of sperm. Recanalization can occur early or late. Early recanalization can be picked up on PVSA that shows high numbers of motile sperm. Late recanalization occurs after a man is declared sterile by PVSA, and is usually identified after occurrence of a pregnancy. The risk of pregnancy consequent to late recanalization (known as late vasectomy failure) is approximately 1 in 2000.[18,45,63–65]

The optimal timing of the PVSA remains controversial. The rationale for early tests is that men can stop using other forms of contraception sooner, whereas later testing will have a greater chance of showing azoospermia and decrease the number of tests. Sperm clearance rates vary across studies, but the majority show azoospermia in more than 80% of men at 12 weeks.[20,21,66–70] The authors prefer obtaining the PVSA at 12 weeks, but any time from 8 to 16 weeks after vasectomy is appropriate as per the most recent AUA guidelines.[45] Some have tried irrigation of the vas deferens with saline or water to decrease time to azoospermia, but only 1 of 4 randomized studies showed a benefit with vas irrigation.[69,71–73]

Some physicians base the timing of the PVSA on the number of ejaculations (eg, 20 ejaculations) since vasectomy. The literature is inconclusive on this matter, and one group's prospective study reported only 44% of patients with azoospermia after 20 ejaculations, with a great degree of variability.[33] Time since vasectomy may therefore be a better parameter for predicting vasectomy success.

Clearance of motile sperm occurs more rapidly than that of nonmotile sperm. When mucosal cautery is used with fascial interposition, motile sperm are mostly absent by 5 to 6 weeks.[26,74] Nonmotile sperm can persist in the semen for months after vasectomy because they can reside in the distal vas deferens or seminal vesicles. If a PVSA reveals high numbers of motile sperm, this is due to either early recanalization or technical error. Patients with signs of recanalization may eventually develop azoospermia (vasectomy success) or may have persistently high numbers of sperm, and eventually are deemed a vasectomy failure.

The PVSA can be either given in a laboratory or collected at home and delivered to the physician or laboratory within 1 hour. The sample should then be analyzed within 1 hour of delivery. Only 16% of samples show a decrease in motility between the first and second hour after collection.[75] Because centrifugation may reduce motility, World Health Organization guidelines (2010) state that centrifugation of the sample should be avoided.[76] The PVSA can be performed by a laboratory with quantitative analysis, or can be performed by the surgeon in the office setting with high-powered light microscopy. In the case of persistent sperm in the PVSA, determination of sperm concentration is difficult to achieve with office examination.

The presence of nonmotile sperm on PVSA can be troubling for the surgeon. It has been shown, however, that nonmotile sperm in concentrations of less than 100,000/mL on PVSA carry a risk of pregnancy similar to a PVSA with azoospermia.[40,77] Therefore, patients can discontinue other contraception after one PVSA shows either azoospermia or rare nonmotile sperm ($\leq$100,000/mL).

If motile sperm are present on semen analysis, this indicates either recanalization or technical failure. In this case, repeat testing should be performed every 4 to 6 weeks until azoospermia or rare nonmotile sperm is seen, at which time vasectomy can be considered successful. At 6 months postoperatively, motile sperm on PVSA indicate vasectomy failure, and repeat vasectomy should be offered. If greater than 100,000 nonmotile sperm per milliliter are present after 6 months, the decision to repeat the vasectomy is based on clinical judgment and patient preference.

SUMMARY

Vasectomy has proved to be a safe and effective form of sterilization. It is underutilized in comparison with tubal ligation, even though vasectomy is simpler, faster, safer, and less expensive. The preoperative visit prior to vasectomy is important for discussion of expectations and risks, including the less than 1% risk of vasectomy failure and

the need for contraception after the procedure until the PVSA shows successful vas occlusion. The no-scalpel vasectomy technique of vas isolation and its minimally invasive variations have decreased the complication rates for vasectomy. The vas occlusion technique determines the chance of vasectomy success, although there is a lack of high-quality, randomized studies for comparison. Based on the current literature, fascial interposition increases efficacy when combined with another method of vas occlusion, and mucosal cautery seems to be the most effective method of occlusion, resulting in failure rates of less than 1%. Further research comparing these techniques is needed to more clearly identify which methods result in the most desirable vasectomy outcomes.

REFERENCES

1. Martinez GM, Chandra A, Amba JC, et al. Fertility, contraception, and fatherhood: data on men and women from cycle 6 (2002) of the 2002 National Survey of Family Growth. Vital Health Stat 23 2006;(26): 1–142.
2. Trussell J, Lalla AM, Doan QV, et al. Cost effectiveness of contraceptives in the United States. Contraception 2009;79:5–14.
3. Trussell J. Update on and correction to the cost-effectiveness of contraceptives in the United States. Contraception 2012;85:611.
4. Bartz D, Greenberg JA. Sterilization in the United States. Rev Obstet Gynecol 2008;1:23–32.
5. Anderson J, Jamieson D, Warner L. Contraceptive sterilization among married adults: national data on who chooses vasectomy and tubal sterilization. Contraception 2012;85:552–7.
6. Anderson JE, Warner L, Jamieson DJ, et al. Contraception sterilization use among married men in the United States: results from the male sample of the National Survey of Family Growth. Contraception 2010;82:230–5.
7. Cooper TP. Use of EMLA cream with vasectomy. Urology 2002;60:135–7.
8. Thomas AA, Nguyen CT, Dhar NB, et al. Topical anesthesia with EMLA does not decrease pain during vasectomy. J Urol 2008;180:271–3.
9. Li S. Ligation of vas deferens by clamping method under direct vision. Chin Med J 1976;4:213–4.
10. Sokal D, McMullen S, Gates D, et al. A comparative study of the no scalpel and standard incision approaches to vasectomy in 5 countries. The male sterilization investigator team. J Urol 1999;162: 1621–5.
11. Cook LA, Pun A, van Vliet H, et al. Scalpel versus no-scalpel incision for vasectomy. Cochrane Database Syst Rev 2007;(2):CD004112.

12. Labrecque M, Dufresne C, Barone MA, et al. Vasectomy surgical techniques: a systematic review. BMC Med 2004;2:21.

13. Li SQ, Goldstein M, Zhu J, et al. The no-scalpel vasectomy. J Urol 1991;145:341–4.

14. Engender Health. No-scalpel vasectomy an illustrated guide for surgeons. 3rd edition. 2003. Available at: http://www.engenderhealth.org/pubs/family-planning/vasectomy.php. Accessed March 2013.

15. Chen KC, Peng CC, Hsieh HM, et al. Simply modified no-scalpel vasectomy (percutaneous vasectomy)—a comparative study against the standard no-scalpel vasectomy. Contraception 2005;71:153–6.

16. Edwards IS. Follow up after vasectomy. Med J Aust 1973;2:132–5.

17. Practice Committee of the American Society for Reproductive Medicine. Practice Committee of the American Society for Reproductive Medicine: Vasectomy reversal. Fertil Steril 2006;(86):S268–71.

18. Philp T, Guillebaud J, Budd D. Complications of vasectomy: review of 16,000 patients. Br J Urol 1984;56:745–8.

19. O'Brien TS, Cranston D, Ashwin P, et al. Temporary reappearance of sperm 12 months after vasectomy clearance. Br J Urol 1995;76:371–2.

20. Barone MA, Irsula B, Chen-Mok M, et al. Effectiveness of vasectomy using cautery. BMC Urol 2004;4:10.

21. Sokal D, Irsula B, Hays M, et al. Vasectomy by ligation and excision, with or without fascial interposition: a randomized controlled trial [ISRCTN77781689]. BMC Med 2004;2:6.

22. Marmar JL, Kessler S, Hartanto VH. A minimally invasive vasectomy with the no suture, inline method for vas occlusion. Int J Fertil Womens Med 2001;46:257–64.

23. Moss WM. Sutureless vasectomy, an improved technique: 1300 cases performed without failure. Fertil Steril 1976;27:1040–5.

24. Schmidt SS, Free MJ. The bipolar needle for vasectomy. I. Experience with the first 1000 cases. Fertil Steril 1978;29:676–80.

25. Schmidt SS. Vasectomy by section, luminal fulguration and fascial interposition: results from 6248 cases. Br J Urol 1995;76:373–4.

26. Labreque M, Hays M, Chen-Mok M, et al. Frequency and patterns of early recanalization after vasectomy. BMC Urol 2006;6:25.

27. Nazerali H, Thapa S, Hays M, et al. Vasectomy effectiveness in Nepal: a retrospective study. Contraception 2003;67:397–401.

28. Alderman PM. Complications in a series of 1224 vasectomies. J Fam Pract 1991;33:579–84.

29. McGuinness BW. Vasectomy—a review of 100 cases. J R Coll Gen Pract 1976;26:297–302.

30. Jackson P, Phillips B, Prosser E, et al. A male sterilization clinic. Br Med J 1970;4:295–7.

31. Kotwal S, Sundaram SK, Rangaiah CS, et al. Does the type of suture material used for ligation of the vas deferens affect vasectomy success? Eur J Contracept Reprod Health Care 2008;13:25–30.

32. Lucon AM, Pasqualotto FF, Schneider-Monteiro ED, et al. Spontaneous recanalization after vasectomy. ScientificWorldJournal 2006;6:2366–9.

33. Barone MA, Nazerali H, Cortes M, et al. A prospective study of time and number of ejaculations to azoospermia after vasectomy by ligation and excision. J Urol 2003;170:892–6.

34. Kumar V, Kaza RM. A combination of check tug and fascial interposition with no-scalpel vasectomy. J Fam Plann Reprod Health Care 2001;27:100.

35. Farrokh-Eslamlou HR, Eslami M, Abdi-Rad I, et al. Evaluating success of no-scalpel vasectomy by ligation and excision with fascial interposition in a large prospective study in Islamic Republic of Iran. East Mediterr Health J 2011;17:517–22.

36. Barone MA, Hutchinson PL, Johnson CH, et al. Vasectomy in the United States, 2002. J Urol 2006;176:232–6.

37. Labreque M, Nazerali H, Mondor M, et al. Effectiveness and complications associated with 2 vasectomy occlusion techniques. J Urol 2002;168:2496–8.

38. Bennett AH. Vasectomy without complication. Vasectomy without complication. Urology 1976;7:184–5.

39. Chawla A, Bowles B, Zini A. Vasectomy follow-up: clinical significance of rare nonmotile sperm in postoperative semen analysis. Urology 2004;64:1212–5.

40. Korthorst RA, Consten D, Van Roijen HJ. Clearance after vasectomy with a single semen sample containing < than 100 000 immotile sperm/mL: analysis of 1073 patients. BJU Int 2010;105:1572–5.

41. Moss WM. A comparison of open-end versus closed-end vasectomies: a report on 6220 cases. Contraception 1992;46:521–5.

42. Denniston GC, Kuebi L. Open-ended vasectomy: approaching the ideal technique. J Am Board Fam Pract 1994;7:285–7.

43. Shapiro EI, Silber SJ. Open-ended vasectomy, sperm granuloma, and postvasectomy orchalgia. Fertil Steril 1979;32:546–50.

44. Black TR, Gates DS, Lavely K, et al. The percutaneous electrocoagulation vasectomy technique—a comparative trial with the standard incision technique at Marie Stopes House, London. Contraception 1989;39:359–68.

45. Sharlip I, Belker A, Honig S, et al. Vasectomy: AUA Guideline. American Urological Association (AUA) Guideline. J Urol 2012;188(Suppl 6):2482–91.

46. Kendrick JS, Gonzales B, Huber D, et al. Complications of vasectomies in the United States. J Fam Pract 1987;25:245–8.

47. Arellano Lara S, Gonzalez Barrera JL, Hernandez Ono A, et al. No-scalpel vasectomy: review of the first 1,000 cases in a family medicine unit. Arch Med Res 1997;28:517–22.

48. Kumar V, Kaza RM, Singh I, et al. An evaluation of the no-scalpel vasectomy technique. BJU Int 1999; 83:283–4.

49. Viddeleer AC, Lycklama GA. Lethal Fournier's gangrene following vasectomy. J Urol 1992;147: 1613–4.

50. Morris C, Mishra K, Kirkman RJ. A study to assess the prevalence of chronic testicular pain in post-vasectomy men compared to non-vasectomised men. J Fam Plann Reprod Health Care 2002;28: 142–4.

51. Leslie TA, Illing RO, Cranston DW, et al. The incidence of chronic scrotal pain after vasectomy: a prospective audit. BJU Int 2007;100:1330–3.

52. Chloe JM, Kirkemo AK. Questionnaire-based outcomes study of nononcological post-vasectomy complications. J Urol 1996;155:1284–6.

53. McMahon AJ, Buckley J, Taylor A, et al. Chronic testicular pain following vasectomy. Br J Urol 1992;69:188–91.

54. Dennis LK, Dawson DV, Resnick MI. Vasectomy and the risk of prostate cancer: a meta-analysis examining vasectomy status, age at vasectomy, and time since vasectomy. Prostate Cancer Prostatic Dis 2002;5:193–203.

55. Bernal-Delgado E, Latour-Perez J, Pradas-Arnal F, et al. The association between vasectomy and prostate cancer: a systematic review of the literature. Fertil Steril 1998;70:191–200.

56. Holt SK, Salinas CA, Stanford JL. Vasectomy and the risk for prostate cancer. J Urol 2008;180:2565–7.

57. Weintraub S, Fahey C, Johnson N, et al. Vasectomy in men with primary progressive aphasia. Cogn Behav Neurol 2006;19:190–3.

58. Han C, Kim H, Kwon D, et al. Lack of association between antisperm antibodies and language dysfunction in Alzheimer's disease. Arch Gerontol Geriatr 2010;50:338–40.

59. Goldacre MJ, Wotton CJ, Seagroatt V, et al. Immune related disease before and after vasectomy: an epidemiological database study. Hum Reprod 2007;22:1273–8.

60. Goldacre MJ, Wotton CJ, Seagroatt V, et al. Cancer and cardiovascular disease after vasectomy: an epidemiological database study. Fertil Steril 2005; 84:1438–43.

61. Coady SA, Sharrett AR, Zheng ZJ, et al. Vasectomy, inflammation, atherosclerosis and long-term followup for cardiovascular diseases: no associations in the atherosclerosis risk in communities study. J Urol 2002;167:204–7.

62. Hewitt G, Logan CJH, Curry RC. Does vasectomy cause testicular cancer? Br J Urol 1993;71:607–8.

63. Philp T, Guillebaud J, Budd D. Late failure of vasectomy after two documented analyses showing azoospermic semen. Br Med J 1984;289:77–9.

64. Aldermann PM. The lurking sperm. JAMA 1988; 259:3142–4.

65. Black T, Francome C. The evolution of the Marie Stopes electrocautery no-scalpel vasectomy procedure. J Fam Plann Reprod Health Care 2002; 28:137–8.

66. Alderman PM. General and anomalous sperm disappearance characteristics found in a large vasectomy series. Fertil Steril 1989;51:859–62.

67. Dhar NB, Bhatt A, Jones JS. Determining the success of vasectomy. BJU Int 2006;97:773–6.

68. Poddar AK, Roy S. Disappearance of spermatozoa from semen after vasectomy. J Popul Res 1976;3: 61–70.

69. Singh D, Dasila NS, Vasudeva P, et al. Intraoperative distal vasal flushing—does it improve the rate of early azoospermia following no-scalpel vasectomy? A prospective, randomized, controlled study. Urology 2010;76:341–4.

70. Griffin T, Tooher R, Nowakowski K, et al. How little is enough? The evidence for post-vasectomy testing. J Urol 2005;174:29–36.

71. Eisner B, Schuster T, Rodgers P, et al. A randomized clinical trial of the effect of intraoperative saline perfusion on postvasectomy azoospermia. Ann Fam Med 2004;2:221–3.

72. Mason RG, Dodds L, Swami SK. Sterile water irrigation of the distal vas deferens at vasectomy: does it accelerate clearance of sperm? A prospective randomized trial. Urology 2002;59:424–7.

73. Pearce I, Adeyoju A, Bhatt RI, et al. The effect of perioperative distal vasal lavage on subsequent semen analysis after vasectomy: a prospective randomized controlled trial. BJU Int 2002;90:282–5.

74. Edwards IS. Earlier testing after vasectomy, based on the absence of motile sperm. Fertil Steril 1993; 59:431–6.

75. Schulte RT, Keller LM, Hiner MR, et al. Temporal decreases in sperm motility: which patients should have motility checked at both 1 and 2 hours after collection? J Androl 2008;29:558–63.

76. World Health Organization. WHO laboratory manual for the examination and processing of human semen. 5th edition. Geneva (Switzerland): World Health Organization; 2010.

77. World Health Organization Task Force on Methods for the Regulation of Male Fertility. Contraceptive efficacy of testosterone-induced azoospermia and oligozospermia in normal men. Fertil Steril 1996; 65:821.

Office-Based Sperm Retrieval for Treatment of Infertility

Kiranpreet K. Khurana, MD,
Edmund S. Sabanegh Jr, MD*

KEYWORDS

- Office-based • Epididymal sperm aspiration • Testicular sperm extraction
- Testicular sperm aspiration • Microdissection

KEY POINTS

- Sperm retrieval is indicated in men with obstructive azoospermia, nonobstructive azoospermia, and in some cases of severe oligospermia.
- For analgesia and anesthesia, local anesthetic infiltration, spermatic cord regional block, or conscious sedation may be used for office-based procedures. Proper personnel training and facility accreditation are needed to use conscious sedation.
- Appropriate discussion before any procedure, including possibility of repeat procedures, must be held, and if indicated, referral to genetic counseling should be provided.
- Success rates of different procedures for nonobstructive azoospermia depend on histopathology, cause, and procedural approach.
- Complication rates of sperm retrieval procedures are low, but rare clinically apparent side effects may be seen.
- Sperm cryopreservation capability is an important component of sperm retrieval procedures.

INTRODUCTION

Minimally invasive sperm retrieval procedures have become increasingly relevant in the last 2 decades as intracytoplasmic sperm injection (ICSI), a technique allowing conceptions from minimal sperm recovery, has revolutionized success rates of assisted reproductive technology (ART). ICSI was described by Palermo and colleagues[1] in 1992, who reported successful pregnancies in 4 couples with severe male infertility using this technique. The success of ICSI has been shown to be better than conventional in vitro fertilization (IVF) in terms of fertilization rates. Bungum and colleagues[2] studied fertilization rates in couples with unexplained infertility who had failed intrauterine insemination. The fertilization rate after ICSI was significantly higher than conventional IVF, at 68% and 46%, respectively. In a randomized study,[3] fertilization rate per oocyte after IVF was 41%, whereas the rate after ICSI was 50%. Before development of ICSI, infertility caused by certain male factors, such as nonobstructive azoospermia (NOA), was difficult to treat and had low success rates. However, ICSI has the ability to surpass some of the most challenging cases of impaired spermatogenesis.

Along with development of more efficient ways of sperm implantation came the need to retrieve sperm successfully. Advanced, more refined and

Funding Sources: None.
Conflicts of Interest: None.
Department of Urology, Glickman Urological & Kidney Institute, Cleveland Clinic, 9500 Euclid Avenue, Q10, Cleveland, OH 44195, USA
* Corresponding author.
E-mail address: sabanee@ccf.org

Urol Clin N Am 40 (2013) 569–579
http://dx.doi.org/10.1016/j.ucl.2013.07.005
0094-0143/13/$ – see front matter © 2013 Elsevier Inc. All rights reserved.

less invasive sperm retrieval techniques have been developed to provide viable sperm for these difficult cases. Anatomically, the main areas for sperm retrieval are the testis, vas deferens, and epididymis. Choice of target for sperm retrieval depends on the cause of infertility and the likelihood of retrieving viable sperm. For example, the epididymis may be aspirated percutaneously in a man with congenital bilateral absence of vas deferens. Surgical sperm retrieval techniques produce quantities of sperm that are insufficient for intrauterine insemination but may be adequate for multiple trials of ICSI.

For cost-effectiveness and efficiency, office-based procedures are becoming increasingly pertinent. A myriad of surgical techniques to retrieve sperm exist, but not all of them may be used in an office-based setting. Successful office-based procedures require adequate training of surgeons as well as staff. The advantages of performing procedures in an office setting include avoidance of general anesthesia, cost benefit, time efficiency, and quicker patient recovery. The goal of this article is to review office-based sperm retrieval procedures for ART. The indications for sperm retrieval from each anatomic target, preoperative considerations and preparation, surgical details, success rates, factors that play a role in success, and complication rates of each procedure are reviewed.

INDICATIONS FOR SPERM RETRIEVAL

Sperm retrieval is often necessary for azoospermia and severe oligospermia with unfavorable viability. Azoospermia is defined as the absence of spermatozoa in the ejaculate, and severe oligospermia is the presence of fewer than 5 million spermatozoa per milliliter of the ejaculate. Azoospermia is classified into obstructive and nonobstructive. Azoospermia is present in 1% of all men, but 15% of infertile men.[4] In 1 study,[5] obstruction caused 40% of azoospermic cases. In obstructive azoospermia (OA), the production of spermatozoa from the testes is normal. However, there is either extrinsic or intrinsic blockage or absence of epididymis, vas deferens, or ejaculatory ducts.

Vasal obstruction may result from previous vasectomy, fibrotic reaction from inguinal hernia repair with mesh, radical prostatectomy, and cystic fibrosis. For men with OA caused by vasal abnormalities, sperm may be retrieved from the vas deferens proximal to the site of obstruction. This procedure is almost always performed in the setting of microsurgical reconstructive surgery, when vasal fluid may be collected and cryopreserved in association with planned vasovasostomy

or vasoepididymostomy. Vasal fluid aspiration may rarely be performed as a separate procedure without reconstruction. Vasal sperm have undergone full maturation as they have traveled through the epididymis.

The epididymis is a more common site used for sperm retrieval. Indications include OA caused by congenital bilateral absence of the vas deferens (CBAVD) or vas deferens occlusion in a setting in which patients are not candidates for or do not desire microsurgical reconstruction. Extraction from the epididymis may be performed percutaneously as well as microsurgically.

Indications for testicular sperm retrieval include NOA, OA with failed reconstructive surgery or epididymal aspiration, and in cases of increased sperm DNA fragmentation and previous unsuccessful IVF/ICSI with ejaculated or epididymal sperm. Testicular sperm extraction may be performed percutaneously, open, or microsurgically.

ANESTHESIA FOR OFFICE-BASED SPERM RETRIEVAL

Office-based procedures require adequate training of all involved personnel, as well as preparedness for emergency situations. Local or regional anesthesia, or conscious sedation, may be used in an office setting. Percutaneous procedures may require only local or regional anesthesia, whereas multifocal, bilateral, or open procedures may need conscious sedation. Patient and physician preference influence final choice of anesthetic.

Local anesthesia involves injecting the skin and subcutaneous tissue with anesthetic medications. It is easy to use, avoids side effects of general anesthesia, and provides adequate local analgesia. Local anesthetics block sodium channels to inhibit the action potential of a neuronal impulse. They can be divided into amide and ester classes. The most commonly used amide is lidocaine, whereas a commonly used ester is tetracaine. If a patient is allergic to lidocaine, an ester class analgesic may be used. Different concentrations of these medications exist, and the lowest concentration needed to provide adequate analgesia should be used. Side effects are a result of intravascular injection and high dose, and include tinnitus, perioral numbness, confusion, seizures, and even cardiovascular collapse.

A spermatic cord block provides regional anesthesia. The block is made by holding the spermatic cord between the thumb and the index finger at the inguinoscrotal junction and injecting 0.5% to 1% lidocaine at 3 different angles around the cord. In addition to a cord block, one must inject the skin at the incision site, because scrotal skin is supplied by pudendal nerve and a perineal branch of the posterior cutaneous nerve of the thigh,[6] which are not blocked by the cord block.

Use of conscious sedation in an office setting requires that the facility be accredited by the Joint Commission, Accreditation Association for Ambulatory Health Care, or the American Association for Accreditation of Ambulatory Surgical Facilities.[7] It also requires appropriate staff training, airway management capability, emergency transfer protocol, and appropriate postprocedural monitoring as well as detailed discharge policies.

PREPROCEDURAL PREPARATION

Before making decisions about the type of procedure for sperm retrieval, it is of the utmost importance to discuss success rates of planned procedure and possible need for additional procedures. In addition, there should be a detailed discussion of possible procedural side effects, including a small risk of clinically apparent hematoma, possibility of changes in testicular volume with a chance of resultant hypogonadism from testicular procedures, infections, hydrocele, and postoperative pain. In addition, the risk of chromosomal abnormalities in offspring from assisted reproductive procedures should be discussed, and if appropriate, genetic counseling should be offered. Any antiplatelet medication should be discontinued 1 week before procedure, unless the risk of discontinuation is exceedingly high. The patient should be advised to abstain from sexual activity for 2 to 3 days to maximize epididymal sperm content. It is advisable to have an accompanying driver on the day of surgery. Close coordination with the andrology laboratory is required both for immediate cryopreservation, and if the specimen is to be used immediately for IVF.

OFFICE-BASED SPERM RETRIEVAL PROCEDURES
Vasal Sperm Aspiration

For all office-based surgeries described later, it is important to provide adequate anesthesia so that the surgical field is stable without any unintended patient movements. For this reason, extensive microdissection procedures are often performed under general anesthesia. Aspiration of vasal fluid is usually performed at the time of microscopic reconstruction (ie, vasovasotomy, vasoepididymostomy), which requires general anesthesia. On rare occasions, vasal fluid may be aspirated without reconstruction; however, this may complicate future reconstructive surgeries.

After administration of adequate anesthesia, the surgical field is prepared and draped in a sterile fashion. A 1.5-cm skin incision is made along the spermatic cord proximal to the area of vasal obstruction. The dartos fascia is divided with electrocautery and the spermatic cord is identified. The vas deferens is dissected free of surrounding tissues. The vas is partially incised perpendicular to its axis with a Beaver blade down to the lumen and the vasal exudate is collected in the appropriate media by aspiration (**Fig. 1**). Vasal fluid is examined under the microscope before cryopreservation. The vasal edges may be reapproximated with fine interrupted sutures such as 8-0 or 9-0 nylon. The vas is returned to its correct anatomic position. Dartos fascia and skin are closed with 4-0 chromic suture.

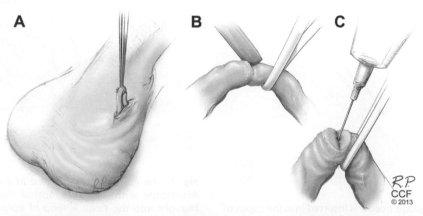

A   **B**   **C**

Fig. 1. A 1.5-cm skin incision is made along the spermatic cord proximal to the area of vasal obstruction and vas deferens is isolated (*A*). The vas is partially incised perpendicular to its axis with a Beaver blade down to the lumen (*B*) and the vasal exudate aspirated (*C*).

Percutaneous Epididymal Sperm Aspiration

Spermatic cord block and local infiltration of analgesic medication, or local anesthesia alone, may be sufficient for percutaneous epididymal sperm aspiration (PESA). If needed, an anxiolytic or conscious sedation may be given. PESA is used for men with OA who make a sufficient quantity of sperm and are likely to have an adequate number of sperm in the epididymis. The testis and epididymis are stabilized by 1 hand, and a 23-gauge needle is inserted into the caput or dilated portion of the epididymis with the dominant hand. Negative pressure up to 60 mL is applied, and aspirate is collected (**Fig. 2**). The aspirate is assessed for presence of sperm, and if needed, the procedure may be repeated on the contralateral side.

Microsurgical Epididymal Sperm Aspiration

Microsurgical epididymal sperm aspiration (MESA) allows direct magnified visualization of the epididymal tubules in an open setting. This procedure allows selection of the most optimal appearing tubules with the highest expected probability of containing sperm. Regional anesthesia and conscious sedation may be used for this procedure if performed in an office setting. It is also appropriate to perform this procedure under general anesthesia in the operating room. After preparing and draping, a 1.5-cm incision is made in the cranial part of a hemiscrotum. The dartos fascia is divided with electrocautery to assure adequate hemostasis. Testicles and epididymis are reached, and the parietal layer of the tunica vaginalis is divided to bring epididymis into the field. After opening the epididymis, the operating microscope with 20 to 25 optical magnification is brought into the field. A loop of epididymal tubule that appears dilated and opalescent is targeted, isolated, and opened. Epididymal fluid is aspirated, examined, and collected (**Fig. 3**). The epididymal tubule and tunica are closed with fine suture before closure of the more superficial layers. The surgery may be repeated on the contralateral side if inadequate sperm are found on 1 side.

Testicular Sperm Aspiration

Testicular sperm aspiration (TESA) may be performed with a fine needle (20–23 gauge), large needle (18–20 gauge), or cutting biopsy needle (14–18 gauge). For fine-needle aspiration biopsy (FNAB) and large-needle aspiration biopsy (LNAB), spermatic cord block and local anesthesia or local anesthesia alone are adequate. However, conscious sedation with local anesthesia or cord block is preferred for large-needle cutting biopsy. The

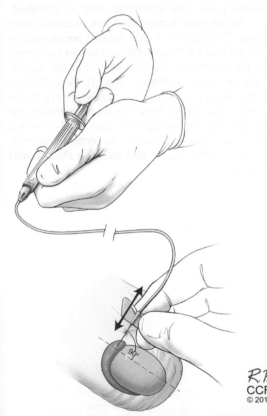

Fig. 2. A 23-gauge needle is inserted into the caput of the epididymis at 90° axis to the testicle. Negative pressure up to 60 mL is applied, and aspirate is collected.

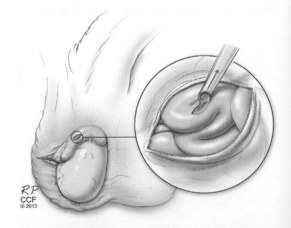

Fig. 3. The epididymis is isolated and the operating microscope with 20 to 25 optical magnification is brought into the field. A loop of epididymal tubule that appears dilated and opalescent is targeted, isolated, and opened, and epididymal fluid is aspirated (*inset*).

testicle is fixed against the scrotal skin and held by the nondominant hand. For FNAB, a 20-gauge to 23-gauge needle is inserted percutaneously into the testicle and negative pressure applied to aspirate and collect sperm. The procedure may be repeated at a different location in the testicle or in the contralateral testicle. For testicular mapping, the upper, mid, and lower poles are sampled several times to assess which area has the best probability of finding viable sperm. The only difference in an LNAB is the use of an 18-gauge to 20-gauge needle. For a cutting biopsy, a biopsy gun with a 14-gauge to 18-gauge needle is used to sample a larger area of the testicle (**Fig. 4**).

Testicular Sperm Extraction

Conventional open testicular sperm extraction (cTESE) may be performed under regional anesthesia with or without conscious sedation; however, microdissection TESE (mTESE) should be performed under general anesthesia. After preparing and draping the genitalia in a sterile fashion, the testicle is held in place to prevent it from moving. A small incision is made in the anterior midportion of the scrotum. The subcutaneous layers are opened with electrocautery to expose the testicle. A small incision is made in the tunica albuginea in an avascular plane, followed by a gentle squeeze to extrude some seminiferous tubules. The tubules are divided sharply, suspended in a sperm-friendly solution such as synthetic human tubular fluid and

sent for andrology laboratory analysis. The tunica albuginea is closed before closure of the subcutaneous tissue and scrotal skin. This procedure may be performed at multiple sites and repeated bilaterally (**Fig. 5**). If there is a discrepancy in testicular size, the larger testicle and the one without varicocele is sampled first for greater likelihood of finding sperm.

SUCCESS AFTER SPERM RETRIEVAL PROCEDURES
OA: Vasal Aspiration, PESA, MESA, TESA

For OA, the American Society of Reproductive Medicine (ASRM) and Society for Male Reproduction and Urology (SMRU) believe that sperm retrieval is equally successful from any anatomic target.[8] All surgeries are acceptable treatment options for patients with OA, including microsurgical reconstruction or sperm retrieval surgeries. The choice between reconstruction and sperm retrieval depends on several factors like female age, need for female reproductive tract reconstruction, or presence of other female infertility factors, as well as likelihood of success with reconstructive procedures. Although the ASRM and SMRU address only PESA and TESA, the success rate of obtaining viable sperm from vasal aspiration ranges from 70% to 100% at first attempt, and 100% at second attempt for OA.[9,10]

Cause of obstruction does not seem to have an impact on sperm retrieval and live birth rates. A study of 1121 men with OA who underwent sperm aspiration via PESA or TESA showed no difference in successful sperm retrieval rates (SRR) because of cause of obstruction when CBAVD was compared with other causes; in addition, the source of sperm did not have any effect on SRR.[11] Similarly, Esteves and colleagues[12] evaluated PESA and TESA in CBAVD, vasectomy, and postinfection patients and found the SRR to be 100%, 96.6%, and 96.3%, respectively. Live birth rates with ICSI were 34.4%, 32.2%, and 34.6%, respectively.

Although the biology of the obstructive process does not influence sperm retrieval, there are certain circumstances when 1 method is preferred over another. The last study showed that PESA was more successful in patients with CBAVD than in vasectomy or postinfectious patients with 96.8%, 69.5%, and 76.4% SRR, respectively. TESA was able to successfully retrieve sperm in the last 2 groups. According to 1 study, PESA is not preferred if there is presence of an epididymal cyst after vasectomy, because the success rate decreases to 20%.[13] In addition, interval since vasectomy has been shown to affect the outcome of

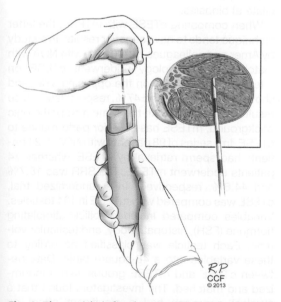

Fig. 4. The testicle is fixed against the scrotal skin and held by the nondominant hand. A biopsy gun with a 14-gauge to 18-gauge needle is inserted percutaneously in a lateral to medial direction (*inset*).

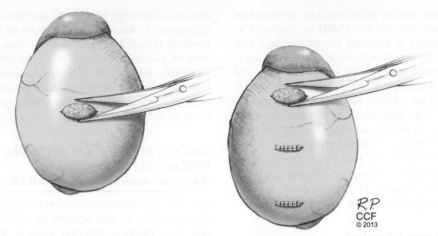

Fig. 5. A small incision is made in the anterior midportion of the tunica albuginea in an avascular plane, followed by a gentle squeeze to extrude some seminiferous tubules (*left*). The tubules are divided sharply. This procedure may be performed at multiple sites (*right*).

microsurgical reconstruction, but it does not seem to alter the success rates in sperm aspiration procedures.[14–16] Moreover, sperm motility does not seem to affect fertilization and pregnancy rates in patients undergoing ICSI.[17] It is important to note and counsel patients on success of sperm retrieval if no sperm is observed intraoperatively. Per 1 study of mTESE, there is still a 7% chance of finding sperm on tissue digestion in the laboratory.[18]

Success rates of PESA range from 61% to 100%.[12,14,19,20] If a percutaneous approach is not successful, sperm may be retrieved by microsurgical techniques. The success rates for MESA for OA are greater than 90%.[20,21] The complications of this procedure are minor.

NOA: TESA, TESE

In addition to the particular technique used for testicular sperm retrieval, success is also dependent on histology and cause of NOA. TESA, as described earlier, may be performed with a fine needle, large needle, or cutting biopsy needle. The success rate of FNAB for sperm retrieval ranges from 10% to 64%,[22–28] a wide range likely attributable to histology, use of multifocal biopsies, and cause of NOA. Cutting needle biopsy has a higher success rate as exemplified by 1 study of 23 men,[29] 21 of whom had NOA, in which cutting needle biopsies with 14-gauge and 16-gauge needles revealed the presence of sperm in 56% of the patients.

In cases of failed percutaneous needle testicular biopsies, open biopsies are more successful.[27] The success of TESE ranges from 41% to 87%.[30] Use of multiple testicular biopsies over

single biopsy is preferred because of higher success rate. Twenty-nine men underwent testicular biopsies in 55 testes at 3 predetermined areas (ie, rete testis, midline, and proximal regions). Overall success rate was 50.9% (28/55 testes). Sperm were retrieved from 3, 2, or 1 region in 53.6%, 17.9%, and 28.6% of the testes.[31] If only 1 area had been biopsied, SRR would have been approximately halved. Another study compared single biopsy from both testicles with 2 to 4 biopsies from each testicle in 316 and 100 patients, respectively. The SRR was 37.5% with single bilateral biopsies compared with 49% with multiple bilateral biopsies.[32]

When comparing cTESE with mTESE, the latter technique tends to have superior results. In a study by Amer and colleagues,[33] 100 men with NOA with matched histopathology underwent cTESE on 1 testicle, and mTESE on the opposing side, and showed SRR of 30% and 47%, respectively. These results showed that with the same histopathologic background, mTESE has superior performance to cTESE. In a series of 98 patients with NOA,[34] 24 patients had sperm retrieval by cTESE, whereas 74 patients underwent mTESE. The SRR was 16.7% and 44.6%, respectively. In a randomized trial, cTESE was compared with mTESE in 194 testicles. Variables compared included follicle-stimulating hormone (FSH), histopathology, and testicular volume. Each testicle was classified according to these variables into a 48-square table. Data between cTESE and mTESE groups were randomized and matched. The investigators found that a surgical approach had a significant effect on finding sperm; however, most of the difference was seen in the Sertoli cell only group (27.5% and 12.5% for mTESE vs cTESE, respectively), whereas other groups had similar rates with both techniques.[35]

Role of Histopathology

Histopathology plays a major role in predicting the success of sperm retrieval in patients with NOA. Hypospermatogenesis has the most success (70%–100%), followed by maturation arrest (MA) (44%–75%), with the least success seen in Sertoli cell only (also known as germinal cell aplasia) syndrome (16%–50%).[30] Some investigators make a distinction between early and late MA. Early MA is defined as arrest in the spermatogonia or spermatocyte phase, whereas late MA is during the spermatid phase.[36,37] In a study of 223 men with NOA,[36] 34 were identified as having MA, of whom 21 had early MA and 13 had late MA. These investigators found that patients with early MA had greater frequency of genetic anomalies, compared with patients with late MA, who had a higher likelihood of a previous testicular insult (varicocele, cryptorchidism, heat exposure, and testicular trauma). Patients underwent cTESE as well as mTESE, although the technique did not seem to influence the SRR in this study. The sperm retrieval in early MA versus late MA was successful in 23.5% and 53.8% of patients, but this difference was not significant, likely because of small number of cases. In another study,[37] 49 of 219 men with NOA were found to have MA. Men with late MA had increased testosterone, lower FSH level, and higher SRR than early MA, 65.5% versus 30%, respectively.

Use of mTESE results in higher success rate in some of these histopathologic diagnoses. Okada and colleagues[34] showed that men with MA treated with cTESE versus mTESE had successful sperm retrieval in 37.5% and 75%, respectively. Superior results were also seen in men with Sertoli cell only syndrome with mTESE compared with cTESE, with the SRR being 33.9% and 6.3%, respectively. Comparison of hypospermatogenesis was not available because no men with that histopathology underwent cTESE, although these men had 100% success with mTESE.

Sperm Retrieval in Patients Who Have Cancer

Retention of fertility is an important issue for cancer survivors. Fewer than half of the physicians treating patients who have cancer refer them for fertility preservation before initiation of therapy.[38] The type and duration of therapy, and pretreatment reproductive function, influence posttherapy fertility potential. In a study by Hsiao and colleagues,[39] 73 men with variable cancer types who received different chemotherapies underwent 84 mTESE procedures. Mean age of the men was 34.5 years, mean FSH level was 21.9 U/L, average testicular volume was 9.1, and average time from chemotherapy to TESE was 19 years. Of the patients who received a diagnostic testicular biopsy, 90% had Sertoli cell disease, whereas the remaining 10% had hypospermatogenesis. The SRR was 43% (36/84 surgeries), with the highest in patients who had testicular cancer and lowest in patients with sarcoma. Other smaller studies have shown similar results, with SRR of 42%[40] and 65%,[41] although in the latter study, frequency of Sertoli cell only histologic type was lower, at 48%.

Klinefelter Syndrome

Another cause that may play a role in sperm retrieval success is the diagnosis of Klinefelter syndrome. The chromosomal abnormality may be caused by meiotic nondisjunction, 47, XXY or mosaicism, 46, XX/47, XXY. Men with mosaicism have a greater chance of having rare sperm in their ejaculate than nonmosaics. These men have small firm testes, and small focal areas of spermatogenesis. TESE has made it possible to retrieve sperm from this cohort, with superior results seen with mTESE. In a study by Vernaeve and colleagues,[42] 50 nonmosaic men underwent cTESE, and SRR was 48%. None of the factors including FSH, testosterone, facial hair pattern, gynecomastia, or testicular volume were predictive of success. In another study, 24 nonmosaic patients with Klinefelter syndrome underwent cTESE with 33% SRR. FSH, inhibin B, and testosterone levels did not have any predictive value; however, age younger than 32 years was predictive of greater success.[43] A larger study using mTESE to extract sperm in 68 men with nonmosaic Klinefelter syndrome found an SRR of 66%.[44]

Y Microdeletions

Another type of chromosomal abnormality that is found in about 10% of men with severe oligospermia or azoospermia is Y chromosome microdeletion. Complete and partial deletions of 3 regions, AZFa, AZFb, and AZFc, have been described. Sperm retrieval has not been successful in patients with complete AZFa or AZFb deletions. Patients with AZFc mutation have better results; mTESE in AZFc patients showed an SRR of 71% in 1 series.[45]

Role of Hormonal Treatment in NOA

To increase the success rate of sperm retrieval in men with NOA, hormonal treatment before the procedure has been attempted. A study by Shiraishi and colleagues[46] evaluated 48 men who had 1 failed mTESE. Twenty-eight men were treated with human chorionic gonadotropin (hCG), whereas 20 men did not undergo any hormonal treatment. There was a significantly greater SRR at second mTESE among men who had hormonal treatment (21%) when compared with those who did not (0%). On the contrary, a larger study of 736 men with NOA consisting of a cohort of men who had testosterone level less than 300 ng/dL and were treated with clomiphene citrate, hCG, or aromatase inhibitors, found no significant difference between those who responded to treatment versus those who did not.[47]

Predictive Models for Sperm Retrieval

Some have attempted to build predictive models to assist in making decisions about pursuing surgical sperm retrieval based on predicted success rate. In a study by Tsujimura and colleagues,[48] 9 preoperative factors were analyzed in a cohort of 100 men with NOA who underwent mTESE. Nine parameters were tested, including age, testicular volume, FSH, luteinizing hormone (LH), inhibin B, total testosterone, free testosterone, and estradiol. These investigators found that FSH, total testosterone, and inhibin B were significantly associated with successful sperm retrieval by mTESE. They developed a formula using these variables that could be used to predict presurgery probability of success. The formula is as follows: $P = [1 + \exp(5.201 - 0.048 \times FSH - 0.449 \times \text{total testosterone} - 0.021 \times \text{inhibin B})]^{-1}$. The correlation between predicted probability and observed success was 0.77. This equation had a sensitivity of 71% and specificity of 71.4%. This study used noninvasive parameters, which makes this equation easy to use. However, it remains to be validated in another cohort before it is used widely.

Another study[49] developed an artificial neural network model incorporating age, FSH, LH, testosterone, prolactin, left and right testicular volume, and duration of infertility for predicting sperm retrieval success after bilateral multiple biopsy conventional TESE. The diagnostic accuracy of this model was 80.8%. In a recent study,[50] a nomogram was developed using a cohort of 1026 men with NOA. The parameters included in their nomogram were patient age, FSH, history of cryptorchidism, Klinefelter disease, left testis volume, and presence or absence of a varicocele. History of cryptorchidism and Klinefelter disease had the biggest role in predicting positivity based on this nomogram. However, on internal validation, the accuracy of the nomogram was only 59.6%. The investigators concluded that the model could not be used to reliably predict presence of sperm on

mTESE. These models are intriguing but require further investigation.

Varicocele and NOA

An issue in NOA is the presence of a varicocele. It is controversial whether a varicocelectomy should be performed in men with NOA. Studies investigating this issue have been retrospective in nature, with mixed results. One study[51] compared a group of men with NOA who underwent varicocelectomy with a group who did not and found that SRR on mTESE was significantly higher in the former group, at 53% versus 30%, respectively. In another study of 96 men,[52] similar results were seen, and sperm retrieval was higher in the group who underwent varicocelectomy (61%) compared with those who did not undergo surgery (38%). However, another study[53] showed equal sperm retrieval success in those who did or did not undergo a varicocelectomy. A meta-analysis[54] of 11 studies including 233 patients who had varicocele repair using a variety of techniques showed that 39% of men had return of motile sperm in their ejaculate, and the resulting pregnancy rate was 10%. The issue of varicocele repair in the setting of NOA remains a matter of debate and requires further research.

COMPLICATIONS

Overall, the complications from surgical sperm retrieval procedures are rare and generally minor. The complication rates for PESA range from 0% to 9%.[55,56] Postoperative pain is the most common complication, whereas hydrocele, hematocele, and epididymitis are less common. Similarly, the complications with MESA are unusual and low in severity.

FNAB of the testis is a safe procedure, with rare possibility of bleeding. In a study by Carpi and colleagues,[57] 387 testicles were sampled with FNAB or LNAB, and there were no clinical complications, no requirement of narcotic pain medications, and no day off work after the procedures. A cutting biopsy with an 18-gauge needle was performed in 31 patients, and only 3 required narcotic pain medication. None developed a hematoma or needed time off work. In a study in which 14-gauge and 16-gauge needles were used,[29] there were no complications except minor pain and swelling.

TESE has been shown to cause structural changes when follow-up testicular ultrasonography is performed. Subclinical hematomas, fibrosis, devascularization, and change in testicular size have been seen after the procedure. Clinically relevant changes are infrequent and may include testicular atrophy and hypogonadism, with need for testosterone replacement therapy. Overall, the complication rate has been shown to be lower in mTESE than cTESE. cTESE results in more changes detected by ultrasonography, as seen in 1 study,[34] which showed that 51% of men treated with the conventional technique had a hematoma on ultrasonography at 1 month compared with 12% with microdissection technique. Clinically, significantly more men with lower testicular volume were seen in the cTESE group than the mTESE group (25% vs 2.5%, respectively). One patient (2.5%) in the former group had bilateral testicular atrophy and subsequently needed testosterone replacement therapy. In contrast, another study[58] did not find a significant difference in the rate of hypogonadism between cTESE and mTESE techniques at 18-month follow-up after the procedures.

SUMMARY

Office-based sperm retrieval procedures are becoming increasingly relevant, because they provide patient and surgeon convenience and are cost-effective. The development of ICSI has introduced an increasing need for sperm recovery in even the most challenging cases of male infertility. Men with azoospermia represent a significant part of the infertile population. Men with OA may undergo vasal or epididymal sperm retrieval, whereas men with NOA require removal of sperm from the testicle. Sperm retrieval may be performed open or microsurgically; the success rate is higher with microsurgery. Other factors that influence success of sperm retrieval in NOA include the histopathology and cause of NOA. Complications are minor; the rate of complications is low with most procedures. Before undertaking any office-based procedures, all office personnel must be fully trained and the facility must be appropriately accredited.

ACKNOWLEDGMENTS

We would like to thank Ross Papalardo, CMI, for assistance with the medical art contained in this article.

REFERENCES

1. Palermo G, Joris H, Devroey P, et al. Pregnancies after intracytoplasmic injection of single spermatozoon into an oocyte. Lancet 1992;340:17–8.
2. Bungum L, Bungum M, Humaidan P, et al. A strategy for treatment of couples with unexplained infertility who failed to conceive after intrauterine insemination. Reprod Biomed Online 2004; 8:584–9.
3. van der Westerlaken L, Naaktgeboren N, Verburg H, et al. Conventional in vitro fertilization versus intracytoplasmic sperm injection in patients with borderline semen: a randomized study using sibling oocytes. Fertil Steril 2006;85:395–400.
4. Practice Committee of American Society for Reproductive Medicine in collaboration with Society for Male Reproduction and Urology. Evaluation of the azoospermic male. Fertil Steril 2008;90:S74–7.
5. Jarow JP, Espeland MA, Lipshultz LI. Evaluation of the azoospermic patient. J Urol 1989;142:62–5.
6. Wakefield SE, Elewa AA. Spermatic cord block: a safe technique for intrascrotal surgery. Ann R Coll Surg Engl 1994;76:401–2.
7. Kurrek MM, Twersky RS. Office-based anesthesia: how to start an office-based practice. Anesthesiol Clin 2010;28:353–67.
8. Practice Committee of American Society for Reproductive Medicine in collaboration with Society for Male Reproduction and Urology. The management of infertility due to obstructive azoospermia. Fertil Steril 2008;90:S121–4.
9. Qiu Y, Wang SM, Yang DT, et al. Percutaneous vasal sperm aspiration and intrauterine insemination for infertile males with anejaculation. Fertil Steril 2003;79:618–20.
10. Levine LA, Fakouri BJ. Experience with vasal sperm aspiration. J Urol 1998;159:1551–3.
11. Kamal A, Fahmy I, Mansour R, et al. Does the outcome of ICSI in cases of obstructive azoospermia depend on the origin of the retrieved spermatozoa or the cause of obstruction? A comparative analysis. Fertil Steril 2010;94:2135–40.
12. Esteves SC, Lee W, Benjamin DJ, et al. Reproductive potential of men with obstructive azoospermia undergoing percutaneous sperm retrieval and intracytoplasmic sperm injection according to the cause of obstruction. J Urol 2013;189: 232–7.
13. Wood S, Vang E, Troup S, et al. Surgical sperm retrieval after previous vasectomy and failed reversal: clinical implications for in vitro fertilization. BJU Int 2002;90:277–81.
14. Bromage SJ, Douglas J, Falconer DA, et al. Factors affecting successful outcome from ICSI in men following previous vasectomy. World J Urol 2007; 25:519–24.
15. Nicopoullos JD, Gilling-Smith C, Almeida PA, et al. Effect of time since vasectomy and maternal age on intracytoplasmic sperm injection success in men with obstructive azoospermia after vasectomy. Fertil Steril 2004;82:367–73.
16. Sukcharoen N, Sithipravej T, Promviengchai S, et al. No differences in outcome of surgical sperm retrieval with intracytoplasmic sperm injection at different intervals after vasectomy. Fertil Steril 2000;74:174–5.

17. Moghadam KK, Nett R, Robins JC, et al. The motility of epididymal or testicular spermatozoa does not directly affect IVF/ICSI pregnancy outcomes. J Androl 2005;26:619–23.

18. Ramasamy R, Reifsnyder JE, Bryson C, et al. Role of tissue digestion and extensive sperm search after microdissection testicular sperm extraction. Fertil Steril 2011;96:299–302.

19. Glina S, Fragoso JB, Martins FG, et al. Percutaneous epididymal sperm aspiration (PESA) in men with obstructive azoospermia. Int Braz J Urol 2003;29:141–5 [discussion: 5–6].

20. Lin YM, Hsu CC, Kuo TC, et al. Percutaneous epididymal sperm aspiration versus microsurgical epididymal sperm aspiration for irreparable obstructive azoospermia–experience with 100 cases. J Formos Med Assoc 2000;99:459–65.

21. Schroeder-Printzen I, Zumbe J, Bispink L, et al. Microsurgical epididymal sperm aspiration: aspirate analysis and straws available after cryopreservation in patients with non-reconstructable obstructive azoospermia. MESA/TESE Group Giessen. Hum Reprod 2000;15:2531–5.

22. Vicari E, Grazioso C, Burrello N, et al. Epididymal and testicular sperm retrieval in azoospermic patients and the outcome of intracytoplasmic sperm injection in relation to the etiology of azoospermia. Fertil Steril 2001;75:215–6.

23. Hauser R, Yogev L, Paz G, et al. Comparison of efficacy of two techniques for testicular sperm retrieval in nonobstructive azoospermia: multifocal testicular sperm extraction versus multifocal testicular sperm aspiration. J Androl 2006;27:28–33.

24. Turek PJ, Ljung BM, Cha I, et al. Diagnostic findings from testis fine needle aspiration mapping in obstructed and nonobstructed azoospermic men. J Urol 2000;163:1709–16.

25. Houwen J, Lundin K, Soderlund B, et al. Efficacy of percutaneous needle aspiration and open biopsy for sperm retrieval in men with non-obstructive azoospermia. Acta Obstet Gynecol Scand 2008; 87:1033–8.

26. Mercan R, Urman B, Alatas C, et al. Outcome of testicular sperm retrieval procedures in non-obstructive azoospermia: percutaneous aspiration versus open biopsy. Hum Reprod 2000;15: 1548–51.

27. Ezeh UI, Moore HD, Cooke ID. A prospective study of multiple needle biopsies versus a single open biopsy for testicular sperm extraction in men with non-obstructive azoospermia. Hum Reprod 1998; 13:3075–80.

28. El-Haggar S, Mostafa T, Abdel Nasser T, et al. Fine needle aspiration vs. mTESE in non-obstructive azoospermia. Int J Androl 2008;31:595–601.

29. Rosenlund B, Kvist U, Ploen L, et al. Percutaneous cutting needle biopsies for histopathological assessment and sperm retrieval in men with azoospermia. Hum Reprod 2001;16:2154–9.

30. Donoso P, Tournaye H, Devroey P. Which is the best sperm retrieval technique for non-obstructive azoospermia? A systematic review. Hum Reprod Update 2007;13:539–49.

31. Hauser R, Botchan A, Amit A, et al. Multiple testicular sampling in non-obstructive azoospermia–is it necessary? Hum Reprod 1998;13:3081–5.

32. Amer M, Haggar SE, Moustafa T, et al. Testicular sperm extraction: impact of testicular histology on outcome, number of biopsies to be performed and optimal time for repetition. Hum Reprod 1999;14:3030–4.

33. Amer M, Ateyah A, Hany R, et al. Prospective comparative study between microsurgical and conventional testicular sperm extraction in non-obstructive azoospermia: follow-up by serial ultrasound examinations. Hum Reprod 2000;15:653–6.

34. Okada H, Dobashi M, Yamazaki T, et al. Conventional versus microdissection testicular sperm extraction for nonobstructive azoospermia. J Urol 2002;168:1063–7.

35. Colpi GM, Colpi EM, Piediferro G, et al. Microsurgical TESE versus conventional TESE for ICSI in non-obstructive azoospermia: a randomized controlled study. Reprod Biomed Online 2009;18: 315–9.

36. Tsai MC, Cheng YS, Lin TY, et al. Clinical characteristics and reproductive outcomes in infertile men with testicular early and late maturation arrest. Urology 2012;80:826–32.

37. Weedin JW, Bennett RC, Fenig DM, et al. Early versus late maturation arrest: reproductive outcomes of testicular failure. J Urol 2011;186:621–6.

38. Quinn GP, Vadaparampil ST, Lee JH, et al. Physician referral for fertility preservation in oncology patients: a national study of practice behaviors. J Clin Oncol 2009;27:5952–7.

39. Hsiao W, Stahl PJ, Osterberg EC, et al. Successful treatment of postchemotherapy azoospermia with microsurgical testicular sperm extraction: the Weill Cornell experience. J Clin Oncol 2011;29:1607–11.

40. Meseguer M, Garrido N, Remohi J, et al. Testicular sperm extraction (TESE) and ICSI in patients with permanent azoospermia after chemotherapy. Hum Reprod 2003;18:1281–5.

41. Damani MN, Master V, Meng MV, et al. Postchemotherapy ejaculatory azoospermia: fatherhood with sperm from testis tissue with intracytoplasmic sperm injection. J Clin Oncol 2002;20:930–6.

42. Vernaeve V, Staessen C, Verheyen G, et al. Can biological or clinical parameters predict testicular sperm recovery in 47, XXY Klinefelter's syndrome patients? Hum Reprod 2004;19:1135–9.

43. Ferhi K, Avakian R, Griveau JF, et al. Age as only predictive factor for successful sperm recovery in

patients with Klinefelter's syndrome. Andrologia 2009;41:84–7.

44. Ramasamy R, Ricci JA, Palermo GD, et al. Successful fertility treatment for Klinefelter's syndrome. J Urol 2009;182:1108–13.

45. Stahl PJ, Masson P, Mielnik A, et al. A decade of experience emphasizes that testing for Y microdeletions is essential in American men with azoospermia and severe oligozoospermia. Fertil Steril 2010;94:1753–6.

46. Shiraishi K, Ohmi C, Shimabukuro T, et al. Human chorionic gonadotrophin treatment prior to microdissection testicular sperm extraction in non-obstructive azoospermia. Hum Reprod 2012;27:331–9.

47. Reifsnyder JE, Ramasamy R, Husseini J, et al. Role of optimizing testosterone before microdissection testicular sperm extraction in men with nonobstructive azoospermia. J Urol 2012;188:532–6.

48. Tsujimura A, Matsumiya K, Miyagawa Y, et al. Prediction of successful outcome of microdissection testicular sperm extraction in men with idiopathic nonobstructive azoospermia. J Urol 2004;172:1944–7.

49. Samli MM, Dogan I. An artificial neural network for predicting the presence of spermatozoa in the testes of men with nonobstructive azoospermia. J Urol 2004;171:2354–7.

50. Ramasamy R, Padilla WO, Osterberg EC, et al. A comparison of models for predicting sperm retrieval before microdissection testicular sperm extraction in men with nonobstructive azoospermia. J Urol 2013;189:638–42.

51. Inci K, Hascicek M, Kara O, et al. Sperm retrieval and intracytoplasmic sperm injection in men with nonobstructive azoospermia, and treated and untreated varicocele. J Urol 2009;182:1500–5.

52. Haydardedeoglu B, Turunc T, Kilicdag EB, et al. The effect of prior varicocelectomy in patients with nonobstructive azoospermia on intracytoplasmic sperm injection outcomes: a retrospective pilot study. Urology 2010;75:83–6.

53. Schlegel PN, Kaufmann J. Role of varicocelectomy in men with nonobstructive azoospermia. Fertil Steril 2004;81:1585–8.

54. Weedin JW, Khera M, Lipshultz LI. Varicocele repair in patients with nonobstructive azoospermia: a meta-analysis. J Urol 2010;183:2309–15.

55. Wood S, Thomas K, Sephton V, et al. Postoperative pain, complications, and satisfaction rates in patients who undergo surgical sperm retrieval. Fertil Steril 2003;79:56–62.

56. Lania C, Grasso M, Fortuna F, et al. Open epididymal sperm aspiration (OESA): minimally invasive surgical technique for sperm retrieval. Arch Esp Urol 2006;59:313–6.

57. Carpi A, Menchini Fabris FG, Palego P, et al. Fine-needle and large-needle percutaneous aspiration biopsy of testicles in men with nonobstructive azoospermia: safety and diagnostic performance. Fertil Steril 2005;83:1029–33.

58. Ramasamy R, Yagan N, Schlegel PN. Structural and functional changes to the testis after conventional versus microdissection testicular sperm extraction. Urology 2005;65:1190–4.

Electrical and Mechanical Office-based Neuromodulation

Ravi Kacker, MD, Aaron Lay, MD, Anurag Das, MD*

KEYWORDS

- Overactive bladder • Neuromodulation • Sacral nerve • Tibial nerve • Electric stimulation therapy

KEY POINTS

- Neuromodulation techniques, such as sacral neuromodulation (SNM) and percutaneous tibial nerve stimulation (PTNS), are treatment options for patients who fail behavioral therapy and pharmacotherapy.
- Neuromodulation may augment inhibitory bladder afferents and lead to cortical plasticity to inhibit bladder reflexes.
- A test sacral stimulation can be performed in the office with temporary leads and may help identify patients who are most likely to succeed with SNM.
- PTNS is an emerging therapy that may improve OAB symptoms in some patients through entirely office-based neuromodulation.

INTRODUCTION

Chronic urinary frequency, urgency, and urge incontinence represent common problems in the urologist's practice. The term overactive bladder (OAB) is defined by the International Continence Society as "urgency or frequency with or without urge incontinence in the absence of other pathologic or metabolic conditions to explain these symptoms."[1] An estimated 34 million people in the United States have OAB,[2] leading to significant impairment in quality of life, a higher risk of falls and other accidents, and lower self-esteem and health perception.[3] Annual cost associated with OAB is estimated at more than $9 billion, including direct care, health consequences, and lost productivity.[4]

For patients with OAB, first-line treatment options include conservative therapies, such as pelvic floor exercises and biofeedback, along with pharmacologic therapy. Although many patients find relief with these therapies, up to 40% of patients are either refractory to primary management or have an unsatisfactory response.[5] Currently, several options exist for these patients, ranging from intradetrusor injection of botulinum toxin to

irreversible surgical therapy, including detrusor myomectomy, augmentation cystoplasty, and urinary diversion. Neuromodulation represents a minimally invasive and reversible treatment with a high rate of success for patients who are refractory to first-line therapies for OAB.

In this review, we focus on office-based neuromodulation, specifically percutaneous tibial nerve stimulation (PTNS) and office-based test procedures for sacral neuromodulation (SNM). SNM refers to electrical stimulation of the S3 (or S4) sacral nerve root to modulate the micturition reflex. Initially, a test procedure is performed using either temporary leads placed in the office or, alternatively, permanent leads placed in the operating room (OR). After a successful test period, permanent leads and a pulse generator are implanted in the OR. PTNS is a less invasive, office-based therapy that applies electrical stimulation in a retrograde fashion through the tibial nerve to achieve neuromodulation of the sacral plexus. PTNS is typically applied weekly in the office for 12 weeks and responders continue with monthly therapies.

Division of Urology, Beth Israel Deaconess Medical Center, Harvard Medical School, 330 Brookline Avenue, Boston, MA 02215, USA
* Corresponding author.
E-mail address: adas@bidmc.harvard.edu

Urol Clin N Am 40 (2013) 581–589
http://dx.doi.org/10.1016/j.ucl.2013.07.002
0094-0143/13/$ – see front matter © 2013 Elsevier Inc. All rights reserved.

Historical Perspective

Neuromodulation therapy for OAB is a recent step in the long history of the use of electrical stimulation for medical purposes. In the nineteenth century, electrical stimulation was used for a broad range of psychiatric disorders and later applied to the bladder, pelvic floor, or sacral roots for neurogenic urinary retention or overactivity. Advances in cardiac pacing led to miniaturization of electrical instruments and the first demonstration of sacral neuromodulation by Drs Tanagho and Schmidt[6] in the early 1980s. In patients with neuropathic voiding dysfunction, they showed that continuous stimulation of sacral root S3 modulated detrusor and sphincter activity, resulting in stabilization of micturition reflexes.

Further pioneering work on the mechanism of action of SNM was performed by Drs Craggs and Fowler in London[7] and Drs DeGroat and Chancellor at the University of Pittsburgh.[8,9] Initial large-scale trials (Medtronic [MDT]-130) demonstrating the efficacy of SNM in patients with non-neuropathic OAB were funded by Medtronic (Minneapolis, MN) in the mid-1990s. On the basis of these trials, the US Food and Drug Administration (FDA) approved SNM for urge incontinence in 1997, then urgency/frequency and nonobstructive urinary retention in 1999. Since then, SNM has been successfully used in about 25,000 patients with OAB.[10]

More recently, PTNS has emerged as a lower-cost, office-based form of neuromodulation after pioneering work in the late 1980s by Dr Stoller at the University of California, San Francisco.[11] Recently, a few randomized controlled trials have demonstrating improvements in urinary symptoms above those of placebo[12] and similar to improvements with tolerodine.[13] Subsequent studies have demonstrated a durable response in some patients.[14] Currently, a commercial neuromodulation system is produced by Uroplasty, Inc (Minnetonka, MN), which received 501(k) FDA marketing clearance for urgency/frequency and urge incontinence in 2005.

Mechanism of Action

The exact mechanism of action of neuromodulation on micturition remains unclear. In theory, neuromodulation acts to augment inhibitory somatic afferents that are deficient in patients with OAB.[15] These bladder afferents project to the pontine micturition center and, with chronic stimulation, lead to changes in suprapontine regions that ultimately modulate micturition reflexes.[16] In SNM, electrical stimulation is directly applied to the sacral nerve root.

Chronic sacral nerve stimulation has been shown to lead to augmented somatosensory cortical responses to evoked potentials along the pudendal and posterior tibial nerves.[17] PTNS aims to achieve an effect similar to SNM on micturition reflexes through electrostimulation of the posterior tibial nerves. Chronic electrostimulation of the pudendal nerve has also been shown to improve OAB symptoms in a few patients with neurogenic OAB.[18]

Through positron emission tomography studies, additional neural plasticity is observed over the course of neuromodulation in cortical areas associated with motor learning and with pelvic floor and abdominal musculature.[19] Thus, an additional theory is that neuromodulation also acts by augmenting of the guarding reflex. In animal models, neuromodulation leads to hypertrophy of striated external sphincter muscle fibers and to increased urethral closure pressures. It is unclear if these changes are due to the proposed neuromodulatory effect or simply due to direct stimulation of motor pathways by Onuf nucleus.[20]

INDICATIONS

Neuromodulation is indicated for the treatment of refractory urge incontinence and urinary frequency/urgency syndromes. Generally, patients who have failed or who could not tolerate pharmacotherapy and conservative therapy are candidates for a trial of neuromodulation. Conservative therapy may include behavioral modification, pelvic floor rehabilitation (including pelvic floor biofeedback/muscular vaginal electrical stimulation). Some physicians exhaust all possible options, including high-dose combinations of antimuscarinics and tricyclic antidepressants, before considering neuromodulation; others will move to neruomodulation earlier. Bladder botox therapy has also been approved for these patients who have failed behavioral and pharmacotherapy.

The recently published American Urologic Association Guidelines include both SNM and PTNS as third-line, FDA-approved treatments for patients with non-neurogenic OAB. The Grade C recommendation applies to carefully selected patients who have severe refractory OAB symptoms or those who are not candidates for pharmacotherapy.[21] In 2009, the International Consortium on Incontinence published an algorithm for the management of patients with OAB. SNM is the only minimally invasive treatment option for refractory OAB with a Grade A recommendation (high level of evidence). These recommendations are based on randomized controlled trials (reviewed later in this article) of SNM for urgency/frequency and urge incontinence demonstrating safety and efficacy along with subsequent follow-up studies demonstrating a durable response. Several randomized trials have shown short-term improvement in OAB symptoms with PTNS,[12–14] although there are fewer data on long-term efficacy. European Association of Urology (EAU) guidelines gave a grade B recommendation to offer PTNS for improvement of urge incontinence in women who have not benefited from antimuscarinic medications.[22]

Painful Bladder Syndrome and Neurogenic Voiding Dysfunction

In the United States, the current approval for SNM is for the treatment of refractory urinary frequency/urgency syndromes, urinary urge incontinence, and nonobstructive urinary retention of a nonneurogenic etiology. However, since the introduction of SNM for OAB, there has been growing recognition of the potential benefit of SNM for a broader range of pelvic disorders that may involve some OAB symptoms. Research is ongoing into the potential use of SNM for interstitial cystitis/painful bladder syndrome (IC/PBS) and neurogenic voiding dysfunction among others.

Patients with IC/PBS may experience an improvement in coexisting urinary symptoms with SNM. One series demonstrated short-term improvement in urinary symptoms along 27 carefully selected patients who had successful test stimulation.[23] In another study of carefully selected patients with IC/PBS managed with SNM, 50% of patients underwent explantation for pain at the implantation site, infection, or other reasons. Of the patients who did not undergo implantation, there was minimal loss of benefit over 59.9 months of follow-up.[24] SNM may be suitable for some patients with primarily urinary symptoms and minimal pain.

Patients with neurologic disease were excluded from the initial industry-sponsored trials and subsequent follow-up studies based on the belief that an intact spinal pathway was necessary for neuromodulation. However, similar success rates are observed in patients with neurogenic OAB[25] and there is some evidence to support early intervention with SNM after spinal cord injury to prevent urinary incontinence.[26] One major practical limitation of SNM for neurologic disorders is the need of many of these patients to undergo magnetic resonance imaging studies.

Psychiatric Considerations

Comorbid psychological disorders are common among patients who are candidates for SNM

therapy. Although many patients will have substantial physical and psychological benefit from successful therapy, a history of psychiatric disorders may influence the rate and duration of a successful response to SNM therapy. In an early study of 36 patients undergoing SNM, patients with a history of mental illness were more likely to fail implantation after a successful test procedure (82% vs 28%). Furthermore, patients with a history of mental illness had a shorter duration of therapeutic effect from SNM compared with patients with no history (12 vs 36 months).[27]

Conversely, voiding symptoms impose a clear burden on quality of life and may contribute to the presence or severity of psychological or mental disorders. Improvement in OAB symptoms through neuromodulation may improve or prevent deterioration of mental health. The MDT-103 trial demonstrated a clear benefit in terms of depression and health-related quality of life after SNM therapy. Of the 89 patients in the trial, 73% had some degree of depression at baseline. Patients assigned to direct implantation showed significant improvement in the Beck Depression Index after SNM therapy at 3, 6, and 12 months after starting therapy, whereas patients in the delayed group showed a slight worsening of depression symptoms.[28]

These data suggest that significant psychological benefit may be gained from successful SNM therapy. However, in some cases, such as when there is concern that preexisting psychological disorders may interfere with response to therapy, a psychiatric evaluation may be warranted.

SACRAL NEUROMODULATION TEST PROCEDURE

A test procedure provides a short-term trial of SNM and is important to patient selection before permanent implantation of an implantable pulse generator (IPG). The response during the test period can be used to select the optimal lead position (left vs right, S3 vs S4) and establish patient expectations for symptomatic improvement. The test procedure can be performed with temporary leads in the office under local anesthesia. Although the pioneers of SNM performed this test procedure without fluoroscopy, most practitioners perform it under fluoroscopic guidance. Alternatively, a test procedure using permanent tined leads can be performed in the ambulatory-surgery unit or operating room.

In either case, the patient performs a 2- to 3-day voiding diary before the test procedure. The test period lasts for a few days up to 1 week for temporary and 2 weeks for permanent tined leads. The wires are attached to an external stimulator. The patient maintains stimulation at a comfortable level (it should not be painful) and completes a voiding diary to provide objective data. Based on the patient's experience and voiding diary, a final decision is made to proceed or not to proceed with permanent implantation. Usually, the patient needs to exhibit significant subjective improvement, and the voiding diary should show at least 50% improvement in voiding parameters to warrant proceeding to implantation of the IPG.

Office-based Procedure

The office-based test procedure sometimes is referred to as percutaneous nerve evaluation. The patient is placed in the prone position with 1 or 2 pillows under the lower abdomen to improve the sacral approach. The sacrum is prepped with antiseptic solution and the sacral notches and coccygeal drop-off are identified by palpation or fluoroscopy. S3 usually is located 1.5 to 2.0 cm lateral to the midline at the level of the sacral notches, or about 9 cm above the coccygeal drop-off. Local anesthesia is achieved from S2 to S4 over the underlying skin and subcutaneous tissue, making certain not to enter the foramen.

Insulated foramen needles are placed percutaneously in the S3 and S4 foramen using the previously mentioned landmarks and fluoroscopic guidance (with primarily lateral imaging). Appropriate sensory and motor responses are identified. Once the appropriate responses have been obtained, an insulated wire is placed through the 18-gauge needle in the foramen and the needle is removed. These temporary wires are inexpensive and easy to place. For patients without a clear optimal site of lead placement, 2 or more such wires can be taped in place and attached to an external stimulator. The patient is taught how to adjust for optimal results and can try out left and right sides of S3 and S4 and decide on the best response. Bilateral test stimulation may be helpful for some patients who fail an initial trial with unilateral placement.[29]

Sensory and Motor Neural Responses

Intraoperative motor and sensory neural responses guide lead positioning during the test stimulation. Sensory responses generally include a tingling, pulling, or vibratory sensation in the vagina and rectum in women and in the scrotum, phallus, and rectum in men. Motor responses include levator tightening (bellows response) and plantar flexion of the big toe. Sometimes at S3, a plantar flexion of the entire foot is noted. In such cases, S4 may be the more appropriate foramen,

as most patients are significantly bothered by such a foot response.

An intraoperative motor response during the test procedure generally is considered to be more predictive of success after IPG implantation than a sensory response. Cohen and colleagues[30] followed 35 patients, 21 of whom progressed to permanent IPG implantation after a test procedure using quadripolar tined leads. A positive motor response was observed in 95% of those progressing to permanent implantation versus only 21.4% of patients who failed the test procedure. Patients with a positive sensory response in the absence of a motor response had only a 4.7% chance of having a positive result after implantation. Another recent study examined the role of sensory testing in patients with both OAB and pain symptoms, a group that might be expected to benefit from sensory testing. There was no difference in the rate of symptomatic improvement or explantation for patients who did or did not have sensory testing.[31]

Although intraoperative motor responses are the primary neural responses used to locate the ideal site of electrode implantation, neuromodulation is usually applied at a level below that needed to stimulate a motor response. The patient may use sensory perception to stimulation as an indicator of continued neuromodulation. Loss of sensory perception after implantation may herald a loss in benefit from neurostimulation.

Office-based Test Procedure Versus 2-Stage Implant

A major consideration for the clinician is whether to pursue an office-based test procedure, which if successful, is followed by a "1-stage" implant of permanent leads and an IPG in the OR. An alternative approach is the "2-stage" procedure, in which the patient has permanent quadripolar tined leads implanted in the OR. The patient undergoes a trial period, and if successful then returns to the OR for tunneling of the leads and placement of an IPG.

Before the development of a test procedure with permanent quadripolar leads, use of a temporary lead was the only means for patient selection for SNM. The test procedure itself is considered safe, and complications at the preimplantation stage are rare; however, lead migration and the risk of infection limit the trial period to about 1 week.[32] Lead migration often presents with pain and decreased efficacy and occurs at a rate of about 10% to 15%. Other complications, including pain, may occur at a lower rate (about 2%–3%).[33] It is not clear if these failures are due to undetected lead migration, infection, or other reasons.

Since the introduction of permanent quadripolar tined leads for test stimulation in 1997, multiple groups have published on the successful use these leads. The major advantage of the 2-stage procedure is that the final lead-nerve interface is established before the test period. In theory, the tines should prevent lead migration and thereby allow a longer test period of up to 2 weeks. A recent meta-analysis of SNM trials found a 16% rate of lead migration.[34] Overall, it appears that the use of tined leads may decrease, but not eliminate the risk of lead migration during the test period, particularly for thin patients.[35] The primary disadvantage of a 2-stage procedure is that this procedure requires 2 trips to the OR and may be associated with a higher cost.

A few studies have directly compared outcomes using temporary leads in the office compared with permanent tined lead placement in the OR. In one recent nonrandomized study, patients undergoing a 3-day test period with temporary leads were less likely to progress to implantation than patients who underwent a test procedure with tined leads. However, among those patients who progressed to implantation, the type of test procedure did not impact failure rates, which were below 3% for both groups over 24 months of follow-up.[36] Similar results were found in a smaller, randomized study involving only women.[37]

A longer trial, up to 2 weeks, appears to increase eligibility for implantation, possibly because it takes some patients a longer time to adjust settings or otherwise achieve therapeutic benefit.[38] Although a trial period of 1 to 2 weeks with tined leads does not seem to increase the specificity of a successful trial compared with an office-based trial, there may be a benefit from very long trial periods. Everaert and colleagues[39] randomized 41 patients to either an office-based test procedure or to a 3-week to 5-week trial period after placement of tined leads in the OR. At 24 months of follow-up after implantation, there was a lower rate of failure for patients undergoing the prolonged test procedure compared with those who had only an office-based test procedure (14% vs 33%). In that study, the costs of an office-based test procedure were about $2,667 less than a test procedure initiated in the OR. Our own data (**Table 1**) suggest that in experienced hands, an office-based fluoroscopically assisted test procedure provides excellent results, and can be performed in most patients at a much reduced cost to the health care system and is also an overall more efficient use of surgeon and OR time.

In practice, trial periods longer than 2 weeks are uncommon, primarily because of the potential for increased risk for infection. Huwyler and colleagues[40] performed a microbiologic examination of explanted tined leads from 20 patients who underwent an unsuccessful test period for 2 weeks or longer and identified *Staphylococcus* species growth in 4 patients. However, these bacteria were susceptible to perioperative antibiotics and only 1 of these patients had clinical signs of infection. Furthermore, the manufacturer recommendation is not to exceed a 2-week trial period.

Overall, it seems that an office-based test procedure remains a reasonable option for most patients, and that a successful test procedure generally portends a good outcome after implantation. A test procedure with tined leads placed in the OR may be more suitable for patients in whom the test procedure is equivocal, patients who may require a longer test period to evaluate efficacy, and for patients in whom lead migration is suspected.

PERCUTANEOUS TIBIAL NERVE STIMULATION

The posterior tibial nerve is a mixed sensory-motor nerve, with axons from L4 to S3 spinal roots. The sacral roots contain peripheral nerves involved in motor and sensory control of the bladder, the same nerves involved in SNM. Electrical

Table 1
Outcomes and rate of progression to IPG implantation after office-based SNM test stimulation for 52 patients at our institution

	Frequency, Urgency (n = 24)	Urge Incontinence (n = 24)	Nonobstructive Retention (n = 4)
>50% Sx improved, n (%)	14 (58)	17 (71)	1 (25)
Permanent IPG, n (%)	13 (54)	13 (54)	1 (25)
Equivocal, n (%)	3 (13)	0 (0)	1 (25)
Permanent IPG, n (%)	2 (8)	0 (0)	0 (0)
Did not respond, n (%)	7 (29)	7 (29)	2 (50)

Abbreviations: IPG, implantable pulse generator; SNM, sacral neuromodulation; Sx, symptoms.

stimulation of these nerves inhibits bladder activity, which then evokes a central inhibition of the micturition reflex pathway in the spinal cord and brain.

McPherson first demonstrated in a cat model in 1966 that stimulation of cut ends of peripheral nerves including the posterior tibial nerve inhibited bladder contractions.[40–42] Then in 1983, McGuire and Morrisey applied electrical stimulation of hindquarter nerves to treat detrusor instability in spinal cord injured nonhuman primates.[43–45] They went on to demonstrate efficacy in humans.[46]

PTNS treatments generally use a 34-gauge needle electrode that is inserted approximately 5 cm cephalad to the medial malleolus and slightly posterior to the tibia. The needle is inserted at a 60° angle. A surface electrode is placed on the calcaneus of the same (ipsilateral) foot. The electrode and needle are connected to the stimulator, which is set at a current of 0.5 to 9.0 mA at 20 Hz, based on motor and sensory responses. The patient generally undergoes treatment for 30 minutes weekly for 12 weeks. This is followed by treatments as needed based on patient symptoms.

EFFICACY AND OUTCOMES
SNM

A recent review of the initial randomized controlled trials of SNM for urgency/frequency and urge incontinence found an overall initial response rate of between 64% and 88%.[13] In a separate review and meta-analysis, 80% of patients had either 90% continence or a 50% improvement in urge incontinence in response to SNM.[34] The response to SNM appears to be durable. In a prospective international trial of 121 patients who had an initial response after 1 year of therapy, 84% of patients with urge incontinence and 71% of patients with urgency/frequency showed a persistent response at 5 years (>50% reduction in symptoms).[43]

Three prospective randomized trials of SNM for urgency/frequency or urge incontinence merit mention. A study by Schmidt and colleagues[46] enrolled 155 patients from 16 international centers with urge incontinence refractory to medications and without pelvic pain or known neurologic conditions. All patients underwent a test period of 3 to 7 days and 98 patients had a greater than 50% improvement in their symptoms. These patients were randomized to undergo either immediate IPG implantation or delayed implantation after 6 months of medical therapy. After 6 months of SNM for the immediate implantation group, 47% of patients were completely dry and 29% had a greater than 50% reduction in incontinence with efficacy retained at 18 months of follow-up.

Urodynamic parameters improved for the immediate versus delayed implantation group at 6 months with a higher percentage demonstrating stable detrusor function (56% vs 16%; $P = .014$). For all patients, 32.5% underwent surgical revision for generator or implant site pain or lead migration.

A second trial on SNM for urge incontinence randomized 44 patients to SNM or medical management with an average reduction of 88% in episodes of incontinence and 90% in leakage severity; 56% of implant patients versus 4% of controls had complete resolution of incontinence, and urodynamics demonstrated a roughly quadrupling of volume at first contraction. Based on long-term follow-up, the 3-year actuarial estimate for treatment failure was 32.4%.[47]

The effectiveness of SNM for urgency/frequency was evaluated in a later multicenter trial that randomized 51 patients after a successful test stimulation to either immediate InterStim (Medtronic, Minneapolis, MN, USA) implantation or a control group. In the treatment group, 56% of patients achieved either a 50% reduction in symptoms or achieved fewer than 7 voids per day; 8% of patients had no improvement in voiding symptoms at all. After 6 months, voiding diary, quality of life, and urodynamic parameters were significantly improved on average in the implant group versus no improvement in the control group. After 6 months of therapy, the neurostimulator was turned off and symptoms returned to baseline.[48]

Older age and the presence of comorbidities appear to decrease the rate of treatment success with SNM. This was evaluated in one study involving 105 patients, including those with known neurologic conditions. Patients older than 75 years had a 30% symptom response rate. In comparison, 80% of patients younger than 45 responded to SNM. No patients with 3 or more comorbidities had complete resolution of symptoms.[49] Similarly, patients with pelvic pain or neuropathy may be more likely to fail SNM. A case series of patients failing SNM found that pudendal neuropathy was common, and that many patients benefited from a pudendal nerve block.[50]

Percutaneous Tibial Nerve Stimulation

An early, uncontrolled observational study demonstrated objective urodynamic reduction in detrusor overactivity in 44 patients with OAB.[51] More recently, 3 randomized controlled trials have assessed the efficacy of PTNS. In the Study of Urgent PC vs Sham Effectiveness in Treatment of Overactive Bladder Symptoms (SUmiT) trial, 220 patients with OAB were randomized to receive either PTNS or a sham therapy. Patients did not use pharmacotherapy during the course of the trial. PTNS or a validated sham procedure was performed weekly for 30 minutes over 12 weeks. Outcomes were assessed using a voiding diary and global response assessment questionnaires at baseline and again 1 week after completing treatment. Compared with patients receiving sham therapy, patients who received PTNS had significant improvements in urinary frequency, urgency, urge incontinence episodes, and nocturia; 54.5% of patient receiving PTNS compared with 20.9% of patients receiving sham therapy reported moderate to marked improvements in global response assessment.[12]

These findings were confirmed in a European study randomizing 35 women with medication refractory OAB to either PTNS or placebo (electrical stimulation of the gastrocnemius muscle). In that study, 71% of patients receiving PTNS reported improvement compared with 0% in the placebo group.[52] Both studies are important in that the placebo effect is well documented for patients with OAB[53] and demonstrates short-term efficacy of the procedure. Importantly, although these studies show improvement in symptoms with PTNS, the magnitude of the improvement is generally small and falls short of a "cure."

In the Overactive Bladder Innovative Therapy trial, 100 patients were randomized to either 12 weeks of PTNS without pharmacotherapy or tolterodine extended release 4 mg. A global response assessment demonstrated significantly more patients reporting substantial improvement with PTNS compared with tolterodine (79.5% vs 54.8%). However, both treatments led to similar objective improvements in terms of urinary frequency and urge incontinence episodes, leading the investigators to conclude that PTNS offers similar efficacy as tolterodine.[13]

Longer-term observational studies have suggesting a durable response for at least some patients who respond to PTNS. Fifty patients who had responded to 12 weekly PTNS treatments as part of the SUmiT trial were enrolled in a continuing observational study. After 14 weeks of no treatment, patients received approximately 1 treatment a month. Only 1 patient had an adverse event, which was mild bleeding from the needle site. Only 29 of the 50 patients remained in the study after 3 years of follow-up with an estimated 77% maintaining moderate or marked improvement over this period.[14]

Overall, PTNS appears to be an effective treatment for patients with OAB, noting that, in published PTNS trials, only one exclusively involved patients who were nonresponsive to pharmacotherapy. PTNS appears to improve symptoms for most patients similarly to tolterodine; however, few patients are cured or achieve complete relief of symptoms. There do not seem to be any significant adverse events associated with treatment. The treatment effect appears to be durable with monthly "maintenance" procedures, at least for some patients.

COST CONSIDERATIONS

SNM is associated with high initial treatment costs because of device costs, costs related to the test procedure, and OR and anesthesia costs for implantation. SNM must have excellent long-term efficacy to justify initial costs, estimated at $22,226 in 2010.[54] In theory, an office-based test procedure may be useful in identifying patients who are likely to fail implantation. The office-based test procedure is less expensive than an OR procedure with permanent leads[39]; however, permanent lead placement may be a more sensitive screening method for SNM.[36] Cost-effectiveness modeling studies have not yet demonstrated the cost-effectiveness of either test procedure.[55]

Although no head-to-head trials have been performed, overall success rates are similar for PTNS and an SNM test stimulation. A recent Markov cost-effectiveness study used estimated success rates as 67% for PTNE versus 55.4% for an SNM test stimulation. Based on 2013 reimbursement rates, initial costs are also similar for the 2 treatments ($1857 for SNM vs $1773 for PTNS). A slightly higher percentage (90% vs 71%) remained on therapy with SNM versus PTNS after a successful initial treatment, but at a significantly higher cost ($24,342 vs $4867).[56]

SUMMARY

OAB affects many, with profound effects on quality of life with high economic costs. Although antimuscarinic drugs can reduce voiding symptoms, many patients do not tolerate the side effects, and some do not experience sufficient relief. Modulation of bladder reflex pathways with office-based procedures, such as SNM and PTNS, have proven to be efficacious. They are minimally invasive and are important options in the treatment armamentarium for patients with OAB.

REFERENCES

1. Abrams P, Cardozo L, Fall M, et al. The standardisation of terminology of lower urinary tract function: report from the Standardisation Subcommittee of the International Continence Society. Neurourol Urodyn 2002;21(2):167–78.

2. Stewart WF, Van Rooyen JB, Cundiff GW, et al. Prevalence and burden of overactive bladder in the United States. World J Urol 2003;20(6):327–36.

3. Tyagi S, Thomas CA, Hayashi Y, et al. The overactive bladder: epidemiology and morbidity. Urol Clin North Am 2006;33(4):433–8, vii.

4. Hu TW, Wagner TH. Health-related consequences of overactive bladder: an economic perspective. BJU Int 2005;96(Suppl 1):43–5.

5. Basra RK, Wagg A, Chapple C, et al. A review of adherence to drug therapy in patients with overactive bladder. BJU Int 2008;102(7):774–9.

6. Tanagho EA, Schmidt RA, Orvis BR. Neural stimulation for control of voiding dysfunction: a preliminary report in 22 patients with serious neuropathic voiding disorders. J Urol 1989;142(2 Pt 1):340–5.

7. Sheriff MK, Shah PJ, Fowler C, et al. Neuromodulation of detrusor hyper-reflexia by functional magnetic stimulation of the sacral roots. Br J Urol 1996;78(1):39–46.

8. Lavelle JP, Teahan S, Kim DY, et al. Medical and minimally invasive treatment of incontinence. Rev Urol 1999;1:111–20.

9. deGroat WC. Neuroanatomy and neurophysiology: innervation of the lower urinary tract. In: Raz S, editor. Female Urology. Philadelphia: WB Saunders Company; 1996. p. 28–42.

10. Van Kerrebroeck PE, Marcelissen TA. Sacral neuromodulation for lower urinary tract dysfunction. World J Urol 2012;30(4):445–50.

11. Cooperberg MR, Stoller ML. Percutaneous neuromodulation. Urol Clin North Am 2005;32(1):71–8.

12. Peters KM, Carrico DJ, Perez-Marrero RA, et al. Randomized trial of percutaneous tibial nerve stimulation versus sham efficacy in the treatment of overactive bladder syndrome: results from the SUmiT trial. J Urol 2010;183(4):1438–43.

13. Peters KM, Macdiarmid SA, Wooldridge LS, et al. Randomized trial of percutaneous tibial nerve stimulation versus extended-release tolterodine: results from the overactive bladder innovative therapy trial. J Urol 2009;182(3):1055–61.

14. Peters KM, Carrico DJ, MacDiarmid SA, et al. Sustained therapeutic effects of percutaneous tibial nerve stimulation: 24-month results of the STEP study. Neurourol Urodyn 2013;32(1):24–9.

15. Fall M, Lindstrom S. Electrical stimulation. A physiologic approach to the treatment of urinary incontinence. Urol Clin North Am 1991;18(2):393–407.

16. Amend B, Matzel KE, Abrams P, et al. How does neuromodulation work. Neurourol Urodyn 2011; 30(5):762–5.

17. Malaguti S, Spinelli M, Giardiello G, et al. Neurophysiological evidence may predict the outcome of sacral neuromodulation. J Urol 2003;170(6 Pt 1): 2323–6.

18. Spinelli M, Malaguti S, Giardiello G, et al. A new minimally invasive procedure for pudendal nerve stimulation to treat neurogenic bladder: description of the method and preliminary data. Neurourol Urodyn 2005;24(4):305–9.

19. van der Pal F, Heesakkers JP, Bemelmans BL. Current opinion on the working mechanisms of neuromodulation in the treatment of lower urinary tract dysfunction. Curr Opin Urol 2006;16(4):261–7.

20. Bazeed MA, Thuroff JW, Schmidt RA, et al. Effect of chronic electrostimulation of the sacral roots on the striated urethral sphincter. J Urol 1982;128(6): 1357–62.

21. Gormley EA, Lightner DJ, Burgio KL, et al. Diagnosis and treatment of overactive bladder (non-neurogenic) in adults: AUA/SUFU guideline. J Urol 2012;188(Suppl 6):2455–63.

22. Lucas MG, Bosch RJ, Burkhard FC, et al. EAU guidelines on assessment and nonsurgical management of urinary incontinence. Eur Urol 2012; 62(6):1130–42.

23. Comiter CV. Sacral neuromodulation for the symptomatic treatment of refractory interstitial cystitis: a prospective study. J Urol 2003;169(4):1369–73.

24. Powell CR, Kreder KJ. Long-term outcomes of urgency-frequency syndrome due to painful bladder syndrome treated with sacral neuromodulation and analysis of failures. J Urol 2010;183(1): 173–6.

25. Lay AH, Das AK. The role of neuromodulation in patients with neurogenic overactive bladder. Curr Urol Rep 2012;13(5):343–7.

26. Sievert KD, Amend B, Gakis G, et al. Early sacral neuromodulation prevents urinary incontinence after complete spinal cord injury. Ann Neurol 2010; 67(1):74–84.

27. Weil EH, Ruiz-Cerda JL, Eerdmans PH, et al. Clinical results of sacral neuromodulation for chronic voiding dysfunction using unilateral sacral foramen electrodes. World J Urol 1998;16(5):313–21.

28. Das AK, Carlson AM, Hull M, et al. Improvement in depression and health-related quality of life after sacral nerve stimulation therapy for treatment of voiding dysfunction. Urology 2004;64(1):62–8.

29. Marcelissen TA, Leong RK, Serroyen J, et al. The use of bilateral sacral nerve stimulation in patients with loss of unilateral treatment efficacy. J Urol 2011;185(3):976–80.

30. Cohen BL, Tunuguntla HS, Gousse A. Predictors of success for first stage neuromodulation: motor versus sensory response. J Urol 2006;175(6): 2178–80 [discussion: 2180–1].

31. Peters KM, Killinger KA, Boura JA. Is sensory testing during lead placement crucial for achieving positive outcomes after sacral neuromodulation? Neurourol Urodyn 2011;30(8):1489–92.

32. Koldewijn EL, Rosier PF, Meuleman EJ, et al. Predictors of success with neuromodulation in lower urinary tract dysfunction: results of trial stimulation in 100 patients. J Urol 1994;152(6 Pt 1): 2071–5.

33. Siegel SW, Catanzaro F, Dijkema HE, et al. Long-term results of a multicenter study on sacral nerve stimulation for treatment of urinary urge incontinence, urgency-frequency, and retention. Urology 2000;56(6 Suppl 1):87–91.

34. Brazzelli M, Murray A, Fraser C. Efficacy and safety of sacral nerve stimulation for urinary urge incontinence: a systematic review. J Urol 2006;175(3 Pt 1):835–41.

35. Hijaz A, Vasavada S. Complications and troubleshooting of sacral neuromodulation therapy. Urol Clin North Am 2005;32(1):65–9.

36. Leong RK, De Wachter SG, Nieman FH, et al. PNE versus 1st stage tined lead procedure: a direct comparison to select the most sensitive test method to identify patients suitable for sacral neuromodulation therapy. Neurourol Urodyn 2011; 30(7):1249–52.

37. Borawski KM, Foster RT, Webster GD, et al. Predicting implantation with a neuromodulator using two different test stimulation techniques: a prospective randomized study in urge incontinent women. Neurourol Urodyn 2007;26(1):14–8.

38. Kessler TM, Madersbacher H, Kiss G. Prolonged sacral neuromodulation testing using permanent leads: a more reliable patient selection method? Eur Urol 2005;47(5):660–5.

39. Everaert K, Kerckhaert W, Caluwaerts H, et al. A prospective randomized trial comparing the 1-stage with the 2-stage implantation of a pulse generator in patients with pelvic floor dysfunction selected for sacral nerve stimulation. Eur Urol 2004;45(5):649–54.

40. Huwyler M, Kiss G, Burkhard FC, et al. Microbiological tined-lead examination: does prolonged sacral neuromodulation testing induce infection? BJU Int 2009;104(5):646–50 [discussion: 650].

41. McPherson A. The effects of somatic stimuli on the bladder in the cat. J Physiol 1966;185(1): 185–96.

42. McPherson A. Vesico-somatic reflexes in the chronic spinal cat. J Physiol 1966;185(1):197–204.

43. van Kerrebroeck PE, van Voskuilen AC, Heesakkers JP, et al. Results of sacral neuromodulation therapy for urinary voiding dysfunction: outcomes of a prospective, worldwide clinical study. J Urol 2007;178(5):2029–34.

44. McGuire E, Morrissey S, Zhang S, et al. Control of reflex detrusor activity in normal and spinal injured non-human primates. J Urol 1983;129(1):197–9.

45. McGuire E, Zhang S, Horwinski E, et al. Treatment of motor and sensory detrusor instability by electrical stimulation. J Urol 1983;129(1):78–9.

46. Schmidt RA, Jonas U, Oleson KA, et al. Sacral nerve stimulation for treatment of refractory urinary urge incontinence. Sacral Nerve Stimulation Study Group. J Urol 1999;162(2):352–7.

47. Weil EH, Ruiz-Cerda JL, Eerdmans PH, et al. Sacral root neuromodulation in the treatment of refractory urinary urge incontinence: a prospective randomized clinical trial. Eur Urol 2000;37(2):161–71.

48. Hassouna MM, Siegel SW, Nyeholt AA, et al. Sacral neuromodulation in the treatment of urgency-frequency symptoms: a multicenter study on efficacy and safety. J Urol 2000;163(6):1849–54.

49. Amundsen CL, Romero AA, Jamison MG, et al. Sacral neuromodulation for intractable urge incontinence: are there factors associated with cure? Urology 2005;66(4):746–50.

50. Antolak SJ Jr, Antolak CM. Therapeutic pudendal nerve blocks using corticosteroids cure pelvic pain after failure of sacral neuromodulation. Pain Med 2009;10(1):186–9.

51. Amarenco G, Ismael SS, Even-Schneider A, et al. Urodynamic effect of acute transcutaneous posterior tibial nerve stimulation in overactive bladder. J Urol 2003;169(6):2210–5.

52. Finazzi-Agro E, Petta F, Sciobica F, et al. Percutaneous tibial nerve stimulation effects on detrusor overactivity incontinence are not due to a placebo effect: a randomized, double-blind, placebo controlled trial. J Urol 2010;184(5):2001–6.

53. van Leeuwen JH, Castro R, Busse M, et al. The placebo effect in the pharmacologic treatment of patients with lower urinary tract symptoms. Eur Urol 2006;50(3):440–52 [discussion: 453].

54. Watanabe JH, Campbell JD, Ravelo A, et al. Cost analysis of interventions for antimuscarinic refractory patients with overactive bladder. Urology 2010;76(4):835–40.

55. Leong RK, de Wachter SG, Joore MA, et al. Cost-effectiveness analysis of sacral neuromodulation and botulinum toxin A treatment for patients with idiopathic overactive bladder. BJU Int 2011; 108(4):558–64.

56. Martinson M, MacDiarmid S, Black E. Cost of neuromodulation therapies for overactive bladder: percutaneous tibial nerve stimulation versus sacral nerve stimulation. J Urol 2013;189(1):210–6.

Infusion Therapy and Implantables for the Urologist

Jennifer Rothschild, MD, MPH[a], Ian M. Thompson III, MD[b],
Raoul S. Concepcion, MD[c],*, Neal D. Shore, MD[d]

KEYWORDS

- Urology • Infusion • Treatment • Therapy • Implantables

KEY POINTS

- Urology has historically adapted to the changing health care environment.
- The urology practice is in the position to deliver many novel and unique therapies across multiple disease states.
- Urologists have been quick to adopt new technology, therapeutics, and devices to deliver state-of-the-art patient care with improved clinical outcomes.
- As urologists move toward less invasive, outpatient-friendly procedures, it is incumbent on the specialty that urologists offer comprehensive care to patients.

Historically, the practicing urologist has received classic surgical training. This has usually involved 1 to 2 years of general surgery and 3 to 4 years of urology residency, often times with a research component. The amount of out patient clinical experience may vary by program, with most educational instruction being based within the operating room. When a chief resident matriculates into clinical practice, he or she may spend upward of 50% of the time in the clinic setting. Urology represents a hybrid specialty, where most patients seen are symptom driven and may not have a defined diagnosis. There is a cognitive requirement to properly evaluate and determine an appropriate treatment plan for every patient, pending the result of the work-up. Currently, depending on the number of providers in the practice, geographic area, and scope of practice, accounting for some of the variables, the revenues generated from the nonsurgical portion of a practice may range from 30% to 65% of collections.[1]

Medicine, in general, is changing rapidly. Most practices are faced with continued decreases in reimbursement, rising group overhead, and sweeping health insurance reform at the federal level that threatens the very existence of independent community practice. The field of urology has been morphing with regard to its historical clinical and practice patterns. The pharmaceutical management of benign prostatic hyperplasia has reduced the number of surgical interventions.[2] The advent of minimally and noninvasive procedures continues to grow and the number of "open cases" is diminishing in training programs and in practice. There is an increasing amount of time now required for office therapeutics, because many of the treatments that have evolved can be delivered and administered in an outpatient setting. The busy urology practice is now in the position to deliver many novel and unique therapies across multiple disease states. As a result, clinicians can provide state-of-the-art care in a clinic setting and potentially reduce the overall costs of health care delivery. This article reviews some of these potential new opportunities available to the practicing urologist.

Disclosures: The authors have nothing to disclose.
a Department of Urology, University of California at Davis Medical Center, 4806 Y Street, Suite 2200, Sacramento, CA 95817, USA; b Department of Urology, University of Texas Health Science Center at San Antonio, San Antonio, TX 78229, USA; c Urology Associates, Nashville, TN 37209, USA; d Carolina Urologic Research Center, Myrtle Beach, SC 29572, USA
* Corresponding author.
E-mail address: rsconcepcion@ua-pc.com

HORMONE-REPLACEMENT THERAPY

As the life expectancy in the United States has significantly increased over the past century, men have increasingly encountered hypogonadism as they age. The Nobel Prize was awarded to Butenandt and Ruzicka in 1939 for their work in isolating testosterone. In men, testosterone is produced primarily by the testes with smaller amounts produced by the adrenal glands. Testosterone is converted to dihydrotestosterone by 5α-reductase and within androgen target cells. About 98% of circulating testosterone is bound, of this approximately 30% is bound to sex hormone-binding globulin and the rest is bound to albumin and other serum proteins; the remainder represents free testosterone. Bioavailable testosterone is made up by free testosterone and that which is bound to albumin.[3]

There are several different assays used for measuring testosterone with different normal ranges for each. Measuring testosterone levels is not an exact science because circulating testosterone levels can be affected by many factors including medical conditions, diurnal variation, changes in SHBG, age, body mass index, and more. The definition of hypogonadism is controversial and to this point the American Urological Association released a white paper titled "The Laboratory Diagnosis of Testosterone Deficiency" in 2013. The position statement at the end of this document is as follows:

> Based on the extensive review of published data and input from professional organizations, the members of this panel believe that, for now, diagnosis of hypogonadism should be based as much on the presence of signs and symptoms as on serum T measurement. Based on overall poor quality of T testing in most clinical laboratories and age bias of published reference ranges, no patient should be denied coverage for treatment based solely on payer defined cut-off points if need for such treatment is established by a health professional. The AUA works closely with regulatory and professional agencies to improve assay performance and normal range, and as literature accumulates, this position will be reevaluated.

Symptoms of hypogonadism include decreased libido, fatigue, erectile dysfunction (ED), decreased muscle mass, irritability, decreased motivation, and hot flashes. Men are becoming increasingly aware of hypogonadism as a diagnosis and of treatment options for this condition. This is caused in part by increased advertising in many communities by nonurologic practitioners.

Testosterone replacement can be administered in several different forms. Oral preparations are available but are rarely used in the United States because much of the drug undergoes first-pass metabolism by the liver and carries with it a higher incidence of primary hepatoma.[3] Testosterone can be administered by intramuscular injections and there are different formulations for this available. Testosterone cypionate injection is available in two strengths: 100 and 200 mg/mL. The half-life of testosterone cypionate is approximately 8 days. Ninety percent of a dose is excreted in the urine, 6% in the feces, and inactivation of testosterone occurs mostly in the liver. Testosterone cypionate, 100 and 200 mg/mL, is manufactured in 10-mL multidose vials. Intramuscular (IM) injections of testosterone cypionate should be administered in the gluteus. Dosing varies based on patient's symptoms and serum testosterone levels. In general, 50 to 400 mg can be administered every 2 to 4 weeks for testosterone replacement in hypogonadal men.

Testosterone can also be applied topically. Testosterone gels available include Androgel, Testim, Fortesta, and Axiron. In addition, there is the once daily transdermal patch (Androderm). Testopel is a testosterone pellet, manufactured by Slate pharmaceuticals, that is implanted into the subcutaneous (SC) fat in the outer quadrant of the hip. This requires a short procedure in the clinic every 3 to 6 months. Each pellet contains 75 mg of testosterone.

There are several contraindications for use of testosterone replacement common to all methods and formulations of replacement therapy, including allergy or hypersensitivity to the drug; males with breast cancer; history or suspicion of prostate cancer; women who are or may become pregnant; and patients with serious cardiac, hepatic, or renal disease.

Men receiving replacement testosterone therapy should have hemoglobin/hematocrit checked periodically given the risk of polycythemia. Lipid panels should be checked regularly because of risk of hyperlipidemia while on replacement therapy and serum testosterone levels should be checked to assess efficacy of treatment. Baseline complete blood count and lipid panel should be checked before initiating testosterone-replacement therapy.

ERECTILE DYSFUNCTION

The incidence of ED increases with age and the prevalence of ED has increased in the United States alongside increasing life expectancies. In the Massachusetts Male Aging Study, which surveyed men between 40 and 70 years of age in the Boston area, Feldman and colleagues[4] demonstrated a 52% prevalence of ED and that the prevalence of complete ED increased from 5% to 15% between subject ages 40 and 70 years old. In their analysis of the US adult male population, Selvin and colleagues[5] found the overall prevalence of ED in men greater than or equal to 20 years of age at 18.4%, with prevalence positively related to age, hypertension, cardiovascular risk factors, diabetes, and lack of physical activity.

The most important component of evaluation of a patient with ED is a thorough history and physical examination. Evaluation often includes the use of questionnaires, examples of which include the International Index of Erectile Function, the Erectile Dysfunction Inventory for Treatment Satisfaction, and the Brief Males Sexual Function Inventory.[6–8] These questionnaires are also often used to monitor patient response to treatment.

Nonsurgical interventions for ED include lifestyle changes, pelvic floor muscle therapy, oral PDE5-inhibitor therapy, and use of a vacuum-erection device.[9,10] Dr Giles Brindley, famous for presentation of his research results at the 1983 American Urological Association annual meeting, demonstrated the success of intracavernosal injection of phenoxybenzamine.[11] Options for intracavernosal injection therapy include papaverine; alprostadil; papaverine + phentolamine (Bi-Mix); and papaverine + phentolamine + alprostadil (Tri-Mix). Initiation of therapy with intracavernosal injection requires initial administration in clinic for patient education and to ascertain the effective dosing.

ADVANCED PROSTATE CANCER
Androgen-Deprivation Therapy

In 1966, Charles Huggins received the Nobel Prize for Physiology and Medicine for his work in discovering the hormonal control of prostate cancer growth.[12] His work ultimately led to the development of androgen-deprivation therapy (ADT). Before the advent of pharmacologic castration, bilateral orchiectomy had been the gold standard for androgen deprivation because the testes produce 90% to 95% of testosterone.

Luteinizing Hormone–Releasing Hormone Agonists

Luteinizing hormone–releasing hormone (LHRH) agonist therapy was first administered for the treatment of prostate cancer in 1980. LHRH agonists work by stimulating the LHRH receptors in the pituitary gland to cause increased secretion of LH and follicle-stimulating hormone (FSH),

initially causing an increased production of testosterone. Continued LHRH agonism causes subsequent decreased LH/FSH production and hence decreased levels of testosterone result. The initial rise in testosterone can cause a flare response in patients with advanced prostate cancer. Antiandrogens can be administered before initiation of LHRH agonist therapy to prevent a flare response. LHRH agonists include the following:

Lupron (leuprolide acetate)
- 7.5 mg IM q month
- 22.5 mg IM q 3 months
- 30 mg IM q 4 months
- 45 mg IM q 6 months

Eligard (leuprolide acetate)
- 7.5 mg SC q month
- 22.5 mg SC q 3 months
- 30 mg SC q 4 months
- 45 mg SC q 6 months

Viadur (leuprolide acetate): 65-mg implant placed SC in the inner aspect of the upper arm q 12 months. The implant must be removed at the end of the 12 months. This was removed from the market by the manufacturer (Bayer).

Vantas (histrelin): 50-mg implant placed SC in the inner aspect of the upper arm q 12 months. The implant must be removed at the end of the 12 months.

Zoladex (goserelin acetate)
- 3.6 mg SC q month
- 10.8 mg SC q 3 months

Trelstar (triptorelin)
- 3.75 mg IM q month
- 11.25 mg IM q 3 months
- 22.5 mg IM q 6 months

Gonadotropin-Releasing Hormone Antagonists

Gonadotropin-releasing hormone antagonists reduce the secretion of LH, FSH, and testosterone by blocking the gonadotropin-releasing hormone receptors in the pituitary gland. There is no flare response associated with gonadotropin-releasing hormone antagonist therapy. Firmagon (Degarelix), an initial dose of 240 mg SC (2 × 120 mg injections), is administered in the abdomen and then an 80-mg SC injection is given every 28 days going forward. Ninety-six percent of men have castrate levels of testosterone by Day 3, and 99% by Day 7.

Additional ADTs available but not necessarily administered in clinic include estrogens (diethylstilbestrol, Premarin, estradiol); progestins (Megace); antiandrogens (flutamide, nilutamide, bicalutamide); and androgen synthesis inhibitors (ketoconazole, aminoglutethimide).

There has been debate as to the optimal use of androgen deprivation for the treatment of advanced prostate cancer and much of this has to do with the potential side effects of therapy. Long-term androgen deprivation can lead to increased risk of cardiovascular events, diabetes, hyperlipidemia, anemia, osteoporosis, and fatigue. The benefit of long-term androgen deprivation for prostate cancer treatment must be weighed against the risk of increased risk of death from other causes and this requires individual assessment of each patient. To mitigate some of these risks, many practitioners advocate the use of intermittent ADT.

Provenge

Provenge (sipuleucel-T) is an immunotherapy approved by the Food and Drug Administration (FDA) for the treatment of men with asymptomatic or minimally symptomatic metastatic castrate-resistant prostate cancer. Provenge is the result of culturing a patient's own antigen-presenting cells with the recombinant antigen PAP-GM-CSF. When administered to the patient, Provenge potentiates the patient's T cells to attack prostate cancer cells.

Treatment with Provenge starts with patients undergoing leukopheresis at an approved blood collection center. The result of the collection is then sent to a Provenge manufacturing facility, which then cultures the patient's immune cells with the recombinant antigen. Provenge is administered by peripheral or central intravenous (IV) access during a 1-hour infusion, usually 2 to 3 days after the leukopheresis. Approximately 30 minutes before initiation of infusion, patients are pretreated with acetaminophen and an antihistamine to reduce risk of an infusion reaction.

The IMPACT trial, a phase 3, randomized, double-blind, multicenter, controlled trial of 512 men with asymptomatic or minimally symptomatic castrate-resistant prostate cancer, demonstrated a 4.1-month improvement in overall survival at 24 months after treatment.[3] The most common side effects experienced by patients receiving Provenge include fatigue, fever, chills, nausea, headache, and joint pain.

Xofigo (Radium-223 Dichloride)

Xofigo (radium-223 dichloride, formerly known as Alpharadin) is an IV-administered radiopharmaceutical that targets bone metastases with alpha radiation from radium-223 decay. A phase III study of radium-223 dichloride in patients with symptomatic hormone-refractory prostate cancer with skeletal metastases is ongoing with estimated completion date of December, 2013. Preliminary results have demonstrated improved overall survival and increased time to first skeletal-related event (SRE).[13]

Radium-223 has been the first radiopharmaceutical to demonstrate increased overall survival and it was approved by the FDA in May of 2013 for the treatment of men with castrate-resistant prostate cancer and symptomatic bone metastases, and no known visceral metastases.[14] The dose of Xofigo is 50 kBq per kilogram bodyweight and it is injected intravenously once every 4 weeks for a total of six injections. Radium-223 is usually administered by a radiation oncologist or nuclear medicine radiologist.

There are some urologists that will manage the infusion of chemotherapy, such as docetaxel and cabazitaxel, for advanced prostate cancer. The number of urologic providers administering such therapy might increase with time as comfort grows with administering systemic therapies, because this is a dynamic and growing area in urology.

BENIGN PROSTATIC HYPERPLASIA THERAPIES

The gold standard for traditional treatment of benign prostatic hyperplasia has been transurethral resection of the prostate. Since the advent of medical therapy in the mid-1980s, including α-adrenergic blockers and 5α-reductase inhibitors, there has been an ever increasing movement toward medical therapy and minimally invasive procedures.[2]

Transurethral Microwave Thermotherapy

Transurethral microwave thermotherapy involves the placement of a specially designed catheter, containing a microwave coil, within the urethra. After the catheter is properly in place it is connected to the energy source and the prostate is treated. During treatment cooling fluid is cycled through the catheter to reduce risk of thermal injury to surrounding urethral tissue. This can be done with conscious sedation and local anesthesia in the office or outpatient setting.

Transurethral Needle Ablation of Prostate

The transurethral needle ablation of prostate catheter used for treatment includes a fiberoptic scope that allows for visual guidance of needle placement. The generator produces low-level monopolar radiofrequency waves that generate temperatures up to 100°C in the tissue around the needles. Depending on the practice of the urologist, this procedure can be performed in the clinic or in an operating room setting. The patient is placed in the dorsal lithotomy position with a grounding pad placed over the sacrum. Anesthesia options include from local with lidocaine jelly, conscious IV sedation, to general sedation.

INJECTABLE THERAPIES FOR INCONTINENCE
Intradetrusor Injection of Botulinum Toxin

Injectable agents for the treatment of overactive bladder (OAB) remain limited; however, recent data for one injectable therapy, botulinum toxin, demonstrate exceptionally promising results. Botulinum toxin, previously approved by the FDA for the treatment of neurogenic detrusor overactivity, has recently gained indication for medication refractory OAB. Clinically, botulinum toxin is expected to gain rapid acceptance as a therapy for severe OAB, which has been refractory to standard management.

A potent neurotoxin, botulinum toxin is derived from anaerobic bacterium *Clostridium botulinum*. Although several structural serotypes have been identified (A–G), types A and B are the primary serotypes with clinical significance. Type A is the most common subtype used because of duration of effect when compared with type B.[3] Botulinum toxin induces detrusor muscle relaxation by inhibiting the release of acetylcholine from the presynaptic nerve terminal. It is postulated that symptomatic relief is experienced because of reduction/suppression of involuntary detrusor contractions, leading to a reduction in many of the symptoms of OAB. Studies continue to investigate the action of botulinum toxin in more detail, including the possible contribution of afferent signaling in the urothelium leading to sensory suppression. For example, there may be an action on afferent C-fibers, which are postulated to contribute to the mechanism underlying the reduction of urgency.[15,16]

Evolving literature provides robust evidence that intradetrusor injection of onabotulinum toxin A is effective, well tolerated, and safe.[3] A clinical response may be seen in up to 60% of the women who receive botulinum toxin,[17] although the duration of effect has been reported to vary widely because of variation in dosage and outcome measures.[3] Benefits usually last between 3 and 12 months depending on indication and dosage.[17,18] Studies have concluded that injection of botulinum toxin results in a significant increase in maximum cystometric capacity.[19,20]

Preoperatively, patients must be able and willing to return for postvoid residual evaluations and have the ability to perform self-catheterization. In addition, patients should also be counseled that the effects of intradetrusor botulinum toxin diminishes over time, thus requiring repeat injections. Postoperatively, patients should be monitored closely for transient urinary retention and urinary tract infections.[7]

Botulinum toxin can be injected into the bladder wall using either a rigid or flexible cystoscope and is often done as an outpatient procedure, using general, spinal, or local anesthesia. Multiple injection needles are commercially available and the intricacies of the procedure are outside the scope of this review. Ultimately, the botulinum toxin is injected into the detrusor muscle at multiple sites (generally 10–30 sites), avoiding the trigone because of a theoretical risk of vesicoureteral reflux. Interestingly, some studies suggest that suburothelial injections may have comparable efficacy to intradetrusor injections.[3]

Much attention has been given to what dose safely balances the symptomatic benefits with the postvoid residual urine volume related safety profile for use in medication-refractory OAB. In regards to botulinum toxin, less may prove to be more. Lower doses of botulinum toxin (100–150 U) have been shown to have beneficial effects, and larger doses (300 U), although they may be more effective and longer lasting, have more side effects, such as urinary retention, particularly in the neurogenic population.[3] Indeed, depending on indication, a lower dose of 100 U may have comparable efficacy and improved safety over 200- and 300-U dosages.[18] Doses of 100 U have demonstrated durable efficacy in the management of idiopathic OAB and urinary urgency incontinence.[21,22]

Injectable Therapies for the Treatment of Stress Urinary Incontinence

Injectable agents for the treatment of stress urinary incontinence (SUI) represent a commonly used and minimally invasive therapeutic option. Although injectable agents for incontinence have been used for more than 100 years, their diminished success rate when compared with open procedures has often dampened enthusiasm as a durable treatment.[23] Therefore, injectable therapies are usually reserved as second-line treatment options or for women who prefer less invasive procedures or are more medically suited for them.[24]

In addition to a second-line treatment option, other possible indications include elderly patients, patients with high anesthetic risks, patients who must remain on anticoagulants at all times, women who are young and desire more children in the future, or have mild persistent SUI after an incontinence procedure.[25–27] Careful patient selection is important to the success of bulking therapies. Patients should ideally have urethral hypermobility of less than 30 degrees and have adequate urethral mucosal blood supply (and estrogen effects).[28]

Literature suggests that efficacy and duration are inferior to surgery and patients are often appropriately counseled that injectable therapies may offer an improvement rather than a cure for their SUI symptoms.[24,29] Patients should be advised that injection therapy is a process and not a one-time procedure; sometimes two or three injections (4 weeks apart) are required to achieve continence; and that periodic repeat injections may be necessary to maintain continence.[27] Active urinary tract infection, hypersensitivity to the injectable material, and presence of urethral diverticula are the major contraindications.

Ideally, a urethral bulking agent should be biocompatible, durable, cost effective, and nonimmunogenic, but despite enormous medical advances, the perfect bulking agent remains elusive.[15] Clinical concerns regarding long-term efficacy, cost effectiveness, and patient safety remain a persistent challenge.[23] In general, glutaraldehyde cross-linked bovine collagen (Contigen) is the biomaterial most commonly injected worldwide with a cure rate of up to 53%.[29] More recently, a study from Europe has demonstrated that polyacrylamide hydrogel (Bulkamid) resulted in a subjective response rate (cured or improved) of 64% and a significant decrease in urine leakage after 24 months.[30] Patients should be counseled that limited data exist with which to assess the long-term safety and efficacy of injectable agents.[31] Multiple additional agents are commonly used and are gaining traction for women wishing to avoid surgical interventions. Currently available injectable agents for SUI include gluteraldehyde cross-linked bovine collagen (Contigen); carbon beads (Durasphere); silicone particles (Macroplastique); and calcium hydroxyapatite (Coaptite). New agents undergoing development include polyacrylamide hydrogel (Bulkamid), autologous chondrocytes, and autologous muscle-derived cells.

Depending on the injected material used, the goal is not to coapt the urethral mucosa but to obtain "static increase in resistance in the urethral outlet" and thus avoid overinjection.[28] The agent can be either injected periurethral or transurethral, such that the agent is adequately injected into the bladder neck or proximal urethra, preferably into the submucosa or lamina propria. Different injection sites can be used, such as the 3- and 9-o'clock position or the 4- and 8-o'clock position.[32] Risks generally include urinary retention, urinary tract infection, hematuria, and transient dysuria. Although urethral bulking agents have a lower cure rate than open surgery, they are generally associated with fewer complications.

BONE-TARGETING THERAPY

Since the Nobel Prize winning discovery by Huggins and Hodges of the role of circulating androgens in patients with prostate cancer,[12] ADT remains the mainstay of advancing prostate cancer in patients with metastatic and nonmetastatic disease. As many as 200,000 patients in 2008, both Medicare and commercially insured, received ADT for greater than 6 months.[33,34] However, it has long been recognized that one of the potentially serious and undertreated complications of ADT is bone mineral density loss (BMD). It has been estimated that BMD loss in men on ADT may be as high as 4% per year once therapy has been instituted.[35] Contrast this with the recognized loss in the postmenopausal woman, which is commonly reported and treated, of 1.5% to 2%.[36] This is an underrecognized medical problem that the urology community needs to address.

Normal bone turnover is a coordinated dance between osteoblasts and osteoclasts, resulting in formation and resorption, mediated by receptor activator of nuclear factor kappa (RANK) ligand.[37] It is thought that estrogens have a protective effect by increasing osteoblast proliferation (increased bone formation) and decreasing RANK ligand production by the cells (decrease resorption).[38] When ADT is initiated, the lowering of serum testosterone, which is peripherally converted to estrogen by aromatase, results in lowering of peripheral estrogen levels and results in decreasing osteoblast production and increased RANK ligand activity, favoring resorption over formation with resultant BMD loss and increased risk to male osteoporosis.[37] This castration treatment–induced bone loss (CTIBL) in the patient with nonmetastatic prostate cancer is associated with a 45% excess risk of fracture compared with patients not on ADT.[39] This increased fracture rate results in a higher mortality, especially if the patient requires hospitalization.[40]

A National Comprehensive Cancer Network Task Force Report in 2009 emphasized the need for bone health management in cancer care.[41] Strategic to this push to preserve BMD and decrease fracture risk is supplemental calcium, vitamin D, lifestyle modification, and pharmacologic therapy. Oral bisphosphonates (alendronate, ibandronate) are pyrophosphate analogs that are directly taken up by the osteoclasts, which results in decreased bone resorption and may have an apoptotic effect.[42] However, bisphosphonate therapy is not approved for CTIBL.

In September of 2012, the FDA approved denosumab, a fully human monoclonal antibody that binds RANK ligand, which results in a decrease in bone resorption, a 6.7% increase in BMD at the lumbar spine at 2 years, and a reduction in new vertebral fractures compared with placebo.[43] The dose is 60 mg SC every 6 months with an increase risk of hypocalcemia, arthralgia, back pain, osteonecrosis of the jaw, and cataracts.[44] This dose is packaged and marketed as Prolia (Amgen) and is indicated for patients with nonmetastatic prostate cancer on high-risk drug (ADT) for the prevention of CTIBL.

Patients that unfortunately progress despite being on ADT and develop castration-resistant prostate cancer (CRPC) with bone metastasis are at an increased risk of developing SRE, defined as a patient that requires palliative radiation to the bone for pain control and surgical stabilization for a fracture, and that experiences a pathologic fracture or spinal cord compression.[45] An SRE can be a devastating event, altering quality of life in patients with already limited survival.[3] Zoledronic acid (ZA), an intravenous bisphosphonate, has been approved in the patient with CRPC for SRE prevention. It delayed SRE by a median time of 17.1 months, compared with the control arm, which may have included patients on supplemental calcium and vitamin D, at 10.7 months.[45] Many urologists, however, were reluctant to administer ZA in the office because it required a 1-hour infusion and monitoring of renal function. The former was not necessarily what most offices were or are set up to do, unlike medical oncology clinicians, and many patients went untreated.

In November of 2010, XGEVA (Amgen) was approved for the prevention of SRE in patients with bone metastasis from any malignancy except multiple myeloma.[46] XGEVA is the same molecule as Prolia, denosumab, but at a SC dose of 120 mg monthly. It was shown to be superior to ZA in a head-to-head study for the prevention of first and subsequent SRE with an 18% risk reduction compared with ZA. The median time to the first SRE was 20.7 months. Because of denosumab's SC route of delivery, it can and should be incorporated into the typical urology practice. The National Comprehensive Cancer Network recommends bone targeting therapy for patients with CRPC.[47]

SUMMARY

The specialty of urology has historically adapted to the changing health care environment. It has been quick to adopt new technology and new therapeutics and devices to render state-of-the-art patient care with improved clinical outcomes. As the field moves toward less invasive procedures that are outpatient friendly, it is incumbent on the specialty, especially within the potentially changing reimbursement environment, that clinicians offer comprehensive care to patients.

REFERENCES

1. Internal Data, Urology Associates, P.C., Nashville TN, 2009-2011.
2. Elliott SP, Sweet RM. Contemporary surgical management of BPH. Curr Prostate Rep 2009;7(1):19–24.
3. Kantoff PW, Higano CS, Shore ND, et al. Sipuleucel-T immunotherapy for castration-resistant prostate cancer. N Engl J Med 2010;363(5):411–22.
4. Mooradian AD, Morley JE, Korenman SG. Biological actions of androgens. Endocr Rev 1987;8(1):1–28.
5. Feldman HA, Goldstein I, Hatzichristou DG, et al. Impotence and its medical and psychosocial correlates: results of the Massachusetts Male Aging Study. J Urol 1994;151(1):54–61.
6. Selvin E, Burnett AL, Platz EA. Prevalence and risk factors for erectile dysfunction in the US. Am J Med 2007;120(2):151–7.
7. Rosen RC, Riley A, Wagner G, et al. The international index of erectile function (IIEF): a multidimensional scale for assessment of erectile dysfunction. Urology 1997;49(6):822–30.
8. Althof SE, Corty EW, Levine SB, et al. EDITS: development of questionnaires for evaluating satisfaction with treatments for erectile dysfunction. Urology 1999;53(4):793–9.
9. O'Leary MP, Fowler FJ, Lenderking WR, et al. A brief male sexual function inventory for urology. Urology 1995;46(5):697–706.
10. Esposito K, Giugliano F, Di Palo C, et al. Effect of lifestyle changes on erectile dysfunction in obese men: a randomized controlled trial. JAMA 2004;291(24):2978–84.
11. Dorey G, Speakman M, Feneley R, et al. Randomised controlled trial of pelvic floor muscle exercises and manometric biofeedback for erectile dysfunction. Br J Gen Pract 2004;54(508):819–25.
12. McDougal WS, Wein AJ, Kavoussi LR, et al. Campbell-Walsh urology. 10th edition review, 1e. 10th edition. Saunders; 2011.
13. Brindley GS. Cavernosal alpha-blockade: a new technique for investigating and treating erectile impotence. Br J Psychiatry 1983;143:332–7.
14. FDA. Radium Ra 223 dichloride. 2013. Available at: http://www.fda.gov/Drugs/InformationOnDrugs/ApprovedDrugs/ucm352393.htm.
15. Harrison MR, Wong TZ, Armstrong AJ, et al. Radium-223 chloride: a potential new treatment for castration-resistant prostate cancer patients with metastatic bone disease. Cancer Manag Res 2013;5:1–14.
16. Duthie JB, Vincent M, Herbison GP, et al. Botulinum toxin injections for adults with overactive bladder

syndrome. Cochrane Database Syst Rev 2011;(12):CD005493.

17. Shaban AM, Drake MJ. Botulinum toxin treatment for overactive bladder: risk of urinary retention. Curr Urol Rep 2008;9:445–51.

18. Khera M, Somogyi GT, Salas NA, et al. In vivo effects of botulinum toxin A on visceral sensory function in chronic spinal cord-injured rats. Urology 2005;66:5.

19. Brubaker L, Richter HE, Visco A, et al. Refractory idiopathic urge urinary incontinence and botulinum A Injection. J Urol 2008;180:217–22.

20. Kuo HC. Will suburothelial injection of small dose of botulinum A toxin have similar therapeutic effects and less adverse events for refractory detrusor overactivity? Urology 2006;68:5.

21. Sahai A, Khan MS, Dasgupta P. Efficacy of botulinum toxin-A for treating idiopathic detrusor overactivity: results from a single center, randomized, double-blind, placebo controlled trial. J Urol 2007;177:6.

22. Kuo HC. Clinical effects of suburothelial injection of botulinum A toxin on patients with nonneurogenic detrusor overactivity refractory to anticholinergics. Urology 2005;66:94–8.

23. Dmochowski RR, Chapple CC, Nitti VW, et al. Efficacy and safety of onabotulinumtoxin A for idiopathic overactive bladder: a double-blind, placebo controlled, randomized, dose ranging trial. J Urol 2010;184:7.

24. Keegan PE, Atiemo KK, Cody JJ, et al. Periurethral injection therapy for urinary incontinence in women. Cochrane Database Syst Rev 2007;(3):CD003881.

25. Davis NF, Kheradmand F, Creagh T. Injectable biomaterials for the treatment of stress urinary incontinence: their potential and pitfalls as urethral bulking agents. Int Urogynecol J 2013;24(6):913–9.

26. Leach GE, Dmochowski RR, Appell RA, et al. Female stress urinary incontinence clinical guidelines panel summary report on surgical management of female stress urinary incontinence. J Urol 1997;158:6.

27. Reynolds WS, Dmochowski RR, Penson DF. Epidemiology of stress urinary incontinence in women. Curr Urol Rep 2011;12:370–6.

28. Cespedes RD, Serkin FB. Is injection therapy for stress urinary incontinence dead? No. Urology 2009;73:3.

29. Dmochowski RR, Blaivas JM, Gormley EA, et al. Update of AUA guideline on the surgical management of female stress urinary incontinence. J Urol 2010; 183:9.

30. Corcos J, Collet JP, Shapiro S, et al. Multicenter randomized clinical trial comparing surgery and collagen injections for treatment of female stress urinary incontinence. Urology 2005;65:7.

31. Reynolds WS, Dmochowski RR. Urethral bulking: a urology perspective. Urol Clin North Am 2012;39: 279–87.

32. Toozs-Hobson PP, Al-Singary WW, Fynes MM, et al. Two-year follow-up of an open-label multicenter study of polyacrylamide hydrogel (Bulkamid®) for female stress and stress-predominant mixed incontinence. Int Urogynecol J 2012;23:1373–8.

33. Huggins C, Hodges C. Studies on prostate cancer. The effect of castration, of estrogen and of androgen injection on phosphatases in metastatic carcinoma of the prostate. Cancer Res 1941;1:293–7.

34. Smith MR, Lee WC, Brandman J, et al. GnRH agonist and fracture risk. J Clin Oncol 2005;23(31): 7897–903.

35. Gilbert SM, Kuo YF, Shahinian VB. Prevalent and incident use of ADT among men with prostate cancer in the U.S. Urol Oncol 2011;29(6):647–53.

36. Cetin K, Li S, Blaes AH, et al. Prevalence of patients with nonmetastatic prostate cancer on ADT in U.S. Urology 2013;81(6):1184–9.

37. Higano CS. In: Figg WD, et al, editors. Drug management of prostate cancer. 2010. p. 321.

38. Lipton A, Smith MR, Ellis GK, et al. Treatment induced bone loss and fracture in cancer undergoing hormone ablation therapy: efficacy and safety of denosumab. Clin Med Insights Oncol 2012;6: 287–303.

39. Chin KY. Sex Steroids in bone health. Int J Endocrinol 2012;2012:298719.

40. Shahinian VB, Kuo YF, Freeman JL, et al. Risk of fracture after ADT for prostate cancer. N Engl J Med 2003;352:154–64.

41. Beebe-Dimmer JL, Cetin K, Shahinian V, et al. Timing of ADT use and fracture risk among elderly men with prostate cancer in the United States. Pharmacoepidemiol Drug Saf 2012;21(1):70–8.

42. Gralow JR, Biermann JS, Farooki A, et al. NCCN task force report: bone health in cancer care. J Natl Compr Canc Netw 2009;7(Suppl 3):S1–32.

43. Corey E, Brown LG, Quinn JE, et al. Zoledronic acid exhibits inhibitory effects in osteoblast and osteolytic metastases of prostate cancer. Clin Cancer Res 2003;9:295.

44. Smith MR, Cook R, Lee KA, et al. Disease and risk characteristics as predictors of time and bone metastases and death in men with progressive castration resistant prostate cancer. Cancer 2011; 117(10):2077–85.

45. Prolia. Package Insert. Thousand Oaks. CA: Amgen Inc; 2010.

46. Fizazi K, Carducci M, Smith M, et al. Denosumab versus zoledronic acid for treatment of bone metastases in men with castration resistant prostate cancer: A randomized double-blind study. Lancet 2011;377(9768):813–22.

47. Mohler JL, et al. National Comprehensive Cancer Network Guidelines in Oncology. Prostate Cancer. Version 2 2013.

Coding for Urologic Office Procedures

Robert A. Dowling, MD[a],*, Mark Painter[b]

KEYWORDS

- Coding and reimbursement • Urology office procedures • Urology CPT codes
- Coding for office procedures

KEY POINTS

- The American Medical Association is the steward of Current Procedural Terminology (CPT), and the Centers for Medicare and Medicaid Services (CMS) often implements that terminology in rules and regulations that are followed by most insurance payers.
- CPT codes are highly specific, and there is a code or set of codes to fit all office urology procedures and common scenarios.
- Many resources are available to assist in complex coding scenarios.
- Coding for urologic office procedures is founded in proper documentation in the medical record.
- Urologic office procedures often involve expensive drugs or disposables, and recovery of acquisition costs depends on a detailed understanding of coding rules and nuances.

INTRODUCTION AND PURPOSE

Typical urologists today generate a significant portion of practice revenue performing procedures in the office, and a detailed knowledge of documentation and coding guidelines is necessary to insure appropriate, compliant, and optimal reimbursement. Several recent trends have highlighted the importance of coding, billing, and collecting payment correctly for office-based procedures. Diagnostic and therapeutic procedures, once commonly requiring facility-based anesthesia services, can now be performed in a urologist's office. The stewards of procedural terminology have introduced more codes with more specificity to replace general codes in the urinary and male genital sections and, in some cases, deleted once

commonly used codes. Advances in technology have introduced new office-based procedures into the armamentarium of urologists—for example, in the treatment of benign prostatic hypertrophy—demanding new codes. Worker salaries and other practice expenses for urologists continue to rise, while allowable charges for procedures have remained flat or even decreased. Employers and insurance companies are asking patients to shoulder more responsibility for health care expenses; patients in turn are demanding more transparency in their bills. The emergence of value-based payment systems and the passage of health care reform legislation are predicted to result in savings primarily by reducing payments to hospitals and surgical specialists. Commercial

Conflict of Interest: (Dr Dowling) Principal, Dowling Medical Director Services LLC; Consultant, Healthtronics Information Technology Solutions. (Mr Painter) Principal, Physician Reimbursement Systems; Principal, PRS Urology SC; Principal, PRS Consulting, LLC; Principal, Relative Value Studies, Inc; Consultant, Dendreon; Consultant, Photocure; Consultant, Watson Pharma.
Disclaimer: Best efforts to provide accurate information, codes, and descriptions have been made in development of this information. Rules and regulations are subject to interpretation and change, however. Variation by payer, region, and contract are common. Advice and direction on coding and reimbursement are based primarily on Medicare rules with general advice for private payers included where relevant.
a Dowling Medical Director Services LLC, 6387 Camp Bowie Boulevard, Suite B-339, Fort Worth, TX 76116, USA;
b PRS Network, 12301 North Grant Street, Unit 230, Thornton, CO 80241, USA
* Corresponding author.
E-mail address: rdowling@dowling-consulting.com

payers are attempting to control rising costs by managing utilization of high cost procedures, thereby increasing the number of office-based procedures that require preauthorization. Finally, federal agencies have signaled their interest in recovering overpayments made to providers for high-volume, high-cost procedures with an emphasis on medical necessity and appropriate documentation. In this complex and changing landscape, it is imperative that urologists document and bill correctly for office procedures.

This article first reviews some general principles of proper documentation, coding, and getting paid for procedures performed in a urologist's office. Then, specific coding and billing issues for each of the most common diagnostic and therapeutic procedures are examined. By the end of this article, readers should have a tool for their practice that should optimize reimbursement and ensure standard and compliant documentation and coding.

GENERAL PRINCIPLES
Definition of a Procedure

Although many factors may determine the setting in which a procedure is performed, for the purposes of this article, office-based urologic procedures are defined as those urinary or genital tract procedures that do not require services only available in an operating room and that are commonly performed in a urologic office setting in the United States. The procedure may be diagnostic or therapeutic in nature, may be invasive or noninvasive, and usually includes the professional service to perform the procedure, any same-day evaluation and management (E&M) services related to the procedure, and the supplies necessary to conduct the procedure. Most office-based urologic procedure codes and their descriptions can be located in the surgery section of the American Medical Association CPT manual, urinary system subsection (50010-53899) or male genital subsection (54000-55899).[1]

Documentation

Proper documentation of office procedures is at the foundation of good clinical care, licensure in most states, risk management, compliant coding, and optimal reimbursement. All urologists should be familiar with an axiom used by utilization review companies, payers, state and federal regulators, and malpractice experts and quoted in the American Medical Association CPT manual: "if something is not documented in the medical record, then the procedure was not performed and therefore is not subject to reimbursement." The

components of procedural documentation are standard, often routine, and lend themselves well to paper forms or electronic templates. The indication for the procedure should be clearly listed to support medical necessity. The place of service (office and examination room) should be clearly specified, not simply inferred from the name of a provider and a date. The normal and abnormal findings of the procedure, and any complications, should be described separately from the procedure itself because they are always unique to a patient and procedure. The procedure note itself should be descriptive enough to support the relevant procedure code and specific enough to support a standard of care but not contain unnecessary detail that obscures the important content. Finally, the procedure note should be separate and clearly distinguishable from documentation of any other services performed during the same visit.

Documenting common procedures presents an opportunity for efficiency by designing and using paper forms or electronic templates, but a careful balance must be struck between benefit and risk. With the adoption of electronic health records in group practices, the person who designs the templates is often not the only person who uses the templates; furthermore, many electronic medical records do not easily allow users to view the data entry screen and the output screen at the same time. Finally, the ability to "copy forward" procedural notes, such as surveillance cystoscopy for bladder cancer, can result in "cloned notes" and unintentionally perpetuate documentation that is not appropriate. These factors can introduce significant risk of inaccurate documentation that can be mitigated with careful template design. For example, a male cystoscopy template might contain default content for preparation of the genitals, insertion of the scope, and systematic inspection of the bladder—but should not contain text, settings, or other content, such as "all findings were normal," that could be inserted inappropriately and inadvertently. A well-designed template should allow users to be efficient, thorough, and accurate in the creation of a compliant yet readable note. The ideal procedure template should also make clear the contents of the note output to minimize inadvertent documentation.

Coding for Office-Based Procedures

Office procedures are described and classified in CPT 5-digit codes, a system copyrighted by the American Medical Association, mandated by federal law for government insurance programs, and accepted as the standard nomenclature by commercial insurance payers. The most relevant codes in the CPT manual for office-based urology procedures are in the surgery subsections of urinary system (50010-53899) and male genital system (5400055899).[1] The CPT codes are revised once a year, and it is essential that the urology practice keep current with additions, deletions, and changes to the CPT manual. Causes for claim denial include use of an outdated code, failure to use a new code, reporting the wrong code, and use of a nonspecific unlisted code when a specific one exists. Whenever possible, the provider or staff member performing the office procedure should be the same person who assigns or approves the code submitted for billing. Urologic procedures performed in an office setting should always be billed with the place of service code 11 (office facility).

Multiple procedures

Although CPT codes for most office-based urology procedures are specific and inclusive, some office procedures (transrectal ultrasound–guided prostate biopsy, for example) require more than 1 CPT code for compliant coding and optimal reimbursement. The rules governing which codes can be paired with other codes are administered by the CMS and are called the National Correct Coding Initiative (NCCI) (also known as CCI). This system was implemented in 1996 by the CMS "to promote national correct coding methodologies and to control improper coding leading to inappropriate payment. NCCI code pair edits are automated prepayment edits that prevent improper payment when certain codes are submitted together for Part B-covered services."[2] For example, the NCCI edits permit submitting a prostate biopsy (55700) and a transrectal ultrasound (76872) but never allow the submission of cystoscopy (52000) and complex catheterization (51703) on the same date of service. Most commercial insurers include NCCI edits, and the CMS updates this list quarterly.

When multiple codes are necessary and appropriate, it is best practice to report the procedure with the highest fee first, the additional procedures on separate lines of the claim form with a -51 modifier attached, and to submit full fees for each procedure. Most insurance payers reduce the reimbursement of the second and additional procedures by at least 50%. The practice of itemizing multiple CPT codes when only 1 code is "needed" is referred to as "unbundling," and systematic unbundling may invite the scrutiny of auditors and regulators. In some circumstances, it is appropriate to report multiple codes considered bundled under current CCI data sets—a modifier may be used when conditions warrant separate reporting

(decision for surgery, left or right laterality for example). Later in this article, the best practice for coding common procedures that require more than 1 CPT code is discussed.

Global period

In order to process claims quickly and accurately, most payers have developed specific definitions for a global surgical package, including time frames (the global period) during which other professional services are considered included in the payment of the procedure. Most payers follow the definition of the global surgical package developed by the CMS, and most procedural CPT codes on the Medicare fee schedule are associated with a global period of 0, 10, or 90 days. The global surgical package specifically includes the procedure itself, all services that are a "usual and necessary" part of the procedure, local anesthesia, the treatment of any minor complications related to the procedure, E&M services performed on the day of the procedure (exceptions discussed later), and, in cases of 90-day global packages services, the day of and day prior to the procedure. Diagnostic urology procedures performed in the office generally have a 0-day global period, but some therapeutic procedures—including vasectomy—have a 90-day global period. Urologists should also understand when it is permissible to bill for an office procedure when it is performed in the global period of another earlier procedure, such as cystoscopy and stent removal after *extracorporeal shock wave lithotripsy*. Submitting claims for services normally included during the global period is considered unbundling. The global period for each CPT code is generally listed on the insurance company fee schedule and can also be found at the CMS Web site.[3]

Supplies

CPT and Healthcare Common Procedure Coding System (HCPCS) level II codes also form the basis of the resource-based relative value system used by the CMS and most commercial payers to set fees. Most codes contain component relative value units that consider physician work, practice expense, and malpractice cost for that particular procedure. For this reason, the cost of supplies and equipment used during an office-based procedure are usually factored into the fee and are generally not billed or reimbursed separately.

Modifiers

A urologist's coding staff should be familiar with CPT code modifiers. When used appropriately, modifiers may increase reimbursement and, when used inappropriately, may result in claim denial or payer audits. Although a comprehensive discussion of modifiers is beyond the scope of this article, some examples of modifiers that might be appropriate for some office-based procedures are found in **Table 1**.

Incident to Services

Office-based urology procedures may be performed under the supervision of a physician and, therefore, reimbursed under "incident to" rules. The CMS defines "incident to services" as those that are provided "as part of" a physician's professional services in the office and directly supervised by the treating physician. To qualify as "incident to," a service must be rendered to a patient who was initially seen by a treating physician, and the supervising provider must remain actively involved in the care of that patient; the supervising (billing) provider must be physically present in the facility and immediately available when the service was provided. Medical assistants, nurses, and others have long provided "incident to services" in a urology office: examples include injections, catheterizations, and measurement of residual urines. The increased presence of nurse practitioners (NPs) and physician assistants (PAs) in urology practices has created some confusion about "incident to" rules for several reasons:

- NPs and PAs are licensed professionals credentialed by insurance companies and may bill under their own identification (ID) number (including the CMS) for services performed independently. When doing so, physician extenders are generally reimbursed by the CMS at 85% of the fee schedule amount. These services are not billed "incident to."

- NPs and PAs may also perform services "incident to" a physician service and, therefore, bill under a physician's ID number. When doing so, the physician is reimbursed at 100% of the fee schedule amount.

- NPs and PAs enjoy a scope of practice broader than medical assistants and nurses and narrower than physicians, defined by a state licensing authority and subject to modification by a supervising physician of record (who is also licensed by the state).

- Private payers may allow "incident to" reporting for NPs and staff without a physician's physical presence in the office

Subject to any limitations on the scope of practice imposed by state licensure, many urologists have trained NPs and PAs to perform routine procedures, including cystoscopy, prostate biopsy, and vasectomy under direct supervision in the office. In order to qualify under "incident to" rules, patients must have been seen for an initial evaluation by a supervising physician and the supervising physician must be physically present within the office suite while the procedure is performed by the employed extender. Assuming these conditions are met, claim forms are submitted just as if physicians themselves had performed the procedure. The increased volume of services performed when both a physician and an extender are billing under the physician provider ID number could invite auditing activity by payers, and records should be maintained (calendars and schedules) to prove that the physician was physically present in the office on the date of such claims.

Evaluation and Management Services

As described previously, the CMS and other payers consider the procedure CPT code inclusive of all visit charges for that day, and charges for E&M codes are generally not paid separately for the same date of service. CPT coding guidelines do provide for billing for an E&M service, as long as it is separate and distinct from the procedure itself. In these cases, the modifier, -25, is appended to the E&M service, not the procedure code. For example, a patient who travels a great distance for care may be scheduled for follow-up of bladder cancer and prostate cancer during the same visit. During that visit, the urologist may perform surveillance cystoscopy (for the bladder cancer) and separately perform a digital rectal examination, review recent prostate-specific antigen results, and schedule further testing for prostate cancer follow-up. The claim form should reflect 52000 linked to bladder cancer and the appropriate level E&M code with a -25 modifier linked to prostate

Table 1
Examples of CPT code modifiers

22	Unusual procedural services (example, repeat vasectomy)
26	PC only (example, urodynamics interpretation)
51	Multiple procedures (example, transrectal ultrasound biopsy)
58	Related procedure during postoperative period (example, stent removal)
59	Distinct procedure
76	Repeat procedure by same physician
77	Repeat procedure by another physician
78	Unplanned return to the operating/ procedure room
79	Unrelated procedure during postoperative period

cancer. Coding guidelines do not require 2 separate diagnoses in order to bill a separate significant E&M service, but separate diagnoses help justify the additional service.

A related but separate scenario commonly occurs when a patient is seen primarily for an E&M service and a decision is made to perform an office-based procedure the same day. For example, a patient referred for the initial evaluation of gross hematuria may receive a recommendation to have cystoscopy the same day. In that scenario, the appropriate coding includes a 52000 and a modifier attached to the appropriate E&M code. This example highlights that the CMS frequently develops rules and definitions that differ from the CPT directives. CPT guides physicians to append the modifier, -57, to the E&M code in this circumstance because this modifier alerts payers that a decision for the procedure was made during the E&M service. Medicare, however, considers the decision for surgery part of the global surgical package for minor procedures (defined as procedures having a 0-day or 10-day global period); therefore, the modifier, -57, is not appropriate; because Medicare does allow for E&M services that are clearly separate and identifiable to be reported and paid on the same day as a minor procedure, the modifier, -25, is appropriate for this payer and others that follow Medicare policy.

Finally, as discussed previously, documenting procedures separate from any E&M services performed the same day help support correct coding and justify claims that are audited for any reason.

Laboratory and Radiology Services

Urology practices are increasingly performing their own laboratory and radiology services, and coding for these services requires a detailed understanding of the specific codes, the circumstances under which they can be billed, and the concept of professional component (PC), technical component (TC), and global service (PC and TC). Just as with other CPT codes, the description of the laboratory or radiology service is specific and it is crucial to match the service to the correct code.

Specimen collection

Physicians are permitted to bill and collect a fee for collecting blood via venipuncture and urine specimens via catheterization in addition to other services performed in the office. The proper codes for the CMS are G0001—routine venipuncture for collection of specimen(s) and P9612—catheterization for collection of specimen(s); most private payers use a different code for venipuncture 36415. A separate specimen collection fee cannot be charged for simple urines, swabs, or biopsies

(as it is considered included in the procedural code).

PC TC global

Pathology, radiology, urodynamic, and some other diagnostic services may be billed globally by urologists or split into PCs and TCs. For example, a urologist who performs a renal ultrasound in the office and renders the official interpretation bills 76775, and the provider is reimbursed for the equipment, supplies, and technical support as well as the interpretation of the results and the report. It is important when billing globally for a diagnostic study that the report is documented separately from any other services performed that day. A practice that owns an in-office pathology laboratory may bill for the TC (equipment, supplies, and labor) of preparing surgical pathology and prostate biopsy (88305-TC) and send the slides to an independent pathologist for interpretation; some practices contract with pathologists and bill globally. Finally, there may be some circumstances where a urologist performs only the professional interpretation of a test and another supplier bills for the TC; in those circumstances, the modifier, -26, should be appended (ie, urodynamics 51726-26).

Resources and Reference Materials

Coding for medical services is a complex and rapidly changing subject area and it is important that a urology practice performing procedures maintain current competency or expertise in this field. As discussed previously, the American Medical Association is the steward of the CPT manual.[1] Additions, deletions, and revisions are published in October and are effective January 1 of the following calendar year. The CPT manual is a reference work and general guide, but often the answers to coding and reimbursement questions are found in or from CMS manuals, local coverage determinations, subject matter experts in specialty societies, online forums, or even individual explanations of benefits that accompany payments for claims. The complexity of this field has created a demand for credentialed professionals, and organizations, like the American Academy of Professional Coders and the American Health Information Management Association, certify thousands of professional coders for careers in physician offices. The American Academy of Professional Coders offers a specialty certification in urology, the Certified Urology Coder, which is specifically designed for urologic procedures, ancillary procedures performed in the office, and other urology-specific scenarios. Many large urology practices employ such professionals to optimize reimbursement and mitigate the risk of incorrect coding. In addition to these valuable resources, the American Urologic Association's Office of Practice Management offers both free and purchased access to subject matter experts in urology coding.[4]

COMMON UROLOGY OFFICE PROCEDURES

In the following sections, common urology office procedures are described by groupings that generally reflect their common association. A description of the codes in each family is followed, when pertinent, by special considerations for documentation and best practices for using these codes.

Urinalysis Procedures

Documentation
The distinction between these 4 codes lies in whether an automated reader was used and whether microscopy was performed; therefore, the documentation should clearly state whether an automated reader was used and ideally incorporate the output from that automated reader. If microscopy is performed, the results should be documented separately from the other constituents and conform to a standard format (ie, red cells, white cells, crystals, bacteria, and other). Urinalysis is commonly performed as part of routine patient intake, and ideal documentation should clearly reflect an order associated with a clear indication (Table 2).

Post Void Residual Procedures

Documentation
Determining the amount of urine remaining in the bladder after a patient has voided is typically measured in a urology office with ultrasound or by inserting a catheter in the bladder and measuring the urine volume drained. Payment for these procedures has become a specific target of payers and auditors, and the advent of noninvasive testing may have broadened the indications for urologists and their patients. Most payers do not reimburse for this procedure when it is only used as a screening tool. Office documentation should clearly address the indication for measurement of residual urine and state which method is used (including the size of the catheter, if used) (Table 3).

Coding best practice
CPT 51701 has a global period of 000, and billing of E&M services on the same date requires use of modifiers for the E&M service code. The 51701 is included in the NCCI listing for most urology service codes with an indicator that does not allow unbundling with a modifier. Therefore, it is not appropriate to report code 51701 for dates of service in which other urologic services are reported (for example, cystoscopy) (Table 4). Furthermore, the 51701 is considered a minor surgery and is included in the postoperative period of other surgical services.

Cystoscopy Procedures

Documentation
This closely related group of CPT codes underscores that the correct code can only be applied with the correct and specific description of the procedure performed; also, urologists may start the procedure intending to perform a simple diagnostic cystoscopy but based on findings perform a different closely related procedure/code. Many electronic medical record templates are built in a fashion to link templates to generation of specific CPT codes; in those cases, it is important to choose the template/begin the documentation after knowing the final code to be applied in order to avoid generating the wrong code. When performing biopsy, fulguration, or treatments, the exact number, size, and location of the lesions should be documented because this may determine the appropriate code. When removing a foreign body from the bladder, it is prudent to document whether or not the foreign body is intact or remnants remain.

Table 2
Urinalysis

Code	Global	Description
81000	XXX	Urinalysis, nonautomated, with microscopy
81001	XXX	Urinalysis, automated, with microscopy
81002	XXX	Urinalysis, nonautomated, without microscopy
81003	XXX	Urinalysis, automated, without microscopy

Table 3
Post void residual

Code	Global	Description
51798	XXX	Measurement of postvoiding residual urine by ultrasound, nonimaging
51701	000	Insertion of nonindwelling bladder catheter

Table 4		
Cystoscopy procedures		
Code	Global	Description
52000	000	Cystourethroscopy (separate procedure)
52001	000	Cystourethroscopy with irrigation and evacuation of multiple obstructing clots
52204	000	Cystourethroscopy, with biopsy(s)
52214	000	Cystourethroscopy, with fulguration (including cryosurgery or laser surgery) of trigone, bladder neck, prostatic fossa, urethra, or periurethral glands
52224	000	Cystourethroscopy, with fulguration (including cryosurgery or laser surgery) or treatment of MINOR (less than 0.5 cm) lesion(s) with or without biopsy
52281	000	Cystourethroscopy, with calibration and/or dilation of urethral stricture or stenosis, with or without meatotomy, with or without injection procedure for cystography, male or female
52287	000	Cystourethroscopy, with injection(s) for chemodenervation of the bladder (ie, botox)
52310	000	Cystourethroscopy, with removal of foreign body, calculus, or ureteral stent from urethra or bladder (separate procedure); simple

Table 5		
Transrectal ultrasound–guided biopsy of the prostate		
Code	Global	Description
55700	000	Biopsy, prostate; needle or punch, single or multiple, any approach
76872	XXX	Ultrasound, transrectal
76942	XXX	Ultrasonic guidance for needle placement (eg, biopsy, aspiration, injection, localization device), imaging supervision and interpretation

Coding best practice

These codes are generally bundled with the other codes in this list and usually cannot be billed together on the same date of service. For example, it is not appropriate to bill for a biopsy (52204) and fulguration (52224) of the base of the same site (**Table 5**). Coding of biopsy in conjunction with other services may be allowed with modifiers if the biopsies are taken from sites other than lesions sites being treated. Diagnostic cystoscopy may not include a discussion of treatment of the findings; therefore, an E&M code can be billed separately for that discussion (with the appropriate modifier) with some payers. Finally, cystoscopy with treatment of multiple lesions should be coded according to the method and size of the largest lesion.

Transrectal Ultrasound Guided Biopsy of the Prostate

Documentation

Many urologists perform a diagnostic ultrasound at the same time as performance of a transrectal ultrasound–guided biopsy of the prostate. The documentation for the diagnostic ultrasound should include a description of the equipment and the technique, separate documentation of the findings, including the dimensions of the prostate, and an image of the prostate; the image serves as an important record of the technical portion of the radiology procedure and the findings constitute the PC/interpretation included in the global code. The biopsy procedure should be distinct from the diagnostic ultrasound in the office documentation and should include a description of the equipment used and the location of the biopsy sites. Although a statement that ultrasound guidance was used is prudent, no image is necessary to support the use of the code 76942.

Coding best practice

When billed together, the codes should be listed in the order shown and no modifiers are necessary; 55700 does have a 0 global, and appropriate modifiers should be attached to any additional services billed the same day. The concept of global period does not apply to radiology codes.

Vasectomy Procedures

Documentation

If a vasectomy is performed on the same day as the consultation (E&M visit), it is critical to document the consultation and procedure separately (**Table 6**). Vasectomy is a high-volume routine office procedure and, as such, lends itself well to standard documentation templates. As discussed previously, this presents both opportunity for

Table 6
Vasectomy procedures

Code	Global	Description
55250	090	Vasectomy, unilateral or bilateral (separate procedure), including postoperative semen examination(s)
55450	010	Ligation (percutaneous) of vas deferens, unilateral or bilateral (separate procedure)

Table 7
Bladder catheterization and irrigation and instillation procedures

Code	Global	Description
51102	000	Aspiration of bladder; with insertion of suprapubic catheter
51700	000	Bladder irrigation, simple, lavage and/or instillation
51701	000	Insertion of nonindwelling bladder catheter (eg, straight catheterization for residual urine)
51702	000	Insertion of temporary indwelling bladder catheter; simple (eg, Foley)
51703	000	Insertion of temporary indwelling bladder catheter; complicated (eg, altered anatomy, fractured catheter/balloon)
51705	000	Change of cystostomy tube; simple
51710	000	Change of cystostomy tube; complicated
51720	000	Bladder instillation of anticarcinogenic agent (including retention time)
P9612	000	Catheterization for collection of specimen, single patient, all places of service

efficiency if the procedure is routine and risk for inaccuracy if the procedure is not routine. By requiring separate documentation of the procedure and the findings, most mistakes can be avoided. It is important to document the method of occlusion and whether or not a segment of vas was removed during the procedure because there is more than 1 possible CPT code for vasectomy.

Coding best practice

There are 3 CPT codes for vasectomy, and they differ in 2 important respects. First, 1 code specifically refers to vasectomy, which the authors interpret to mean removal of a segment of vas. If a segment of vas is removed, the most appropriate code is 55250; if a ligation procedure is performed without removal of vas, then 55450 may be more appropriate. Second, 1 code has a 90-day global and the other a 10-day global period. If a decision to perform 55250 is made the day of (same-day consult) or the day prior to the procedure, it is necessary to append a -57 modifier to the E&M code. If a decision to perform 55450 is made the same day as the procedure, during the process of a separate significant identifiable E&M services, modifier -25 should be appended to the E&M code; otherwise, no modifiers are necessary. In summary, the date of the consultation and the type of the procedure performed are the key variables in determining which codes and which modifiers are best applied.

Bladder Catheterization, Irrigation and Instillation Procedures

Documentation

Catheterization of the bladder is a common urologic procedure with different indications, and one of the challenges in documentation is that it is often performed by nonphysicians (**Table 7**). The best documentation practices call for the provider who performs a procedure to be the provider who documents the procedure. Therefore, it is important to train ancillary staff in proper documentation to support this family of codes.

Documentation should include the indication for catheterization, the method used, the equipment used, and the findings (such as residual urine). A common scenario in a urology office is that a physician may become involved in catheterizing a patient after several failed attempts by staff; those failed attempts should be documented in addition to a successful attempt in order to support a higher level of complexity for the procedure. This pertains to urethral catheterization (51702 and 51703) and to catheterization through an established suprapubic tract (51705 and 51710).

Insertion of a nonindwelling catheter to determine postvoid residual (51701) or to obtain a specimen for testing (P9612, Medicare) requires only a brief description but should include the exact amount of urine obtained and, if pertinent to the indication, the appearance of the urine. When a temporary catheter is inserted for irrigation or instillation of various agents, a more complete description of the indication, the findings, and patient tolerance is advised. Best practice calls for documenting dosage, lot number, expiration date, and even National Drug Code (NDC) for office-administered drugs and biologics. The administration procedure note should clearly explain whether the drug/biologic was acquired and provided by the physician office or by the patient (for example, a prescription or specialty pharmacy shipment).

Many urologists perform suprapubic trochar cystostomy in the office (51102). Appropriate documentation should include informed consent, the indication for the procedure (failed attempts at urethral catheterization, for example), the technique and equipment used, and the findings/results.

Coding best practice

Each of the codes in this family has a global period of 000 and, as such, any E&M services rendered separately on the same day require the appropriate modifiers (and documentation). These codes are bundled in to most office procedures and generally cannot be billed with those procedures (for example, cystoscopy 52000) or with each other unless a clear and separate indication is carefully documented.

Medications used during a catheterization procedure are billed using HCPCS code (for example, J codes) only if acquired and provided by the physician office and so documented. Many medications have different codes for different dosage/formulations with different reimbursement schedules, and careful attention to detail, supported by documentation, is necessary for optimal reimbursement.

The costs of the catheter, insertion kit, collection bag, and other supplies (except drugs) associated with this family of procedures are considered by most payers to be included in the payment for the procedure and, therefore, are not separately reported in most circumstances. Medicare allows for billing of catheters and leg bags supplied to patients for in-home use only if the billing entity has the appropriate supplier number and the supplies are provided to patients who are permanently incontinent.

Urodynamics Procedures

Documentation

The number of different procedures that constitute "office urodynamics" highlights the importance and application of principled documentation to support optimal coding and reimbursement (**Table 8**). The indication for and medical necessity of the procedure should be clearly documented. Like radiology services, the technical portion of the procedure may be performed on a different

Table 8 Urodynamics procedures		
Code	Global	Description
51725	000	Simple cystometrogram (eg, spinal manometer)
51726	000	Complex cystometrogram (ie, calibrated electronic equipment)
51727	000	Complex cystometrogram (ie, calibrated electronic equipment); with urethral pressure profile studies (ie, urethral closure pressure profile), any technique
51728	000	Complex cystometrogram (ie, calibrated electronic equipment); with voiding pressure studies (ie, bladder voiding pressure), any technique
51729	000	Complex cystometrogram (ie, calibrated electronic equipment); with voiding pressure studies (ie, bladder voiding pressure) and urethral pressure profile studies (ie, urethral closure pressure profile), any technique
51736	XXX	Simple uroflowmetry (eg, stop-watch flow rate, mechanical uroflowmetry)
51741	XXX	Complex uroflowmetry (eg, calibrated electronic equipment)
51784	000	EMG studies of anal or urethral sphincter, other than needle, any technique
51785	000	Needle EMG studies of anal or urethral sphincter, any technique
51792	000	Stimulus evoked response (eg, measurement of bulbocavernosus reflex latency time)
51797	ZZZ	Voiding pressure studies, intra-abdominal (ie, rectal, gastric, intraperitoneal) (list separately in addition to code for primary procedure)

day, in a different location, and by a different provider than the professional interpretation; it is, therefore, critical that these variables be carefully documented not only in the billing records but in the medical record as well.

Uroflowmetry is a common diagnostic test that can be performed alone or in conjunction with some of the other codes within this family. Simple uroflowmetry requires observation of patients, offers limited information, requires limited documentation, and is rarely performed in the contemporary urologic practice. Complex uroflowmetry can be performed with limited staff involvement and, because it requires a full bladder, is often performed during routine nursing intake of patients as a standing order (for example, at the same time as collection of a urine specimen). Optimal documentation includes an indication based on medical necessity and an order for the test; this may be accomplished by indication-based protocol, but the medical record should clearly reflect the reason—for example, "uroflowmetry ordered today to assess response to α-blocker therapy after urinary retention."

Cystometry (cystometrogram) in the contemporary urology practice is usually performed by calibrated electronic equipment, and in some cases the equipment also generates the documentation of the technical portion of the procedure(s). Machine-generated documentation should be imported into the medical record when possible and not stored separately from other records used to support coding and reimbursement. Documentation should include the indication for the procedure(s), the equipment and supplies used (for example, the size of the catheter), the method (for example, rate of bladder filling or type of electromyography [EMG] electrode used), and the raw observations of the person conducting the test (for example, "first urge to void"). If additional procedures are performed at the same setting, each component of the procedure should be documented clearly in order to support coding; for example, in order to support 51729, the document should indicate that cystometry, voiding pressure, and urethral pressure studies were conducted separately. A statement that a patient was able to void should be included, and studies that depend on patient voiding (for example 51729) cannot be supported if the patient was unable to void. The professional interpretation of the urodynamic testing requires a summative narrative, should address the observations made during the technical performance of the procedure, and should be separate and distinct from documentation of the actual procedure. If multiple procedures are performed, each component's interpretation should be readily identifiable in the summation.

Coding best practice

As discussed previously, if the TC is performed on a different day, by a different provider, and/or in a different location from the professional interpretation, it is necessary to split the services and append the appropriate modifiers (TC, 26) to each of the selected codes. "Incident to" rules of coding may apply if the technical portion of the procedure is performed by supervised personnel; care should be taken to bill under the supervising provider's ID and follow other "incident to" rules. The date of service, not the ordering provider, determines the proper place of service and billing provider in those circumstances.

Note also that all codes with the exception of uroflowmetry codes have global periods of 000 assigned. As such, E&M codes reported on the same date as the -TC, -26, or global service (neither -TC or -26 appended) requires appropriate use of modifier -25.

Injection Procedures

Documentation

Injection or implantation of medication in the urology office is a common and minor procedure that lends itself well to template documentation (**Table 9**). Many electronic medical records have robust modules for medication administration, and these should be used whenever possible to take advantage of clinical decision support and structured data entry; these templates also drive best documentation practices. The medical record should contain a discrete indication and order for the medication procedure. The document should include exact injection site, laterality if pertinent, drug, dosage, NDC, lot number, expiration date, and absence or presence of complications. The administration procedure note should clearly explain whether the drug/biologic was acquired and provided by the physician office or by the patient (for example, a prescription or specialty pharmacy shipment).

Coding best practice

The injection/implantation procedure and medication are typically coded separately with CPT codes and appropriate HCPCS (J) codes. Injections are often provided by staff under "incident to" guidelines and this is allowed without physician contact for the injection visit as long as the injection is part of the treatment plan developed and periodically reviewed by a qualified provider; this underscores the importance of documenting a physician order. Note the specificity of the injection codes and that antineoplastic medications are coded with 96402 despite the subcutaneous or intramuscular route. Medications often have different J codes for different dosage forms and it is sometimes necessary to append "units" to the J code in order to receive proper reimbursement. Reporting of the

Table 9
Injection procedures

Code	Global	Description
11980	000	Subcutaneous hormone pellet implantation (implantation of estradiol and/or testosterone pellet)
11981	XXX	Insertion, nonbiodegradable drug delivery implant
11982	XXX	Removal, nonbiodegradable drug delivery implant
11983	XXX	Removal with reinsertion, nonbiodegradable drug delivery implant
54200	010	Injection procedure for Peyronie disease
54235	000	Injection of corpora cavernosa with pharmacologic agent(s) (eg, papaverine, phentolamine)
96372	XXX	Therapeutic, prophylactic, or diagnostic injection (specify substance or drug); subcutaneous or intramuscular
96402	XXX	Chemotherapy administration, subcutaneous or intramuscular; hormonal antineoplastic
J0270	XXX	Injection, alprostadil, 1.25 µg
J0900	XXX	Injection, testosterone enanthate and estradiol valerate, up to 1 mL
J1060	XXX	Injection, testosterone cypionate and estradiol cypionate, up to 1 mL
J1070	XXX	Injection, testosterone cypionate, up to 100 mg
J1080	XXX	Injection, testosterone cypionate, 1 mL, 200 mg
J2440	XXX	Injection, papaverine hydrochloride, up to 60 mg
J2760	XXX	Injection, phentolamine mesylate, up to 5 mg
J3120	XXX	Injection, testosterone enanthate, up to 100 mg
J3130	XXX	Injection, testosterone enanthate, up to 200 mg
J3140	XXX	Injection, testosterone suspension, up to 50 mg
J3150	XXX	Injection, testosterone propionate, up to 100 mg
S0189	XXX	Testosterone pellet, 75 mg
J9219	XXX	Leuprolide acetate implant, 65 mg
J3315	XXX	Injection, triptorelin pamoate, 3.75 mg
J9202	XXX	Goserelin acetate implant, per 3.6 mg
J9217	XXX	Leuprolide acetate (for depot suspension), 7.5 mg

amount of drug is allowed up to full amount in the vial.

Most of the codes in this family are assigned a global period of XXX; however, current CCI bundling edits include E&M codes so E&M services provided on the same date of service require the use of modifier -25 and the appropriate documentation to support use of the modifier. Billing of E&M codes in conjunction with injection codes are a historical target of payer audits and must be medically necessary.

Intracorporal injection of vasoactive medications deserves separate mention for several reasons. First, the CPT code 54235 has a 000 global period and E&M services thus require appropriate modifiers. Second, the procedure typically administering 2 or 3 medications in different dosages; as such, careful attention to proper J codes and units is recommended. The most common medications and their codes are J2440

papaverine, J2760 phentolamine, and J0270 alprostadil—a combination often referred to as Trimix by compounding pharmacies. Finally, because Medicare considers this a procedure to train a patient for self-injection and typically allows billing 54235 once in a patient's lifetime, it is important to ensure the patient has not received a previous injection (and to so document).

Transurethral Microwave Thermotherapy (TUMT) and Transurethral Needle Ablation (TUNA) of Prostate

Documentation
Ablative treatments for BPH performed in the office are invasive procedures, involve expensive disposable items, and require careful and thorough documentation (**Table 10**). Special considerations include the importance of documenting the treatment setting, the equipment used,

Table 10
Transurethral microwave thermotherapy and transurethral needle ablation of prostate

Code	Global	Description
53850	090	Transurethral destruction of prostate tissue; by microwave thermotherapy
53852	090	Transurethral destruction of prostate tissue; by radiofrequency thermotherapy

Table 11
Pelvic floor therapy and biofeedback

Code	Global	Description
90911	XXX	Biofeedback training, perineal muscles, anorectal or urethral sphincter, including EMG and/or manometry
97032	XXX	Application of a modality to 1 or more areas; electrical stimulation (manual), each 15 min
G0283	XXX	Electrical stimulation (unattended), to 1 or more areas for indication(s) other than wound care, as part of a therapy plan of care
G8990	XXX	Other physical or occupational primary functional limitation, current status, at therapy episode outset and at reporting intervals
G8991	XXX	Other physical or occupational primary functional limitation, projected goal status, at therapy episode outset, at reporting intervals, and at discharge or to end reporting
G8992	XXX	Other physical or occupational primary functional limitation, discharge status, at discharge from therapy or to end reporting

the energy settings and times of treatments, and the monitoring and supervision involved. The treatment equipment often provides a log of energy and times, and this should be made a part of the permanent medical record.

Coding best practice

Note that these procedures include a global period of 90 days (including the first preoperative day) and, as such, require that additional services be appended with appropriate modifiers. Supplies used during the procedure, including the treatment catheters, bladder catheters, and other disposables, are considered included and generally not reimbursed separately.

Pelvic Floor Therapy (PFE) and Biofeedback

Documentation

Many payers require that patients fail other therapy (timed voiding or pelvic floor exercises at home, for example) prior to reimbursing for biofeedback and physical therapy, so it is important to document previous unsuccessful therapies and the indications for the procedure (**Table 11**). Many payers require that a clear plan of treatment, including measurable goals, be included in the patient record. Each treatment session should include documentation of the session number, time spent during treatment, equipment used, and findings, including interim assessments of progress toward goals.

Coding best practice

These procedures are often provided by staff under "incident to" guidelines and this is allowed without physician contact for the injection visit as long as the therapy is part of the treatment plan developed and periodically reviewed by a qualified provider. Medicare may require use of quality reporting CPT II codes for pelvic floor exercise treatment series. Space does not permit full discussion of proper use of G codes; the authors recommend that readers review current Medicare

guidelines for quality reporting methods required for payment. EMG diagnostic services may be used in conjunction with biofeedback or pelvic floor exercise but can only be reported if performed to determine baseline readings or to record measurement of progress. Finally, many payers, including Medicare, have benefit caps related to total amount that are paid for physical therapy services, underscoring the importance of predetermination of benefits for patients.

SUMMARY

Adherence to some general principles of documentation and coding serves as a firm foundation for urologists committed to compliant billing of most office procedures. Complex and new procedures can be coded correctly with the assistance of readily available subject matter experts and other resources. Maintaining current competency in this rapidly changing field is imperative to optimize reimbursement, meet regulatory requirements, and minimize risk.

REFERENCES

1. CPT plus 2013: a comprehensive guide to current procedural terminology. Los Angeles (CA): Practice Management Information Corporation; 2012.
2. Centers for Medicare and Medicaid Services Website. Available at: http://www.cms.gov/Outreach-and-Education/Medicare-Learning-Network-MLN/MLN Products/Downloads/How-To-Use-NCCI-Tools.pdf. Accessed April 15, 2013.
3. Centers for Medicare and Medicaid Services Physician Fee Schedule. Available at: http://www.cms.gov/apps/physician-fee-schedule/overview.aspx. Accessed April 15, 2013.
4. Available at: http://www.auanet.org/content/health-policy/practice-management.cfm. Accessed April 15, 2013.

Office-Based Behavioral Therapy for Management of Incontinence and Other Pelvic Disorders

Diane K. Newman, DNP, ANP-BC[a],*, Alan J. Wein, MD[b]

KEYWORDS

- Lower urinary tract symptoms • Behavioral treatment • Lifestyle modification • Timed voiding
- Pelvic floor muscle training • Bladder training

KEY POINTS

- Behavioral treatment with pelvic floor muscle training is the first-line treatment option for patients with lower urinary tract symptoms.
- Urology lends itself to a multidisciplinary model of a Bladder and Pelvic Floor Disorder service that provides comprehensive surgical and medical care.
- Before prescribing a behavioral intervention, assessment of the pelvic floor musculature is performed to evaluate strength, tone, and ability to contract.
- Certain lifestyle practices can cause lower urinary tract symptoms, and changes in these practices arising from evidence-based research can have a positive effect in decreasing symptoms.
- Bladder training is an education program that teaches the patient to restore normal bladder function by gradually increasing the intervals between voiding.
- Pelvic floor muscle training has been shown to decrease urgency, stress, and mixed incontinence in women, and should be offered preoperatively to men undergoing radical prostatectomy surgery.
- The best outcomes with behavioral treatments are achieved when they are provided by a knowledgeable professional in a supervised program, making it an ideal and necessary service in urology.

INTRODUCTION

Behavioral treatment with pelvic floor muscle training (PFMT) is the first-line treatment option for persons with lower urinary tract symptoms (LUTS) including urinary incontinence (UI), overactive bladder (OAB), urgency, frequency, nocturia, incomplete bladder emptying, and pelvic floor muscle (PFM) spasm.[1] These interventions, categorically referred to as conservative management, improve symptoms through pelvic floor muscle strengthening, identification of lifestyle habits, and frequently changing a person's behavior, environment, or activity that are contributing factors or triggers.[2] Such a program can be initiated after simple non-invasive urologic assessment in most patients, and should be considered the mainstay of urology care of men and women with incontinence and related voiding and pelvic floor disorders. The goals of conservative treatment are to correct voiding patterns, improve the ability to suppress urgency, and thereby to increase bladder

---

The authors have nothing to disclose.
a Division of Urology, Penn Center for Continence and Pelvic Health, Perelman School of Medicine, Penn Medicine, University of Pennsylvania, 3rd Floor, West Pavilion, Perelman Center, 34th Street and Civic Center Boulevard, Philadelphia, PA 19104, USA; b Division of Urology, Penn Medicine, Perelman School of Medicine, University of Pennsylvania Health System, Philadelphia, PA, USA
* Corresponding author.
E-mail address: diane.newman@uphs.upenn.edu

Urol Clin N Am 40 (2013) 613–635
http://dx.doi.org/10.1016/j.ucl.2013.07.010
2094-0143/13/$ – see front matter © 2013 Elsevier Inc. All rights reserved.

capacity and to lessen the frequency and amount of both stress and urgency urinary incontinence. Interventions such as bladder training (BT) and PFM rehabilitation attempt to decrease incontinence and OAB symptoms, and aid bladder emptying through increasing awareness of the function and coordination of the PFMs, so as to gain muscle identification, control, and strength and to decrease bladder overactivity. These interventions involve learning new skills through extensive one-on-one patient instruction on techniques for preventing urine loss, urgency, and other symptomatology. These methods have a large body of evidence-based research,[1] and recommended as treatment for UI which supports this type of program in non-neurogenic OAB by multiple organizations[3,4] and international guidelines.[1] The behavioral treatments discussed in this article are the ones commonly provided in urology practice for LUTS, and a behavioral treatment pathway is illustrated in **Fig. 1**. The different interventions are shown in **Fig. 2**, and **Box 1** lists the components.

BEHAVIORAL TREATMENT MODELS FOR LUTS

Urologic diseases encompass a wide scope of illnesses of the genitourinary tract of men and women, including conditions that are congenital and acquired, malignant and benign, medical and surgical. These diseases span all age groups and many conditions (eg, incontinence, voiding dysfunction, benign prostatic hyperplasia) are chronic in nature, and require care for the duration of a patient's life. With the growing shortage of urologists, the difficulty of recruiting them in some regions of the country,[5] and the aging population, many practices are turning to advanced practice providers (APPs), nurse practitioners, or physician assistants to help fill the need to provide adequate and accessible care. An APP (sometimes referred to as a physician extender), when properly trained and deployed, enables practices to provide an increased number and higher quality of services, and allows the urologist to treat more patients in a timely manner. These highly trained "extenders" can assist the urologist by accepting delegated tasks of greater complexity than had previously been delegated to registered nurses and office assistants with less training.[6]

LUTS (both storage and emptying abnormalities) and pelvic floor dysfunction are areas of urologic practice that have seen tremendous growth in the use of APPs. These conditions have been inadequately treated and poorly addressed by the medical community and industry, despite substantial impact on health, self-esteem, and quality of life. APPs providing behavioral treatments

(sometimes referred to as continence nurse practitioners) have emerged in urology practices, specifically to assess and provide nonsurgical treatment of LUTS such as UI, OAB, urgency, frequency, urinary retention, pelvic pain, and interstitial cystitis (**Box 2**). Urology lends itself to a multidisciplinary model of a Bladder and Pelvic Floor Disorder service that provides comprehensive surgical and medical care. These centers are an attractive addition to a hospital or urology practice because they provide secure revenue-generating services, and there are increasing opportunities for billing of APP services. A Bladder and Pelvic Floor Disorder center usually offers the combined knowledge of a multidisciplinary group of experts in UI, voiding, and pelvic floor dysfunction. Changes in reimbursement for nonsurgical treatments such as biofeedback therapy, pelvic muscle electrical stimulation (E-stim), and posterior tibial nerve stimulation have allowed urologists to consider the expansion of current treatments (pharmacologic and surgical) to include alternative treatments such as PFM rehabilitation.

ASSESSMENT BEFORE BEHAVIORAL TREATMENTS

Before initiating nonsurgical treatment a focused and detailed history is essential. History is one of the most important steps in evaluating the patient with LUTS, as findings will direct behavioral treatment. Symptoms include urgency, frequency, and nocturia, stress and urgency-related incontinence, postvoid dribbling, nocturnal enuresis, straining to void, hesitancy, weak stream, and incomplete bladder emptying and retention. Understanding the onset, duration, characteristics, and progression of the LUTS is important. Many patients will report situational antecedents or "triggers."[7]

Appropriate treatment with PFMT should always include an assessment of PFM contraction and relaxation, because the effect of PFMT depends on whether the contractions and relaxations are performed correctly. Digital (eg, vaginal or rectal) PFM assessment is a form of biofeedback performed before starting behavioral therapy. PFM strength can be determined in women by inserting 1 or 2 fingers into the vagina to the level of the first knuckle. Muscular attachments along the pubic arch and the insertion of the levator ani and coccygeus muscles are palpated.[8] The levator ani can be palpated just superior to the hymeneal ring, at the 4- and 8-o'clock positions, to determine strength and whether palpation reproduces any discomfort or tenderness. The patient is asked to contract the PFMs around the examiner's finger with as much force and for as long as able. The

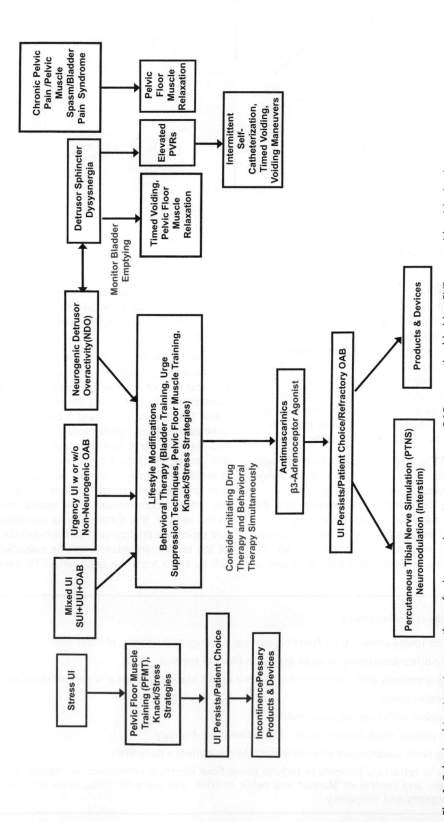

Fig. 1. Behavioral treatment care pathway for lower urinary tract symptoms. OAB, overactive bladder; PVR, postvoid residual volume; SUI stress urinary incontinence; UI, urinary incontinence; UUI, urge urinary incontinence.

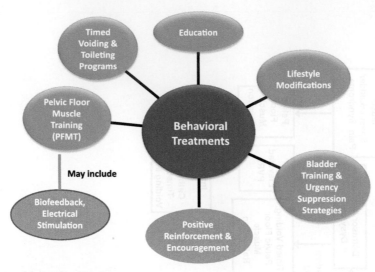

Fig. 2. Components of behavioral treatment.

patient is asked to squeeze or pull in and upward with vaginal muscles in short, fast contractions called "flicks." It is important to realize that when asked to contract the pelvic muscle, women will often use the wrong muscle, strain down, and perform a Valsalva maneuver, or fail to activate all layers of the pelvic musculature. The examiner notes through observation whether accessory muscles (such as gluteal and abdominal muscles) also contract. When assessing PFM strength, 3 criteria should be used[9] and the results noted:

- Pressure: the amount of pressure or strength of the muscle contraction, which can range from imperceptible to a firm squeeze
- Duration: the number of seconds that the examiner feels the muscle contraction
- Alteration in position: in a well-supported PFM, the muscle contraction can lift the base of the examiner's finger. Note use of

accessory muscles (abdominal movement, gluteal lifting). If the patient has a pelvic muscle spasm (inability to relax muscle), note the degree

Assessment of the PFMs in men and women can also be performed by evaluating the contraction and tone of the anal sphincter, and PFM exercises can be taught during the rectal examination. Have the patient relax and bear down. As the sphincter relaxes, gently insert the index finger into the anal canal in a direction pointing toward the umbilicus. Note if the resting sphincter tone is weak, moderate, or strong. Normally, the muscles of the anal sphincter close snugly around the entire circumference of the examiner's finger. In the rectum, the distal external sphincter is felt just inside the anal canal. The puborectalis portion of the levator ani muscle can be palpated about 2.5 to 4 cm from the anal verge. To assess the

---

Box 1
List of behavioral interventions

- Education on lower urinary tract function, normal voiding, and healthy bladder habits
- Behavior modification/coping skills to maximize bladder control
- Monitoring symptoms and outcomes through the use of bladder diaries and patient questionnaires
- Lifestyle modifications
- Bladder training with urgency suppression
- Pelvic floor muscle rehabilitation to include biofeedback therapy
- Ensure long-term transference of skills learned to the patient's daily life
- Stimulation in refractory patients to include pelvic floor electrical stimulation to increase strength, coordination, and control of bladder and pelvic muscles, and posterior tibial nerve stimulation to decrease urgency and frequency

---

Box 2
Bladder and pelvic floor disorder center: specific APP interventions

- Comprehensive evaluation of symptoms and associated disorders
- Analysis of bladder diaries (pre-, during, and posttreatment) and standardized questionnaires
- Instructions on voiding maneuvers (postvoid micturition, improvement in bladder-emptying techniques)
- Pelvic floor muscle assessment using a validated scale (pelvic examination, levator ani palpation, anal sphincter muscle assessment)
- Bladder training and urge-suppression treatments
- Pelvic floor muscle training with the addition of biofeedback and/or pelvic floor muscle electrical stimulation
- Pelvic floor muscle "down-training" for pelvic pain and muscle spasm
- Medication prescribing
- Neuromodulation treatment that includes:
  - Programming and management of Interstim
  - Delivery of posterior tibial nerve stimulation treatments
- Pessary fitting and maintenance
- Catheter management (indwelling catheter [urethral and suprapubic] changes and management, postoperative suprapubic catheter changes, intermittent catheterization teaching and long-term management, urethral stricture catheterization teaching)
- Evaluation, fitting, and education on use of external devices (male external catheter, external pouches, toileting-assistive products)
- Counseling on absorbent containment products

---

strength of the sphincter muscle, ask the patient to tighten the rectum. The examiner should feel a grip, pulling in around entire finger circumference.

Patients are asked to complete a self-monitoring 3-day bladder diary on a daily basis; this is a simple and practical method of obtaining information on voiding behavior.[10] The diary should be constructed in such a way that it provides information regarding sensation of urgency, urine leakage episodes, and the events surrounding these episodes. Before and during treatment, the diary is reviewed to determine voiding patterns: during the day, during the night; frequency of urination; if urine leakage is associated with urgency, or following the ingestion of a bladder irritant such as caffeinated beverages.

Symptoms will direct the interventions. Many providers are interested in the patient noting the type and quantity of absorbent incontinence pads used, and quantifying the amount of urine leakage. An example of a Frequency Volume Bladder Diary is shown in **Fig. 3**. Bladder diaries are also the best noninvasive tools available to objectively monitor the effect of treatment. Keeping a diary is thought to empower patients and make them more aware of their drinking and voiding habits, thus helping them to retrain the bladder more effectively.[11]

BEHAVIORAL TREATMENTS

Education is the initial component of behavioral treatments as patients are taught about the function of the lower urinary tract, the mechanics of bladder storage and emptying, the importance of the urinary sphincter and PFM, and healthy bladder habits.[12] Types of behavior used by women to empty their bladders may be related to the development and worsening of LUTS.[13] These behaviors include:

1. Antecedents: attending to the urge to void, accessing the toilet to empty the bladder, adopting a proper position
2. Micturition: emptying urine into toilet or toilet receptacle, straining
3. Consequences: incomplete bladder emptying, incontinence, bladder control

For example, some women ignore the urge to void and do not urinate while they are at work, delay voiding because of limited work breaks,[14,15] or have a decreased opportunity to leave their work stations to void.[16] As a result, women may develop a habit of voiding at any time (regardless of the presence of the sensation to void), strain or bear down to void quickly, or void on an

NAME:_____DATE:_____

INSTRUCTIONS:

- Column 1: write in the time you void, have an "Accident" or drink a beverage
- Column 2: Next to the time, record if you voided and the amount (in ounces or mL)
- Column 3: Mark every time you have an incontinent episode or urine leakage and circle if **Large** or **Small** amount.
- Column 4: Write the urine leakage, such as *urinary urgency, sneezing, lifting, coughing, laughing, bending, pain, couldn't make it to the bathroom,* and so on.
- Column 5" Write the type of fluid you drank (for example: coffee, water, orange juice, beer) and estimate the amount (for example: one 8-oz cup of coffee).

COLUMN 1 TIME	COLUMN 2 AMOUNT URINATED IN TOILET (OUNCES OR MILLILITERS)	COLUMN 3 LEAKAGE OF URINE (INCONTINENT EPISODE) AT ANY TIME LARGE SMALL	COLUMN 4 REASON FOR URINE LEAKAGE (URGENCY, COUGHING, BENDING)	COLUMN 5 AMOUNT AND TYPE OF FLUID INTAKE
		Large Small		
		Large Small		
		Large Small		
		Large Small		
		Large Small		
		Large Small		
		Large Small		
		Large Small		
		Large Small		
		Large Small		
		Large Small		
		Large Small		
		Large Small		

Circle the product you are using

Write the number of products used:_____

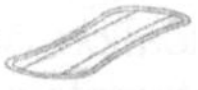

Pantiliners 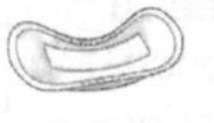　　Pads 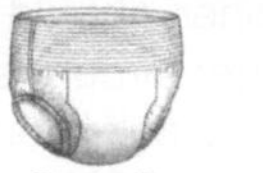　　Protective Underwear 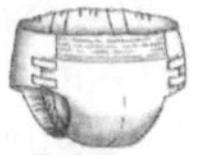　　Briefs or "diapers"

Comments: _____

Fig. 3. Frequency volume bladder diary.

infrequent basis. Too frequent voiding makes the bladder more sensitive to a smaller amount of urine within[17] and may, over time, decrease bladder capacity. Overdistension of bladder may occur as a result of infrequent voiding. Behavioral interventions address optimal voiding behavior, posture, and position, to ensure complete bladder emptying (**Patient Guide 1**).

LIFESTYLE MODIFICATIONS

In many instances, lifestyle practices can contribute or cause LUTS, bladder and/or pelvic pain. Many lifestyle habits are modifiable and these modifications are part of behavioral treatment. Evidence-based research (**Table 1**) has shown that lifestyle changes can decrease LUTS. The following are key elements of a lifestyle modification program:

- Maintaining adequate fluid intake
- Modifying the diet to eliminate possible bladder irritants
- Regulating bowel function to avoid constipation and straining during defecation
- Smoking cessation
- Weight reduction

Altering Fluid Intake and Managing Volume

Individuals may practice either restrictive or excessive fluid intake. Working women often report limitations of fluid intake and avoidance of caffeinated beverages as strategies to avoid urinary symptoms.[14] However, adequate fluid intake may be needed to eliminate irritants from the bladder. Underhydration may play a role in the development of urinary tract infections and may decrease the

---

Patient Guide 1
Lifestyle changes that can improve bladder symptoms

Maintain Healthy Bladder Habits

Here are some tips on good toileting techniques:

- Empty your bladder in a relaxed and private place. Worry and tension can make bladder emptying more difficult.
- You should sit on the toilet seat and not "hover" over the toilet, as sitting relaxes your pelvic floor muscles so you can completely empty your bladder.
- Sit with your feet flat on the floor. If your feet dangle, place a book under your feet for support.
- Breathe gently as you urinate. If possible, minimize bearing down or straining to start your urine stream.
- *Relax your pelvic floor muscles* to start your urine stream.
- *Do not* strain or push down on your bladder with your hands or stomach to help urinate.
- Keep your stomach and pelvic floor muscles relaxed while the bladder empties completely.
- Make sure your bladder feels completely empty before getting off the toilet.

Moderate your liquid and beverage intake

Many people who have bladder problems will drink less, hoping they will need to urinate less often. Although drinking less liquid does result in less urine in your bladder, a much smaller amount of urine may be more highly concentrated and irritate the lining of your bladder. Concentrated urine (dark yellow, strong smelling) may cause you to go to the bathroom more frequently. Also, drinking too little fluids can cause dehydration. Do not limit your fluids to control your bladder symptoms unless your doctor or nurse tells you to.

Other people may increase the amount they drink because they think more urine in the bladder will cause less bladder pain and discomfort. But drinking too much fluid will cause you to go to the bathroom more often. You should avoid extremes in the amount you drink (neither too much nor too little).

Normal fluid intake is 50 to 70 oz (1 oz = 30 mL) of liquid each day. This means that each day, you should consume the equivalent of 6 to 8 8-oz glasses of liquids (any beverages and soups), much of which can be in the form of solid foods. This should produce a healthy 40 to 50 oz of urine in 24 hours. People who work in hot climates or exercise heavily need more fluids because of loss through perspiration, but their urine output should still be approximately 40 to 50 oz. Do not drink large amounts at one time; instead, sip 2 to 3 oz every 20 to 30 minutes between meals. It is very unlikely that you will need to drink more than 2 quarts (or 8 cups) of total fluids each day.

Monitor your diet and medications

Certain food and beverages can irritate the bladder and make symptoms worse. These include alcoholic beverages, caffeinated foods and/or carbonated beverages (soft drinks, coffee or tea, chocolate, energy drinks), tomato-based products, citrus fruits and juices, spicy foods, and artificial sweeteners (eg, Equal). Also some over-the-counter drugs and prescription medications can worsen bladder problems (eg, Excedrin, Midol, Anacin). Do not stop taking prescription drugs without first talking to your health care provider. Keep a record of what you eat and drink and correlate this with lessening or worsening of your symptoms. Here is the caffeine content of some foods and drugs.

	Size	Caffeine Content (mg)
Coffee	8 oz	133 (range 102–200)
Tea	8 oz	53 (range 40–120)
Soft drinks	12 oz	35–72
Energy drinks	8–20 oz	48–300
Chocolate candies	Varies	9–33
Excedrin (extra-strength)	2 tablets	130
Anacin (maximum strength)	2 tablets	64
Vivarin, NoDoz	1 tablet	200

Maintain bowel regularity

Keeping healthy bowel habits may lessen bladder symptoms. Some suggestions include: (1) increase fiber-rich foods in your diet such as beans, pasta, oatmeal, bran cereal, whole wheat bread, fresh fruits and vegetables; (2) exercise to maintain regular bowel movements; (3) drink plenty of nonirritating fluids (water); (4) see your doctor if you have bowel problems.

Maintain a healthy weight

Being overweight can put pressure on your bladder, which may cause leakage of urine when you laugh or cough. If you are overweight, weight loss can reduce pressure on your bladder.

Stop smoking

Cigarette smoking is irritating to the bladder muscle. It can also lead to coughing spasms that can cause urinary leakage.

functional capacity of the bladder. Surveys of community-residing elders with LUTS report self-care practices to include the self-imposed fluid restriction, as they fear UI, urinary urgency, and urinary frequency.[18–20] Excessive fluid intake can also be a problem, as intake of large volumes can trigger incontinence and OAB symptoms of urgency and frequency.[21] Fluid intake averaging greater than 3700 mL/d has been associated with a higher voiding frequency and incidence of UI when compared with an intake of approximately 2400 mL/d.[1] Hashim and Abrams[22] recommend

Table 1
Levels of evidence and recommendations for lifestyle modifications

Lifestyle Practice	Levels of Evidence	Recommendations
Fluid	Fluid intake may play a minor role in the pathogenesis of UI	Minor decrease of fluid intake by 25% may be recommended provided baseline consumption is not less than 30 mL/kg a day *Grade of Recommendation: B*
Caffeine	Caffeine consumption may play a role in exacerbating UI. Small clinical trials do suggest that decreasing caffeine intake improves continence *Level of Evidence: 2*	Caffeine reduction may help in improving incontinence symptoms *Grade of Recommendation: B*
Bowel function	There is some evidence to suggest that chronic straining may be a risk factor for the development of UI *Level of Evidence: 3*	Further research is needed to define the role of straining during defecation in the pathogenesis of UI
Obesity	Massive weight loss (15–20 body mass index points) significantly decreases UI in morbidly obese women *Level of Evidence: 2* Moderate weight loss may be effective in decreasing UI especially if combined with exercise *Level of Evidence: 1*	Weight loss in obese and morbidly should be considered a first-line treatment to reduce UI prevalence *Grade of Recommendation: A*
Smoking		Further prospective studies are needed to determine whether smoking cessation prevents the onset, or promotes the resolution, of UI

Adapted from Moore K. Bradley C, Burgio B, et al. Adult conservative treatment. In: Abrams P, Cardozo L, Khoury S, et al, editors. Incontinence: Proceedings from the 5th International Consultation on Incontinence. Plymouth (United Kingdom): Health Publications; 2013. p. 1101–228; with permission.

decreasing fluid intake by 25% to reduce frequency, urgency, and nocturia, provided baseline consumption is not less than 1 L a day, and that increasing fluid intake by 25% and 50% can result in a worsening of daytime frequency.

Fluid intake should be regulated to 6- to 8-oz (177–236 mL) glasses or 30 mL/kg body weight per day, with a 1500 mL/d minimum at designated times unless contraindicated by a medical condition.

In older adults, there appears to be a strong relationship between evening fluid intake, nocturia, and nocturnal voided volume. Aging causes an increase in nocturia, defined as the number of voids recorded from the time the individual goes to bed with the intention of going to sleep, to the time the individual wakes with the intention of rising. To decrease nocturia precipitated by drinking fluids primarily in the evening or with dinner, the patient is instructed to reduce fluid intake after 6 PM and shift intake toward the morning and afternoon.[23] Wagg and colleagues[24] recommend that late-afternoon administration of a diuretic may reduce nocturia in persons with lower extremity venous insufficiency or congestive heart failure unresponsive to other interventions.

Influence of Dietary Bladder Irritants

Common dietary staples can cause diuresis or bladder irritability, contributing to LUTS. Up to 90% of patients with IC/BPS report sensitivities to a wide variety of comestibles.[25–27] Caffeine intake has been associated with LUTS in both men[28] and women.[29] Caffeine is thought to affect urinary symptoms by causing a significant increase in detrusor pressure and an excitatory effect on detrusor contraction. Daily administration of oral caffeine (150 mg/kg) results in detrusor overactivity and increased sensory signaling in the mouse bladder.[30] The consumption of caffeinated beverages, foods, and medications should not be underestimated. In the United States, more than 80% of the adult population consumes caffeine in the form of coffee, tea, soft drinks, and energy drinks on a daily basis. The Boston Area Community Health[31] reported on beverage intake and LUTS in a large cohort (N = 4144). Women who increased coffee intake by at least 2 servings per day had 64% higher odds of progression of urgency (P = .003). Women who had recently increased soda intake, particularly caffeinated diet soda, had higher symptom scores, urgency, and LUTS progression. Greater coffee or total caffeine intake at baseline increased the odds of LUTS (storage symptoms) progression in men (coffee: >2 cups/d vs none, odds ratio [OR] = 2.09, 95% confidence

interval [CI] 1.29–3.40, P-trend = .01; caffeine: P-trend<.001). Citrus juice intake was associated with 50% lower odds of LUTS progression in men (P = .02). Lohsiriwat and colleagues[32] found that caffeine at a dose of 4.5 mg/kg caused diuresis and decreased the threshold of bladder sensation at filling phase, with an increase in flow rate and voided volume. Other findings suggest that high but not stable caffeine intake is associated with a modest increase in the incidence of frequent urgency incontinence.[33] It has been postulated that one-fourth of the cases of urgency and frequency with the highest caffeine consumption would be eliminated if high caffeine intake were eliminated.[34] Confirmation of these findings in other studies is needed before recommendations can be made.

In addition to caffeine, alcohol is also believed to have a diuretic effect that can lead to increased frequency. A survey conducted by the Interstitial Cystitis Network[35] found that 94% of 535 patients who responded reported that their bladder symptoms worsened when drinking various alcoholic beverages. Anecdotal evidence suggests that eliminating dietary factors such as artificial sweeteners (aspartame) and certain foods (eg, highly spiced foods, citrus juices, and tomato-based products) may contribute to LUTS, especially urgency and frequency. Current questionnaire-based data suggest that citrus fruits, tomatoes, vitamin C, artificial sweeteners, coffee, tea, carbonated and alcoholic beverages, and spicy foods tend to exacerbate LUTS, whereas calcium glycerophosphate and sodium bicarbonate tend to improve IC/BPS symptoms.[27]

Assessment of daily caffeine intake on all patients with LUTS and instructions on the correlation between symptoms and caffeine intake are integral to clinical practice. It is recommended that patients with incontinence and OAB avoid excessive caffeine intake (eg, no more than 200 mg/d or 2 cups). The patient is instructed on an elimination diet by identifying possible irritating products on a one-by-one basis to discern whether symptoms decrease or resolve.

Regulating Bowel Function

Chronic constipation (defined as having less than 3 stools per week) and straining during defecation can contribute to LUTS, specifically UI and OAB. Constipation is associated with impaired bladder emptying and worsening of irritative bladder symptoms.[36] The close proximity of the bladder and urethra to the rectum and their similar nerve innervations make it likely that there are reciprocal effects between them.[37] According to Kaplan and colleagues,[38] animal studies and clinical data support bladder-bowel cross-sensitization, or cross-talk between the bowel and bladder. The Epidemiology of Lower Urinary Tract Symptoms (EpiLUTS) II[39] survey of men and women (N = 2160) aged 40 years or older indicated that OAB is more likely to be reported if either gender had chronic constipation or fecal incontinence, compared with those without OAB. In a case-control study of women with LUTS (n = 820) and matched controls (n = 148), constipation and straining during defecation were significantly more common among the women with LUTS, including detrusor overactivity and urgency, than among the controls.[40] Jelovsek and colleagues[41] reported a 36% overall rate of constipation in women with UI and advanced pelvic organ prolapse.

Lubowski and colleagues[42] reported that denervation of the external anal sphincter and PFMs may occur in association with a history of excessive straining on defecation. Many believe that if these are lifetime habits, they may have a cumulative adverse effect on pelvic floor and bladder function. Patients with LUTS often report self-care practices to cope with LUTS by limiting fluid intake, a strategy that can exacerbate constipation. As combined behavioral and drug therapy is recommended for patients with nonneurogenic OAB,[3] an antimuscarinic can compound the problem. Therefore, as part of the behavioral treatment, an initial approach is to question the patient about bowel habits and, if reported, to manage constipation and normalize defecation. Self-care practices that promote bowel regularity are an integral part of any treatment care plan. Suggestions to reduce constipation include the addition of fiber to the diet, increased fluid intake, regular exercise, external stimulation, and establishment of a routine defecation schedule. High fiber intake must be accompanied by sufficient fluid intake. Improved bowel function can also be achieved by determining a timetable for bowel evacuation so that the patient can take advantage of the urge to defecate.[23]

Smoking and Chronic Obstructive Pulmonary Disease

Conditions exist under which increased intra-abdominal pressure may promote the development of UI and urinary urgency, particularly in women. These conditions include pulmonary diseases such as asthma, emphysema, and chronic coughing, such as seen in persons who smoke and/or have chronic obstructive pulmonary disease (COPD). Coughing causes increased intra-abdominal pressure, which directly increases pressure in the bladder. Usually the sphincter muscle is able to contract tightly to avoid leakage of urine. However, it is thought that persons who cough repetitively cause downward pressure on the pelvic floor resulting in repeated stretch injury to the pudendal and pelvic nerves, and weakening of the ligaments of the PFMs that support the external sphincter, so that incontinence, specifically stress UI (SUI), can occur. Nicotine may contribute to detrusor contractions, and tobacco products may have antiestrogenic hormonal effects that may influence the production of collagen synthesis.

Hrisanfow and Hägglund[43] surveyed 391 women and 337 men (aged 50–75 years) with COPD to determine the prevalence, characteristics, and status of UI. A response rate of 66% was obtained, and most patients had been diagnosed with moderate COPD. The prevalence of UI in this group of men and women with COPD was 49.6% in women and 30.3% in men. Women and men with UI had a significantly higher body mass index (BMI; calculated as weight in kilograms divided by height in meters squared, ie, kg/m^2) than those without UI, and the most common type of UI in women was SUI (52.4%) and in men, postmicturition dribbling (66.3%). A United States population-based cohort study of 2109 women aged 40 to 69 years, including racially and ethnically diverse participants, found an adjusted association between a change in continence status and COPD at baseline but not with other comorbidities.[44] There is a significantly increased risk of UI among nonpregnant female heavy smokers, both former and current, compared with women who have never smoked.[45] A cohort study of 523 American women found that smoking before pregnancy in comparison with not smoking gave the highest independent risk for UI postpartum in multivariable analyses (OR = 2.9, 95% CI 1.4–3.9).[46]

No data have been reported that examine whether smoking cessation in women resolves incontinence. However, in a behavioral treatment practice, women who smoke are educated on the relationship between smoking and UI, and strategies designed to discourage women from smoking are often suggested.

Obesity

Obesity is an independent and modifiable risk factor for LUTS in women. There is a large amount of data, including several systematic reviews, demonstrating positive association between a BMI of 25 or greater and SUI as a high risk factor for other urinary tract symptoms including urgency, frequency, OAB, and urge UI (UUI).[47–49] There is evidence that obesity increases intra-abdominal pressure and places strain and stress on the pelvic floor structures, leading to weakening of the PFM, nerves, and blood vessels,[50,51] while co-existing metabolic syndrome predisposes to UUI. The resultant impact on vascular perfusion and neural innervation may be a contributing cause of OAB symptoms and incontinence.[52] Moreover, increases in waist circumference are associated with new incidence or progression of current UI.[53] In practice, the authors often see women who have stopped exercising because of LUTS. Weight loss is an acceptable treatment option for morbidly obese women. There is ample evidence-based research to support recommendations of weight loss as part of lifestyle interventions in obese patients with and without diabetes.[54–56]

BLADDER TRAINING AND URGENCY REDUCTION STRATEGIES

Men and women who suffer from LUTS will develop abnormal voiding patterns and will practice preemptive or defensive voiding to prevent incontinence or urgency. These patients can benefit from BT, an education program that teaches the patient to restore normal bladder function by gradually increasing the intervals between voiding.[57,58] Mechanisms of action are not well understood, but it is thought that BT:

- Improves cortical inhibition over detrusor contractions
- Facilitates cortical ability over urethral closure during bladder filling
- Strengthens pelvic striated muscles
- Alters behaviors that affect continence (eg, frequent response to urgency)

The main outcomes for a BT program are to:

1. Improve bladder overactivity by controlling urgency and decreasing frequency
2. Increase bladder capacity
3. Reduce urgency incontinence episodes

Detailed components of a BT program are listed in **Box 3**, and **Patient Guide 2** provides information on BT and the control of urgency and frequency. **Table 2** outlines the evidence and recommendations for BT, PFMT, and E-stim.

PELVIC FLOOR MUSCLE TRAINING

The cornerstone of conservative behavioral therapy is PFMT and exercise, with or without biofeedback. The rationale for this is that mastering a voluntary contraction of the PFMs will help to increase urethral pressure, inhibit detrusor contractions, and prevent leakage of urine (**Box 4**). Arnold Kegel introduced PFM exercises, or Kegel exercises, in the late 1940s by developing a comprehensive program of progressive contractions of the levator ani muscle under direct supervision, and incorporating biofeedback technology. Most female patients presenting to a Urology Pelvic Floor Disorders Service have been told to do Kegel exercises and many report that the exercises have not improved their LUTS. However, few have undergone intensive training on how to identify, isolate, and strengthen the PFMs, making this type of behavioral treatment an important component of a specialized urology service.

A Cochrane review of PFM exercise[59] found that these treatments were effective for both SUI and mixed UI, can reduce urgency in comparison with placebo or no treatment, although women with pure SUI may have better outcomes. However, Hay-Smith and colleagues[60] noted in an abridged Cochrane systematic review that the best approach to PFMT has not been well defined with evidence-based research. Evidence from the literature suggests that supervised PFMT is more effective.[1,61] PFMT has no significant side effects; cure rates for PFMT range from 16% to 27% and improvement rates from 48% to 80.7%. Bø and Hilde[62] reported that long-term adherence to PFMT varied between 10% and 70%. Recommendations for PFMT in women and men are shown in **Table 2**.

Not being able to identify the PFMs or to exercise them correctly is probably the most common reason for poor outcomes with this treatment modality. It is a skill that patients seldom master on their first try, but, with repeated training, it can be used successfully and provides significant improvement in reducing LUTS. Confirming that patients have identified and isolated the correct muscles is essential, and often overlooked. In the past, most patients were given a pamphlet or brief verbal instructions on how to do PFM exercises and were told to "lift the pelvic floor," or to interrupt the urinary stream. Although this simple approach may be adequate for some patients, it does not ensure that they understand which muscles to use when they begin a structured exercise program at home. Patients should be cautioned not to perform these exercises during voiding and to not stop and start urine flow as a form of exercising. This exercise has good face-value validity for effectiveness because many patients initially report an inability to stop the urine flow when it begins. However, there is some controversy regarding this practice because it is nonphysiologic and can be harmful.

Box 3
Components of a bladder-training program

- Normal voiding is approximately 5 to 7 times per day. The goal of a bladder-training program is to achieve a comfortable voiding schedule with the least amount of urinary symptoms
- Analyze the bladder diary to determine voiding frequency and presence of urgency
- Set the initial voiding interval using these guidelines:
  - If voiding occurs on average every 30 to 60 minutes, initial voiding interval would be 30 minutes
  - If voiding occurs on average at least every 1 hour or greater, initial voiding interval would be 1 hour
    - Voiding interval is increased by 15 to 30 minutes per week depending on tolerance of the schedule (such as fewer incontinent episodes than the previous week, minimal interruptions to the schedule, and the patient's feeling of control over urgency and confidence to expand the voiding interval)
  - If voiding is missed, the patient should void as soon as he/she remembers or if it is inconvenient, and then void at next scheduled time
    - Goal is for the patient to void "before" the urge sensation of bladder fullness
    - Voiding regimen is only followed while awake
- Education about normal bladder control and methods to control urgency (called urgency-suppression strategies) so that an expanded voiding interval can be adopted. Strategies include:
  - Distraction
  - Relaxation techniques such as slow, deep breathing to consciously relax the bladder to combat a stressful rush to the toilet
  - Pelvic floor muscle contraction, performing 5 or 6 rapid, deliberate, and intense pelvic floor muscle contractions of 2 to 3 seconds in duration
- Patient should not rush or run to the bathroom, as increased anxiety may trigger incontinence
- Use of reminders such as a kitchen timer or stopwatch can be beneficial to helping the patient keep on a schedule
- Self-monitoring of voiding behavior using bladder diaries to determine adherence to the schedule, enhance self-awareness, evaluate progress, and determine whether the voiding interval should be changed
- Supervising health care professional to monitor progress, suggest adjustments to the voiding interval, and provide positive reinforcement to men and women undergoing bladder training at least weekly during the training period

Data from Moore K, Bradley C, Burgio B, et al. Adult conservative treatment. In: Abrams P, Cardozo L, Khoury S, et al, editors. Incontinence: Proceedings from the 5th International Consultation on Incontinence. Plymouth (United Kingdom): Health Publications; 2013. p. 1166; and Newman DK, Wein AJ. Managing and treating urinary incontinence. 2nd edition. Baltimore (MD): Health Professions Press; 2009. p. 260–3.

PFMs have a higher resting tone than other skeletal muscles. Low muscle tone is the impaired ability to isolate and contract the PFMs in the presence of weak and atrophic muscles. Low-tone PFM dysfunction can be seen in patients with pelvic floor denervation, and contributes to pelvic organ prolapse, UI, vaginal laxity, and fecal incontinence. High muscle tone refers to the clinical condition of hypertonic, spastic PFM with resultant impairment of muscle isolation, contraction, and relaxation.[63] A high resting baseline with high variability and occasional spasms may be seen in patients with chronic pelvic pain syndromes (eg, bladder pain syndrome), overactive bladder, or IC, and be associated with LUTS, pelvic pain, and sexual dysfunction with dyspareunia.

To respond to all physiologic needs, the PFM contains approximately 70% Type 1 or slow-twitch muscle fibers, and 30% Type II or fast-twitch muscle fibers.

- Type I fibers maintain static muscle tone, generate less intense, sustained contractions, and provide postural stability over time. Type I muscle fibers are also fatigue resistant.
- Type II fibers provide a mechanism for active, strong muscle contraction during increases

---

Patient Guide 2
Bladder training: controlling urgency and frequency

Frequency is voiding often, usually 8 times or more in a 24-hour period. Frequency can worsen if you get into the habit of voiding "just in case," which means that the bladder never fills completely and holds only a small amount of urine. It is better to wait until the bladder feels full.

Urgency is a sudden need to void immediately that can cause urine leakage on the way to the bathroom. Urgency follows a wave pattern; it starts, grows, peaks, and then subsides until it stops.

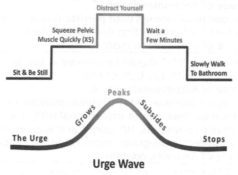

Urge Wave

The key to controlling the urinary urge is *not* to respond by rushing to the bathroom. Rushing causes movement, which jiggles your bladder, which in turn increases the feeling of urge.

Controlling the Urge

The goal is for you to be voiding no more than every _____ hours. If you get the *urge* to void and it is not yet your scheduled voiding time, stop all activity and sit down if possible. Then try one or more of the following techniques that may help the urge to subside allowing the bladder to relax and give you more time to get to the bathroom:

- Take some slow, deep breaths through your mouth, concentrating on your breathing or
- Tighten your pelvic muscle *quickly and hard* several times in a row or
- Use mental distraction strategies such as concentrating on an activity, such as counting backwards from 100 by sevens, or reciting the words of a favorite song or nursery rhyme.

---

in intra-abdominal pressure by contributing to urethral closure, and build pelvic muscle strength. A decrease in the proportion of Type II fibers can occur with inactivity, nerve-innervation damage, and aging.

PFMT consists of repeated, high-intensity PFM contractions of both types of fibers (**Box 5**). Clinicians should provide specific instructions on location and isolation of the PFM, and the following instructions can be helpful:

- Without tensing the muscles of the legs, buttocks, or abdomen, imagine trying to control the passing of gas or pinching off a stool by tightening the ring of muscles around the anus. A closing and lifting sensation should be felt.
- (For men) Imagine moving the penis up and down without moving any other part of the body.

Patients should not overexercise the PFM, as women can develop levator ani myalgia by performing excessive exercises. Supervised PFMT has been shown to give better results than unsupervised exercises,[1] but the degree and type of supervision needed are uncertain. Age should not be a deterrent to PFMT.[64]

Once patients demonstrate the ability to properly contract and relax the PFM, instructions for daily practice and exercise are provided (**Patient Guide 3**). The purpose of daily exercise is not only to increase muscle strength but also to enhance motor skills through practice. Specific exercise regimens vary considerably in frequency and intensity, and the ideal exercise regimen has not yet been determined. The authors recommend at least 45 to 60 pelvic muscle exercises per day, and use an "exercise prescription" as shown in **Box 6** to prescribe the home daily exercise program. Once patients are able to identify the muscle, they are instructed

Table 2
Grade of recommendation: PFMT, BT, E-stim

Treatment	Recommendations
PFMT postpartum	Postnatal women, immediately after delivery: Individually taught PFMT program that incorporates adherence strategies for women who had a vaginal delivery of a large baby (4000 g or more) or a forceps delivery *Grade of Recommendation: C* For postnatal women with persistent symptoms of UI 3 mo after delivery: PFMT is offered as first-line conservative therapy *Grade of Recommendation: A*
PFMT	Supervised PFMT should be offered as first-line conservative therapy to women with SUI, UUI, or MUI *Grade of Recommendation: A* The most intensive PFMT program possible should be provided (in terms of exercise dose, health professional [HP] teaching, and supervision) within service constraints; HP-taught and supervised programs are better than self-directed programs; more HP contact is better than less *Grade of Recommendation: A*
PFMT in women with SUI	PFMT is better than E-stim as first-line conservative therapy, particularly if PFMT is intensively supervised *Grade of Recommendation: B* PFMT is better than BT as first-line conservative therapy *Grade of Recommendation: B*
PFMT in men postprostatectomy	Some preoperative or immediate postoperative instruction in PFMT for men undergoing radical prostatectomy may be helpful *Grade of Recommendation: B* It is not clear whether PFMT taught by digital rectal examination offers any benefit over and above verbal or written instruction in PFMT *Grade of Recommendation: B* The use of BF to assist PFMT is currently a therapist/patient decision based on economics and preference *Grade of Recommendation: B*
PFMT + BT in women with UUI or MUI	PFMT and BT are effective first-line conservative therapy *Grade of Recommendation: B* For women with SUI or MUI, a combination of PFMT/BT may be better than BT alone in the short-term *Grade of Recommendation: C*
BT	BT is an appropriate first-line treatment for UI in women *Grade of Recommendation: A* Either BT or antimuscarinic drug may be effective, although BT may be preferred by some because it does not produce side effects and adverse events associated with drug therapy *Grade of Recommendation: B* There may be no benefit in adding brief written instruction in BT to drug therapy for incontinence, but it may improve episodes of frequency *Grade of Recommendation: B* A combination of PFMT/BT may be better than PFMT alone in the short term for women with symptoms of SUI or MUI *Grade of Recommendation: B* Clinicians and researchers should refer to the operant conditioning and educational literature to provide a rationale for their choice of training parameters or approach *Grade of Recommendation: D* Health Professionals should provide the most intensive BT supervision that is possible within service constraints. *Grade of Recommendation: D*

(continued on next page)

Table 2 (continued)	
Treatment	**Recommendations**
E-stim	E-stim plus PFMT or BF-assisted PFMT program does not appear to add benefit
Grade of Recommendation: B
For men with postprostatectomy incontinence, there does not appear to be any benefit of adding E-stim to a PFMT program
Grade of Recommendation: B

Abbreviations: BT, bladder training; E-stim, pelvic floor electrical stimulation; MUI, mixed urinary incontinence; PFMT, pelvic floor muscle training; SUI, stress urinary incontinence; UUI, urge urinary incontinence.

Adapted from Moore K, Bradley C, Burgio B, et al. Adult conservative treatment. In: Abrams P, Cardozo L, Khoury S, et al, editors. Incontinence: Proceedings from the 5th International Consultation on Incontinence. Plymouth (United Kingdom): Health Publications. 2013; p. 1101–228; with permission.

to perform a series of "quick flicks" or 2-second contractions followed by sustained (endurance contractions) contractions of 5 seconds and longer. It is equally important to relax the muscle completely between each muscle contraction. Patients are encouraged to aim for a high level of concentrated effort with each PFM contraction, as greater contraction intensity is associated with improvement in PFM strength.

A common error in contracting the PFMs is to simultaneously contract the abdominal, gluteal, or adductor muscles, which may mask the strength of the PFM contraction. Abdominal contraction increases intra-abdominal pressure that mechanically elevates bladder pressure, so it is important to measure and prevent concurrent use of abdominal contraction.

To avoid muscle fatigue, it is usually recommended that patients space the exercises across 2 sessions per day. Exercising in the supine position is often recommended at first, because it is the least challenging and facilitates concentration during the learning phase. However, it is important for patients to progress to the more difficult positions (eg, sitting, standing) with time, to become comfortable and skilled in using the muscles and to prevent incontinence in the positions assumed in daily life. Self-monitoring practice through the use of a calendar record and audio taped material that reviews the exercises can improve protocol compliance. Improvement in symptoms may not occur for 2 to 4 months, so patient expectations are important for adherence to these interventions.

In addition to planned exercises, contracting the muscle prior to the event that triggers urine leakage is also taught. This preventive PFM contraction is referred is as the "knack" or stress strategy.[65,66] This technique is an acquired motor skill that requires the patient to anticipate the urine leakage. Contracting the PFMs immediately before a sneeze or cough, or when lifting or changing position can close the sphincter, preventing urine leakage.

Rehabilitating the PFMs can be central in resolving pelvic pain when muscle spasm is present. Using PFMT in patients with high-tone PFM to enhance muscle relaxation is referred to as down-training. Teaching a muscle to relax is often more difficult than teaching it how to contract (up-training). Patients with pain will often benefit from biofeedback-assisted PFMT. The patient can correlate PFM movement with the biofeedback visual signal. Once they are able to feel the muscle release and relax, patients can begin coordination of relaxation following a contraction.

PFMT PREPROSTATECTOMY AND POSTPROSTATECTOMY

UI is a common complication of radical prostatectomy (RP), regardless of the technique used.[67] Continence rate is reported to be 10% to 41% after open RP and between 13.1% and 68.9% after robot-assisted RP.[68] Urology practices have begun to include various levels of PFMT for men undergoing RP; however, translation from research to practice has not been optimum because most men undergoing radical prostatectomy do

---

Box 4
Pelvic floor muscle exercise mechanisms of action

1. Urethral closure through increases in urethral pressure
2. Mechanical pressure increase that causes lifting of the endopelvic fascia, which presses the urethra upward toward the pubic symphysis
3. Pelvic muscle "reflex" contraction that precedes increased bladder pressure and may inhibit bladder overactivity

---

Box 5
Teaching pelvic floor muscle exercises

1. Before exercising, patient should urinate so the bladder is empty. Significant stresses are placed on the pelvic floor muscles as the patient attempts to follow through on the demanding exercise schedule. These weak muscles will rapidly fatigue with all the exercising, and if they must also support a full bladder in addition to being exercised, they then will not receive maximum benefit from the strengthening program.

   - A successful method is to have the patient imagine trying to control the passing of gas or pinching off a stool, or imagine being in an elevator and feeling the urge to pass gas. In these situations, a person will automatically tighten or pull in the ring of muscle around the rectum, which is the posterior pelvic muscle.

2. One exercise consists of both "tightening and relaxing." Patient should be instructed to relax between each muscle tightening.

3. Exercise in 3 positions:

   - Sitting upright in a firm seat and straight-backed chair, knees slightly apart, feet flat on the floor or legs stretched out in front and crossed at the ankles
   - Standing by a chair, knees slightly bent with feet a shoulder-width apart and toes slightly pointed outward. Can also exercise standing and leaning on a counter top
   - Lying down flat or with head slightly elevated, knees bent and feet slightly apart

4. Have patient monitor for accessory muscle (eg, thigh and gluteal) contraction. Often patients will hold their breath; to prevent this, have the patient count out loud.

5. Have patients identify situations that cause urine leakage (eg, coughing, sneezing on way to bathroom) and teach them to purposefully contract the pelvic floor muscles when such a situation is imminent.

Adapted from Newman DK, Wein AJ. Managing and treating urinary incontinence. 2nd edition. Baltimore (MD): Health Professions Press; 2009. p. 271–5; with permission.

---

not receive PFMT. Evidence-based results demonstrate that early biofeedback-assisted PFMT not only hastens the recovery of urinary continence after radical RP but allows for significant improvements in the severity of incontinence, voiding symptoms, and PFMs 12 months postoperatively. **Table 3** reviews some of the recent research in this area of PFMT.

Biofeedback-assisted PFM exercise is a method by which the patient is immediately made aware of the physiologic state of the PFM. This adjunctive technique may be especially helpful in patients who are having difficulty identifying and isolating the correct muscle, or who need encouragement to continue with prescribed treatment. Instruments to provide biofeedback were originally developed by Kegel who used vaginal manometry using an instrument called a perineometer, which measured pressure change occurring during PFM contraction.

Current biofeedback therapy uses either electromyography (EMG) or manometric pressure. EMG measures electrical activity of a muscle in microvolts. The advantage of EMG over manometric pressure is that, provided the machinery is of sufficient sophistication with adequate filtering,

the EMG apparatus can engage the use of the newer types of electrodes that are lightweight and designed to stay in place, hence allowing more functional positions during assessment and treatment. Moreover, EMG can be multichannel, which allows the simultaneous reinforcement of contractions of the PFMs and inhibition of counterproductive accessory muscle contractions (eg, abdominal and gluteal muscle).

Four methods of EMG measurement have been used in the investigation of lower urinary tract dysfunction:

- Vaginal sensor (sEMG)
- Anal sensor or plug electrode (sEMG)
- Skin-surface electrodes (sEMG)
- Needle electrodes

Vaginal and anal electrodes are internal sensors designed to provide a more accurate detection of PFM activity. The accuracy of longitudinal sensing electrodes has been shown to be virtually identical to the gold-standard inserted needle electrodes. However, the use of vaginal or rectal sensors is limited in patients with severe pelvic pain for whom insertion of the sensor causes discomfort,

Patient Guide 3
Pelvic floor muscle exercises

1. What is the Pelvic Muscle? Your pelvic muscle provides support to your bladder and rectum and, in women, the vagina and the uterus. If it weakens, it cannot support these organs and their position can change. This change in position can cause problems with normal function. Keeping the muscle strong can help prevent unwanted urine leakage.

2. Finding the Pelvic Muscle. Without tensing the muscles of your leg, buttocks, or abdomen, imagine that you are trying to control the passing of gas or pinching off a stool. Or imagine you are in an elevator full of people and you feel the urge to pass gas. What do you do? You tighten or pull in the ring of muscle around your rectum: your pelvic muscle. You should feel a lifting sensation in the area around the vagina or a pulling in of your rectum.

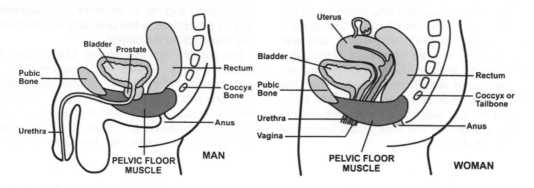

3. Exercise Regimen. One exercise consists of both "tightening and relaxing" the muscle. It is equally important to control when your muscle tightens and relaxes. Be sure to relax completely between each muscle tightening.

4. Types of Exercises. There are 2 types of muscle contractions you will need to practice:
   - *Short* (2 seconds): short or quick muscle contractions.
     - Contract or tighten your pelvic muscle quickly and hard, and immediately relax it.
   - *Quick* contractions and *slow* (3 or 5 or 10 seconds) or *long* contractions.
     - Contract or tighten your pelvic muscle and hold for a count of (3 or 5 or 10 as prescribed) seconds, then relax the muscle completely for the same amount of time.

5. Where to Practice. These exercises can be practiced anywhere and anytime. You can do the exercises in these positions:
   - *Lying down:* Lie on your back, flat or with your head on a pillow, knees bent and feet slightly apart. It is helpful to support your knees with a pillow.
   - *Sitting:* Sit upright in a firm seat and straight-backed chair, knees slightly apart, feet flat on the floor or legs stretched out in front and crossed at the ankles.
   - *Standing:* Stand by a chair, knees slightly bent with feet a shoulder-width apart and toes slightly pointed outward. You can also lean on the kitchen counter with your hips flexed.

6. Times to Use the Muscle. If you experience urine loss in one specific position only, like when you stand, then follow these steps:
   - Increase the number of exercises for that position only, or
   - Add additional exercises per day with focus on doing all the exercises in that position only.

7. Common Mistakes.
   - Concentrate and tighten only the pelvic floor muscle. DO NOT tighten thighs, buttocks, or stomach. If you feel your stomach move, then you are also using these muscles.
   - DO NOT hold your breath. Breathe normally and/or count out loud.

8. Can They be Harmful? No, these exercises cannot harm you in any way. You should find them easy and relaxing. If you get back or stomach pain after you exercise, you are probably trying too hard and using your stomach muscles. If you experience headaches, then you are also tensing your chest muscles and probably holding your breath.

9. When Will I See a Change? After 4 to 6 weeks of daily exercise, you will begin to notice less urine leakage. Make the exercises part of your daily lifestyle. Tighten the muscle when you walk, as you stand up, and on the way to the bathroom.

pregnant patients, those who have undergone recent pelvic or rectal surgery, patients with atrophic vaginitis, and patients who would prefer not to have a device inserted internally. Skin-surface electrodes are relatively noninvasive and well tolerated, and provide qualitative information about muscle activity. Needle electrodes are sometimes used during urodynamic testing. The EMG data are measured in microvolts. The actual threshold of PFM required for maintaining continence is unknown at this time, as are the normal values for PFM strength.

At present, there are sophisticated computerized EMG biofeedback units for muscle evaluation and training (**Fig. 4**), which serve as a diagnostic tool for the clinician while providing visual or auditory feedback to the patient.

The baseline and all follow-up EMG recordings should include 2 sets of measurements of maximum or "short/quick" muscle contractions of 2 seconds' duration with an equal amount of resting muscle activity, and sustained or "long" muscle contractions (5, 10, or 30 seconds) with resting muscle activity for the same length of

---

Box 6
Exercise prescription sample

Please complete the following exercises:

1. Short Quick Exercise

   Contract the muscle Quickly 1 to 2 seconds and immediately relax

2. Long Sustained Exercise:

   Contract the muscle, and hold the contraction for a count of 10 then immediately relax for a count of 10

Exercise Session

Lying Down

    Do 10 exercises holding for 2 seconds

    Do 10 exercises holding for 10 seconds

Sitting

    Do 10 exercises holding for 2 seconds

    Do 10 exercises holding for 10 seconds

Standing

    Do 10 exercises holding for 2 seconds

    Do 10 exercises holding for 10 seconds

3. Be sure to rest your muscle after each muscle contraction for the same length of the contraction or longer

4. When you have completed both types of exercises in all 3 positions, you will have completed one session

Do 2 exercise sessions each day, 1 in the morning and 1 in the evening, for a total of 120 exercises

Special Tips:

- Always empty your bladder before beginning your exercise session.

- Count out loud with sustained or long exercises; remember to keep breathing!

- Keep your stomach, leg, and buttock muscles relaxed. Rest your hand on your stomach, it should not move or tense.

- If it helps, take a deep breath between each exercise to help you keep other muscles relaxed.

Table 3
Evidence base for PFMT in men undergoing surgery for prostate cancer

Authors,[Ref.] Year	N	Intervention	Definition of Continence	Percent Continent: Intervention vs Control Group (%)		
				3 mo	6 mo	1 y
Filocamo et al,[69] 2005	300	PFMT taught with digital anal examination in 3 postoperative sessions, home exercise program, bladder control strategies, the "knack" vs usual care	Pad test, number pads used; Dry on ICS-Male Questionnaire	23 vs 14	77 vs 32	89 vs 68
Burgio et al,[70] 2006	125	Single session of preoperative biofeedback-assisted PFMT and home exercises vs usual care	No leakage reported in bladder diary	48 vs 32	68 vs 48	
Mariotti et al,[71] 2009	60	PFMT via biofeedback and electrical stimulation twice a week for 6 wk postoperatively vs usual care	≤2 g on 24-h pad test and no pad use	80 vs 33	97 vs 67	97 vs 97
Ribeiro et al,[72] 2010	73	Biofeedback-assisted PFMT weekly plus home exercises × 3 mo or until continent vs brief verbal instructions	No pad use	73 vs 39	88 vs 64	96 vs 75
Tienforti et al,[73] 2012	32	Preoperative biofeedback-assisted PFMT, monthly postoperative biofeedback-assisted PFMT vs verbal and written instructions for home exercises	Score of 0 on the ICIQ-SF	50 vs 6	63 vs 6	

Abbreviations: ICIQ-SF, International Consultation on Incontinence Questionnaire, short form; ICS, International Continence Society.

Data from Refs.[69–73]

time as the muscle contraction. The ability to relax one's pelvic muscle following a contraction is of utmost importance if one is to gain control and co-ordination of these muscles.

Manometry is the use of an instrument to detect, assess, and record pressure, and consists of a vaginal or rectal probe with a tube connected to a manometer. The pressure changes can be measured in centimeters of water (cm H_2O) or millimeters of mercury (mm Hg). Although manometry and pressure sensors are available with certain clinical systems and have been used in several clinical trials, they are primarily used for the treatment of rectal dysfunction.

Research in both men and women is extensive, detailing the efficacy of the use of

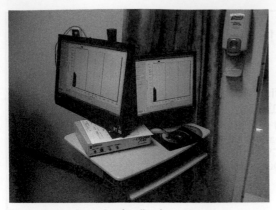

Fig. 4. Prometheus biofeedback equipment.

biofeedback-assisted behavioral therapy for PFMT (see **Table 3**). However, there is debate over the use of adjuncts such as biofeedback therapy.[74] The consensus is that conservative therapy combining lifestyle changes, toileting or bladder retraining programs, and PFMT with or without biofeedback are most effective when provided by a clinician who specializes in the area of pelvic floor dysfunction. Clinician-supervised PFMT with biofeedback is considered to provide the most favorable long-term results,[1] and a multidisciplinary Bladder and Pelvic Floor Disorder Center in urology practice provides this service.

BEHAVIORAL TREATMENT COMBINED WITH DRUG THERAPY

Augmenting drug therapy with a supervised BT program is thought to yield the best outcomes in the treatment of UUI and overactive bladder in women,[1,75–77] may be appropriate in men,[78] and can be effective when combined with an α-blocker in men with nocturia.[79] Usually specific medications are prescribed depending on the predominant symptoms. The Urinary Incontinence Treatment Network BE-DRI study by Burgio and colleagues[76] evaluated whether combined antimuscarinic therapy with behavioral therapy would increase the number of women who could discontinue drug therapy while sustaining a significant reduction in UUI. Although the addition of behavioral therapy did not improve discontinuation of drug therapy, the study found that the combination of behavioral training and drug therapy yielded improved urinary outcomes compared with drug therapy alone.

STIMULATION

E-stim is the application of a low level of electrical stimulation to the PFMs to cause the muscle to contract. E-stim has a twofold action: contraction of PFMs and inhibition of unwanted detrusor contractions. E-stim is usually a component of a urologic behavioral treatment service, and may be prescribed as a home program using a battery-operated home unit. Patients with LUTS secondary to neurologic disease (eg, multiple sclerosis) may benefit from this therapy. Many clinicians institute this treatment in patients who have failed other behavioral treatments.

Patients with urgency and frequency, and who have been unsuccessful with both drug and behavioral therapy, are considered refractory. Posterior tibial nerve stimulation (PTNS) would be indicated in these patients, and is usually a treatment provided by a Bladder and Pelvic Disorders service. The posterior tibial nerve is a branch of the sciatic nerve (L4–S3 nerve roots) and provides innervation to the posterior leg and foot to cause plantar flexion. Although the exact mechanism is unclear, PTNS is thought to work on afferent pathways to activate inhibitory neurons through a direct sacral route. Tibial nerve stimulation is delivered via a 34-gauge needle electrode inserted 3 to 4 cm above the medial malleolus, the medial aspect of the fibula. Stimulation is delivered over 30 minutes, and treatments are performed weekly for 12 weeks. PTNS has been shown to decrease urgency and frequency.

SUMMARY

There are several possible treatments for UI currently available, and for some a combination of several treatment options may be the most successful. Behavioral interventions are usually preferred, as they are noninvasive and low risk. These treatments are indicated for men and women with LUTS, the majority population seen in urology practices. Evidence-based research has shown these interventions to be effective in decreasing LUTS. Specialized services in this practice setting that offer all behavioral treatments and use nurse practitioners and physician assistants are necessary, and constitute a growth service area in urology. The fastest-growing segment of patients seen in urology have pelvic floor disorders. A multidisciplinary approach that includes surgical and nonsurgical treatments is required.

REFERENCES

1. Moore K, Bradley C, Burgio B, et al. Adult conservative treatment. In: Abrams P, Cardozo L, Khoury S, et al, editors. Incontinence: Proceedings from the 5th International Consultation on Incontinence.

Plymouth (United Kingdom): Health Publications; 2013. p. 1101–228.

2. Wyman JF, Burgio KL, Newman DK. Practical aspects of lifestyle modifications and behavioural interventions in the treatment of overactive bladder and urgency urinary incontinence [review]. Int J Clin Pract 2009;63(8):1177–91.

3. Gormley EA, Lightner DJ, Burgio KL, et al, American Urological Association, Society of Urodynamics, Female Pelvic Medicine & Urogenital Reconstruction. Diagnosis and treatment of overactive bladder (non-neurogenic) in adults: AUA/SUFU guideline. J Urol 2012;188(Suppl 6):2455–63. http://dx.doi.org/10.1016/j.juro.2012.09.079.

4. Shamliyan T, Wyman JF, Ramakrishnan R, et al. Systematic review: randomized, controlled trials of nonsurgical treatments for urinary incontinence in women. Ann Intern Med 2008;148(6):459–73.

5. Neuwahl S, Tompson K, Fraher E. HPRI data tracks: urology workforce trends. Bull Am Coll Surg 2012;97(1):46–9.

6. Cooper RA. New directions for nurse practitioners and physician assistants in the era of physician shortages. Acad Med 2007;82(9):827–8.

7. Newman DK. Assessment of the patient with an overactive bladder [review]. J Wound Ostomy Continence Nurs 2005;32(3S):S5–10.

8. Newman DK, Laycock J. Clinical evaluation of the pelvic floor muscles. In: Baessler K, Schussler B, Burgio KL, et al, editors. Pelvic floor re-education: principles and practice. 2nd edition. London: Springer-Verlag; 2008. p. 91–104.

9. Brink CA, Sampselle CM, Wells TJ, et al. A digital test for pelvic muscle strength in older women with urinary incontinence. Nurse Res 1989;38(4):196–9.

10. Sampselle CM, Palmer MH, Boyington AR, et al. Prevention of urinary incontinence in adults: population-based strategies. Nurs Res 2004;53(6 Suppl):S61–7.

11. Vella M, Robinson D, Cardozo L, et al. The bladder diary: do women perceive it as a useful investigation? Eur J Obstet Gynecol Reprod Biol 2012; 162(2):221–3. http://dx.doi.org/10.1016/j.ejogrb.2012.02.012 PMID: 22420997.

12. Burgio KL, Newman DK, Rosenberg MT, et al. Impact of behaviour and lifestyle on bladder health. Int J Clin Pract 2013;67(6):495–504. http://dx.doi.org/10.1111/ijcp.1214.

13. Wang K, Palmer M. Women's toileting behavior related to urinary elimination: concept analysis. J Adv Nurs 2010;66(8):1874–84. http://dx.doi.org/10.1111/j.1365-2648.2010.05341.x.

14. Fitzgerald S, Palmer MH, Berry SJ, et al. Urinary incontinence: impact on working women. AAOHN J 2000;48(3):112–8.

15. Fitzgerald ST, Palmer MH, Kirkland VL, et al. The impact of urinary incontinence in working women:

a study in a production facility. Women Health 2002;35(1):1–16.

16. Palmer MH, Athanasopouos A, Lee K, et al. Sociocultural and environmental influences on bladder health. Int J Clin Pract 2012;66(12):1132–8.

17. Sampselle CM. Teaching women to use a voiding diary. Am J Nurs 2003;103(11):62–4.

18. Diokno AC, Sand PK, Macdiarmid S, et al. Perceptions and behaviours of women with bladder control problems. Fam Pract 2006;23:568–77.

19. Diokno AC, Burgio K, Fultz NH, et al. Medical and self-care practices reported by women with urinary incontinence. Am J Manag Care 2004; 10:69–78.

20. Johnson TM 2nd, Kincade JE, Bernard SL, et al. Self-care practices used by older men and women to manage urinary incontinence: results from the national follow-up survey on self-care and aging. J Am Geriatr Soc 2000;48:894–902.

21. Segal S, Saks EK, Arya LA. Self-assessment of fluid intake behavior in women with urinary incontinence. J Womens Health (Larchmt) 2011;20(12): 1917–21. http://dx.doi.org/10.1089/jwh.2010.2642 PMID: 21970566.

22. Hashim H, Abrams P. How should patients with an overactive bladder manipulate their fluid intake? BJU Int 2008;102:62–6.

23. Newman DK, Wein AJ. Managing and treating urinary incontinence. 2nd edition. Baltimore (MD): Health Professions Press; 2009. p. 245–306.

24. Wagg AS, Chen LK, Kirschner-Hermanns R, et al. Incontinence in the frail elder. In: Abrams P, Cardozo L, Khoury S, et al, editors. Incontinence: Proceedings from the 5th International Consultation on Incontinence. Plymouth (United Kingdom): Health Publications; 2013. p. 1001–228.

25. Herati AS, Moldwin RM. Alternative therapies in the management of chronic prostatitis/chronic pelvic pain syndrome. World J Urol 2013;31(4):761–6.

26. Bassaly R, Downes K, Hart S. Dietary consumption triggers in interstitial cystitis/bladder pain syndrome patients. Female Pelvic Med Reconstr Surg 2011;17:36–9.

27. Shorter B, Lesser M, Moldwin R, et al. Effect of comestibles on symptoms of interstitial cystitis. J Urol 2007;178:145–52.

28. Davis NJ, Vaughan CP, Johnson TM 2nd, et al. Caffeine intake and its association with urinary incontinence in United States men: results from National Health and Nutrition Examination Surveys 2005-2006 and 2007-2008. J Urol 2013;189(6): 2170–4. http://dx.doi.org/10.1016/j.juro.2012.12.061 PMID: 23276513.

29. Gleason JL, Richter HE, Redden DT, et al. Caffeine and urinary incontinence in US women. Int Urogynecol J 2013;24(2):295–302. http://dx.doi.org/10.1007/s00192-012-1829-5.

30. Kershen R, Mann-Gow T, Yared J, et al. Caffeine ingestion causes detrusor overactivity and afferent nerve excitation in mice. J Urol 2012;188(5):1986–92. http://dx.doi.org/10.1016/j.juro.2012.07.010.

31. Maserejian NN, Wager CG, Giovannucci EL, et al. Intake of caffeinated, carbonated, or citrus beverage types and development of lower urinary tract symptoms in men and women. Am J Epidemiol 2013;177(12):1399–410. http://dx.doi.org/10.1093/aje/kws411 PMID: 23722012.

32. Lohsiriwat S, Hirunsai M, Chaiyaprasithi B. Effect of caffeine on bladder function in patients with overactive bladder symptoms. Urol Ann 2011;3(1):14–8. http://dx.doi.org/10.4103/0974-7796.75862.

33. Townsend MK, Resnick NM, Grodstein F. Caffeine intake and risk of urinary incontinence progression among women. Obstet Gynecol 2012;119(5):950–7. http://dx.doi.org/10.1097/AOG.0b013e31824fc604.

34. Jura YH, Townsend MK, Curhan GC, et al. Caffeine intake, and the risk of stress, urgency and mixed urinary incontinence. J Urol 2011;185(5):1775–80. http://dx.doi.org/10.1016/j.juro.2011.01.003.

35. Osborne J. Wine, beer and spirits—do they trigger IC flares? A patient survey reveals surprising results. IC Optimist 2010;7:15–7.

36. Cardozo L, Robinson D. Special considerations in premenopausal and postmenopausal women with symptoms of overactive bladder. Urology 2002;60:64–71.

37. Malykhina AP, Wyndaele JJ, Andersson KE, et al. Do the urinary bladder and large bowel interact, in sickness or in health? ICI-RS 2011. Neurourol Urodyn 2012;31(3):352–8.

38. Kaplan SA, Dmochowski R, Cash BD, et al. Systematic review of the relationship between bladder and bowel function: implications for patient management. Int J Clin Pract 2013;67(3):205–16. http://dx.doi.org/10.1111/ijcp.12028.

39. Coyne KS, Cash B, Kopp Z, et al. The prevalence of chronic constipation and faecal incontinence among men and women with symptoms of overactive bladder. BJU Int 2011;107:254–61.

40. Manning J, Korda A, Benness C, et al. The association of obstructive defecation, lower urinary tract dysfunction and the benign joint hypermobility syndrome: a case-control study. Int Urogynecol J Pelvic Floor Dysfunct 2003;14:128–32.

41. Jelovsek JE, Barber MD, Paraiso MF, et al. Functional bowel and anorectal disorders in patients with pelvic organ prolapse and incontinence. Am J Obstet Gynecol 2005;193:2105Y2111.

42. Lubowski DZ, Swash M, Nicholls RJ, et al. Increase in pudendal nerve terminal motor latency with defaecation straining. Br J Surg 1988;75:1095–7.

43. Hrisanfow E, Hägglund D. The prevalence of urinary incontinence among women and men with chronic obstructive pulmonary disease in Sweden. J Clin Nurs 2011;20(13–14):1895–905. http://dx.doi.org/10.1111/j.1365-2702.2010.03660.x. PMID: 21535273.

44. Thom DH, Brown JS, Schembri M, et al. Incidence of and risk factors for change in urinary incontinence status in a prospective cohort of middle-aged and older women: the reproductive risk of incontinence study in Kaiser. J Urol 2010;184:1394–401.

45. Hannestad YS, Rortveit G, Daltveit AK, et al. Are smoking and other lifestyle factors associated with female urinary incontinence? The Norwegian EPINCONT study. BJOG 2003;110:247–54.

46. Burgio KL, Zyczynski H, Locher JL, et al. Urinary incontinence in the 12-month postpartum period. Obstet Gynecol 2003;102:1291–8.

47. Vaughan CP, Auvinen A, Cartwright R, et al. Impact of obesity on urinary storage symptoms: results from the FINNO study 2013;189(4):1377–82. http://dx.doi.org/10.1016/j.juro.2012.10.058.

48. Subak LL, Richter HE, Hunskaar S. Obesity and urinary incontinence: epidemiology and clinical research update. J Urol 2009;182:S2–7.

49. Dallosso HM, McGrother CW, Matthews RJ, et al, Leicestershire MRC Incontinence Study Group. The association of diet and other lifestyle factors with overactive bladder and stress incontinence: a longitudinal study in women. Leicestershire MRC Incontinence Study Group. BJU Int 2003;92(1):69–77.

50. Hunskaar S, Arnold EP, Burgio K, et al. Epidemiology and natural history of urinary incontinence. Int Urogynecol J Pelvic Floor Dysfunct 2000;11:301–19.

51. Noblett KL, Jensen JK, Ostergard DR. The relationship of body mass index to intra-abdominal pressure as measured by multichannel cystometry. Int Urogynecol J Pelvic Floor Dysfunct 1997;8:323–6.

52. Richter HE, Burgio KL, Clements RH, et al. Urinary and anal incontinence in morbidly obese women considering weight loss surgery. Obstet Gynecol 2005;106:1272–7.

53. Tennstedt SL, Link CL, Steers WD, et al. Prevalence of and risk factors for urine leakage in a racially and ethnically diverse population of adults: the Boston Area Community Health (BACH) Survey. Am J Epidemiol 2008;167(4):390–9. http://dx.doi.org/10.1093/aje/kwm356.

54. Subak LL, Wing R, West DS, et al. Weight loss to treat urinary incontinence in overweight and obese women. N Engl J Med 2009;360:481–90.

55. Subak LL, Whitcomb E, Shen H, et al. Weight loss: a novel and effective treatment for urinary incontinence. J Urol 2005;174:190–5.

56. Wing RR, Creasman JM, West DS, et al. Improving urinary incontinence in overweight and obese women through modest weight loss. Obstet Gynecol 2010;116:284–92.

57. Fantl JA, Wyman JF, McClish DK, et al. Efficacy of bladder training in older women with urinary incontinence. JAMA 1991;265:609–13.

58. Wyman JF, Fantl JA. Bladder training in ambulatory care management of urinary incontinence. Urol Nurs 1991;11:11–7.

59. Dumoulin C, Hay-Smith J. Pelvic floor muscle training versus no treatment, or inactive control treatments, for urinary incontinence in women. Cochrane Database Syst Rev 2010;(1):CD005654.

60. Hay-Smith J, Herderschee R, Dumoulin C, et al. Comparisons of approaches to pelvic floor muscle training for urinary incontinence in women: an abridged Cochrane systematic review. Eur J Phys Rehabil Med 2012;48(4):689–705.

61. Hay-Smith EJ, Herderschee R, Dumoulin C, et al. Comparisons of approaches to pelvic floor muscle training for urinary incontinence in women [review]. Cochrane Database Syst Rev 2011;(12):CD009508. http://dx.doi.org/10.1002/14651858.CD009508.

62. Bø K, Hilde G. Does it work in the long term? A systematic review on pelvic floor muscle training for female stress urinary incontinence. Neurourol Urodyn 2013;32(3):215–23. http://dx.doi.org/10.1002/nau.22292.

63. Fletcher E. Differential diagnosis of high-tone and low-tone pelvic floor dysfunction. J Wound Ostomy Continence Nurs 2005;32(3S):510.

64. Betschart C, Mol SE, Lütolf-Keller B, et al. Pelvic floor muscle training for urinary incontinence: a comparison of outcomes in premenopausal versus postmenopausal women. Female Pelvic Med Reconstr Surg 2013;19(4):219–24. http://dx.doi.org/10.1097/SPV.0b013e31829950e5.

65. Miller J, Aston-Miller J, DeLancey J. The knack: use of precisely-timed pelvic muscle contraction can reduce leakage in SUI. Neurourol Urodyn 1996;15:302–93.

66. Miller JM, Sampselle C, Ashton-Miller J, et al. Clarification and confirmation of the Knack maneuver: the effect of volitional pelvic floor muscle contraction to preempt expected stress incontinence. Int Urogynecol J Pelvic Floor Dysfunct 2008;19(6):773–82.

67. Resnick MJ, Koyama T, Fan KH, et al. Long-term functional outcomes after treatment for localized prostate cancer. N Engl J Med 2013;368:436–45.

68. Campbell SE, Glazener CM, Hunter KF, et al. Conservative management for postprostatectomy urinary incontinence. Cochrane Database Syst Rev 2012;(1):CD001843.

69. Filocamo MT, Li Marzi V, Del Popolo G, et al. Effectiveness of early pelvic floor rehabilitation treatment for post-prostatectomy incontinence. Eur Urol 2005;48:734–8.

70. Burgio KL, Goode PS, Urban DA, et al. Preoperative biofeedback assisted behavioral training to decrease post-prostatectomy incontinence: a randomized, controlled trial. J Urol 2006;175:196–201.

71. Mariotti G, Sciarra A, Gentilucci A, et al. Early recovery of urinary continence after radical prostatectomy using early pelvic floor electrical stimulation and biofeedback associated treatment. J Urol 2009;181:1788–93.

72. Ribeiro L, Prota C, Gomes C, et al. Long-term effect of early postoperative pelvic floor biofeedback on continence in men undergoing radical prostatectomy: a prospective, randomized, controlled trial. J Urol 2010;184:1034–9.

73. Tienforti D, Sacco E, Marangi F, et al. Efficacy of an assisted low-intensity programme of perioperative pelvic floor muscle training in improving the recovery of continence after radical prostatectomy: a randomized controlled trial. BJU Int 2012;110(7):1004–10. http://dx.doi.org/10.1111/j.1464-410X.2012.10948.x. PMID: 22332815.

74. Herderschee R, Hay-Smith EJ, Herbison GP, et al. Feedback or biofeedback to augment pelvic floor muscle training for urinary incontinence in women [review]. Cochrane Database Syst Rev 2011;(7):CD009252. http://dx.doi.org/10.1002/14651858.CD009252.

75. Burgio KL, Kraus SR, Borello-France D, et al, Urinary Incontinence Treatment Network. The effects of drug and behavior therapy on urgency and voiding frequency. Int Urogynecol J 2010;21(6):711–9. http://dx.doi.org/10.1007/s00192-010-1100-x.

76. Burgio KL, Kraus SR, Menefee S, et al, Urinary Incontinence Treatment Network. Behavioral therapy to enable women with urge incontinence to discontinue drug treatment: a randomized trial. Ann Intern Med 2008;149(3):161–9.

77. Burgio KL, Locher JL, Goode PS, et al. Behavioral versus drug treatment for urge incontinence in older women: a randomized clinical trial. JAMA 1998;23:1995–2000.

78. Burgio KL, Goode PS, Johnson TM, et al. Behavioral versus drug treatment for overactive bladder in men: the Male Overactive Bladder Treatment in Veterans (MOTIVE) trial. J Am Geriatr Soc 2011;59(12):2209–16. http://dx.doi.org/10.1111/j.1532-5415.2011.03724.x.

79. Johnson TM 2nd, Markland AD, Goode PS, et al. Efficacy of adding behavioural treatment or antimuscarinic drug therapy to α-blocker therapy in men with nocturia. BJU Int 2013;112(1):100–8. http://dx.doi.org/10.1111/j.1464-410X.2012.11736.x. PMID: 2344828.

Office-Based Ultrasound for the Urologist

Martha K. Terris, MD[a,b,*], Zachary Klaassen, MD[a]

KEYWORDS

- Office ultrasonography • Renal ultrasonography • Bladder ultrasonography
- Scrotal ultrasonography • Penile Doppler ultrasonography • Prostate ultrasonography

KEY POINTS

- Renal ultrasonography allows assessment of a dilated upper urinary tract particularly in pediatric patients, assessment of flank pain during pregnancy, and evaluation of hematuria in patients who are not candidates for intravenous pyelography, contrast computed tomography, or magnetic resonance imaging.
- Bladder ultrasonography allows assessment of postvoid residual in male patients with benign prostatic hyperplasia, particularly during the initial workup.
- Scrotal ultrasonography allows assessment of a scrotal or testicular mass or swelling, assessment of acute scrotal pain, and assessment of male infertility.
- Penile Doppler ultrasonography allows assessment of the cavernosal arteries and their spectral waveform evolution following intracavernosal injection of a pharmacostimulant in patients with erectile dysfunction.
- Transrectal ultrasound of the prostate is the most common modality for imaging the prostate during biopsy; new modalities include color Dopper prostate ultrasonography, three-dimensional ultrasonography, and elastography of the prostate.

INTRODUCTION

Ultrasonography provides the busy office urologist with a minimally invasive, low-risk imaging modality that is easily accessible in the clinic setting. The basic concepts behind ultrasound imaging involve using a frequency (number of sound waves per second, measured in *hertz* [Hz]) too high for the human ear to hear.[1] Ultrasound waves are generated by a transducer, which is housed in an ultrasound probe that is shaped for the desired application. These waves are then transmitted to the tissue of interest and waves that reflect (or echo) after bouncing off the tissue of interest are incorporated by a receiving element in the transducer. Through a process called acoustic-electric conversion, the transducer transforms the sound energy into electrical energy, which is processed by the ultrasound console computer to generate white pixels corresponding to returning signals displayed on a black background.[2] This article reviews the basic applications of ultrasound imaging in the office setting, including renal, bladder, scrotal, penile Doppler, and prostate ultrasonography.

RENAL ULTRASONOGRAPHY

Given a urologist's knowledge of the anatomy of the kidney and retroperitoneum, performing a focused retroperitoneal ultrasound in the office setting can be useful for specific clinical

Funding Sources: None.
Conflict of Interest: None.
[a] Department of Surgery, Section of Urology, Medical College of Georgia-Georgia Regents University, 1120 15th Street, Augusta, GA 30912, USA; [b] Multidisciplinary Genitourinary/Prostate Team, Georgia Regents University Cancer Center, 1411 Laney Walker Boulevard, Augusta, GA 30912, USA
* Corresponding author. Department of Surgery, Section of Urology, Medical College of Georgia-Georgia Regents University, 1120 15th Street, Augusta, GA 30912.
E-mail address: mterris@gru.edu

Urol Clin N Am 40 (2013) 637–647
http://dx.doi.org/10.1016/j.ucl.2013.07.006
0094-0143/13/$ – see front matter © 2013 Elsevier Inc. All rights reserved.

indications. The ultrasound probe and transducer for renal ultrasonography is a 3.5- to 5.0-MHz curved probe; a 6- to 10-MHz transducer may be used for pediatric patients.[3] The patient is placed in the supine position and scanning begins in the midclavicular line for the kidney of interest. In the sagittal plane, the probe is moved laterally until a midsagittal view of the kidney is obtained; when analyzing the image, the upper pole of the kidney is located on the left side of the monitor (**Fig. 1**). Imaging of the kidney in the transverse plane is possible by rotating the probe 90° counterclockwise and the kidney is scanned from upper to lower pole. Important office-based indications for renal ultrasound include follow-up of hydronephrosis on prenatal ultrasound, assessment of a dilated upper urinary tract particularly in pediatric patients, assessment of flank pain and monitoring ureteral stent position during pregnancy, and evaluation of hematuria in patients who are not candidates for intravenous pyelography (IVP), contrast computed tomography (CT), or magnetic resonance imaging (MRI).[3]

Pediatric patients requiring renal imaging represent an important subset of patients for which renal ultrasonography is used. Postoperative follow-up of pediatric patients following ureteroscopic treatment of lithiasis is effective with ultrasound. Resorlu and colleagues[4] found negative and positive predictive values of 97.7% and 100%, respectively, for detecting hydronephrosis at 3 months postoperatively for ureteroscopic manipulation of lithiasis. Similar to postureteroscopy upper tract surveillance, ultrasound is important for surveillance of postpyeloplasty patients and can be used to identify patients who may require a mercaptoacetyltriglycine-3 scan in the setting of postoperative deteriorating renal function.[5]

Recently, 3-dimensional (3D) ultrasonography has been reported when evaluating pediatric patients. 3D ultrasonography improves visualization of complex anatomy and pathologic condition in any plane and allows evaluation of a dilated collecting system with similar specificity to IVP and MR urography.[6]

When assessing a pregnant patient with renal colic, determining whether this is secondary to physiologic hydronephrosis or lithiasis may be challenging. In experienced hands, ultrasonography has a sensitivity of greater than 95% for diagnosis of nephrolithiasis.[7] A review of 300 pregnant patients presenting with renal colic by Andreoiu and MacMahon[8] found that the accuracy of ultrasonography for predicting a calculus improved from 56.2% to 71.9% when features of obstruction were present, such as the absence of a ureteric jet and an elevated resistive index. Although recent studies have suggested that low-dose CT scan may be safe and improve the efficacy of lithiasis diagnosis in pregnant patients,[9] ultrasound remains an important and safe modality for diagnosing nephrolithiasis and monitoring progression of stone passage.

As part of the evaluation for hematuria, the upper urinary tract has historically been evaluated with an IVP and more recently a contrast CT or MRI of the abdomen and pelvis. In patients with an elevated creatinine, a contrasted study risks further worsening of kidney function providing an opportunity for ultrasonography to evaluate the upper urinary tract. In this subset of patients, ultrasonography offers the ability to detect renal masses and cysts (**Fig. 2**). Mucksavage and colleagues[10] analyzed 116 patients who underwent

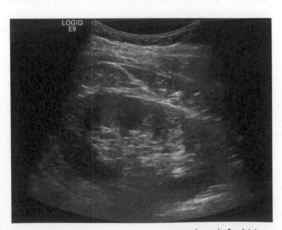

Fig. 1. Normal renal ultrasonography: left kidney measuring 10.8 cm in length demonstrating isoechoic parenchymal echogenicity.

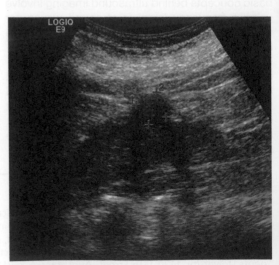

Fig. 2. Renal ultrasonography demonstrating a right 1.72 × 1.80 × 1.78 cm interpolar solid mass (delineated by *red* +).

ultrasound prior to imaging before definitive therapy. Patients also received an MRI or CT scan and they found that the size differences between CT and MRI compared with ultrasound was less than 3.5% and ultrasound correlated well with both MRI and CT (both P<.001). However, diagnosis of upper tract transitional cell carcinoma with ultrasonography is difficult to differentiate from other causes of filling defects of the renal collecting system, such as fungus balls or sloughed papillae.[11] Ultrasound should not replace an IVP or contrasted CT or MRI for the evaluation of the upper urinary tract in the setting of hematuria; however, in select patients with poor kidney function it may be considered a safe alternative.

BLADDER ULTRASONOGRAPHY

Bladder ultrasonography is an important tool for the office urologist, allowing evaluation of the lower urinary tract and prostate in men and the bladder in women. A curved probe set at 3.5 to 5 MHz is used with the patient in the supine position.[3] The bladder should be viewed in the transverse and sagittal planes, angling the probe beneath the pubic bone for optimal bladder assessment (**Fig. 3**). Arguably the most common utilization of bladder ultrasonography in the office setting is assessment of postvoid residual (PVR) in male patients with benign prostatic hyperplasia (BPH). Although the utility of PVR as an objective measure for BPH treatment efficacy and as an indicator for surgical treatment have been

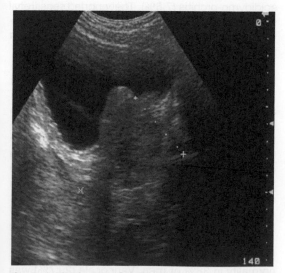

Fig. 3. Sagittal view of the bladder and prostate. The median lobe of the prostate extends into the bladder. (*From* Fulgham PF, Bishoff JT. Urinary tract imaging: basic principles. In: Wein AJ, Kavoussi LR, Novick AC, editors. Campbell-Walsh urology. 10th edition. Philadelphia: Elsevier/Saunders; 2012. p. 122; with permission.)

inconclusive,[12] it is generally accepted that PVR volume be included in the initial assessment of a patient with BPH and during monitoring of patients undergoing conservative treatment regimens.[13] Additional indications for bladder ultrasonography in the office setting may include evaluation of bladder wall configuration and thickness, detection of ureteroceles, assessment for ureteral obstruction, detection of perivesical fluid collections, evaluation of clot retention, confirmation of catheter position, and guidance of suprapubic tube placement.[3]

SCROTAL ULTRASONOGRAPHY

Scrotal ultrasonography provides the urologist with high-quality images when evaluating patients with acute scrotal pain, a palpable scrotal mass, or an enlarged scrotum on physical examination. Ultrasonography is typically performed with high frequency (6–12 MHz) and a 4- or 7.5-cm linear array transducer.[3] Patients should be in the supine position with the scrotum supported by a towel. The penis should be out of the way and adequate conducting gel should be used to circumvent artifact that may result secondary to scrotal hair. Transverse and sagittal images should be obtained paying particular attention to each testis, epididymis, and spermatic cord (**Fig. 4**A). The 2 testes should be compared for echogenicity because certain infiltrative processes (eg, leukemic testicular involvement) may result in subtle changes that are only noticeable when a bilateral comparison is used. Furthermore, Doppler ultrasonography should be used to determine blood flow to each testis particularly when clinical suspicion is concerning for testicular torsion. Indications for in-office scrotal ultrasonography include assessment of a scrotal or testicular mass or swelling, assessment of acute scrotal pain, and assessment of male infertility.

Ultrasonography of the scrotum in the setting of a swollen scrotum or a palpable testis mass allows for delineation between extratesticular (eg, hydrocele) (see **Fig. 4**B) and intratesticular (eg, tumor, infection) causes (see **Fig. 4**C). For medicolegal reasons, evaluation for malignancy should also include a review of the images by a radiologist. Micallef and colleagues[14] retrospectively analyzed 256 patients for scrotal swelling and reported that 75% of cases involved extratesticular causes (most commonly hydrocele) and 25% involved intratesticular causes, most commonly secondary to infection (50%) and tumor (21%). Color Doppler ultrasonography of a testicular nodule is characterized by hypervascularity with irregular branching patterns.[15] Leydig cell tumors often have a unique

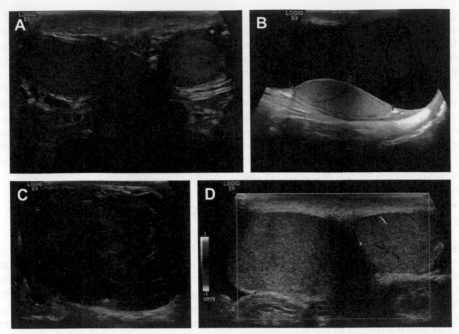

Fig. 4. Scrotal ultrasonography. (*A*) Midtransverse image of left and right testis demonstrating heterogenous parenchymal echogenicity. (*B*) Sagittal image demonstrating a 5.5 × 1.8 × 3.3 cm left testis (delineated by *red* +) and surrounding 9.1 × 5.5 × 6.2 cm hydrocele. (*C*) Sagittal image demonstrating a 6.5 × 4.8 × 4.9 cm right testis tumor encompassing the entire right testis (delineated by *red* +). (*D*) Midtransverse image demonstrating normal flow to the left testis and acute right testicular torsion.

ultrasound finding of hypoechoic nodules with peripheral hypervascularity and no internal flow.[16] When a hydrocele is suspected on physical examination (no nodules, nonpalpable testis, scrotal swelling), ultrasonography may be used to confirm the diagnosis, demonstrating an increased fluid volume around the testis and in increased pulsatility index.

The assessment of the acute scrotum relies on an accurate history and physical examination and, if needed, ultrasonography. Clinical suspicion for testicular torsion obviating scrotal exploration should not be delayed because of ultrasonographic confirmation. The hallmark of testicular torsion on ultrasonography is the absence of intratesticular blood flow (see **Fig. 4**D); paratesticular blood flow secondary to collateral circulation may appear within hours of testicular torsion.[3] Although the paradigm at many tertiary centers is to explore an acute scrotum regardless of ultrasonographic findings for fear of overlooking testicular torsion, a recent report by Altinkilic and colleagues[17] suggests that normal intratesticular perfusion using color-coded duplex sonography (CCDS) obviates scrotal exploration. The authors assessed the diagnostic value of CCDS in 236 patients (median age 13 years) with clinical suspicion of testicular torsion who subsequently underwent exploration whereby

the surgeon was blinded to the ultrasound findings. Testicular torsion was the most common cause of acute scrotum (50.4%), followed by torsion of the testicular appendage (34.8%) and epididymo-orchitis (7.6%). The reported sensitivity, specificity, and positive and negative predictive values of detecting testicular torsion with CCDS were 100%, 75%, 80%, and 100%, respectively.[17]

Scrotal ultrasonography may elucidate pathologic conditions affecting male fertility, including a varicocele (**Fig. 5**), which is the most common abnormality in infertile men with abnormal semen analysis. The degree of testicular size difference that may warrant surgical repair in infertile men has not been defined; however, a 20% size discrepancy has been proposed as a threshold for intervention.[18] Although varicocele is often diagnosed on physical examination of the testis and spermatic cord, accuracy of palpation may be subjective. Pierik and colleagues[19] analyzed 1372 infertile men who were assessed with color Doppler ultrasonography and found a scrotal abnormality in 38% of men. Varicocele (29.7%) was the most common abnormality, followed by epididymal cyst (7.6%), hydrocele (3.2%), testicular microlithiasis (0.9%), testicular cyst (0.7%), and testicular tumor (0.5%). Interestingly, 67% and 60% of overall sonographic findings and

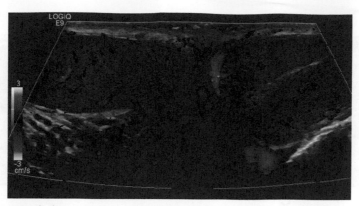

Fig. 5. Midtransverse scrotal ultrasonography demonstrating a large left varicocele.

varicoceles, respectively, were not evident on physical examination.[19]

PENILE DOPPLER ULTRASONOGRAPHY

Penile Doppler ultrasonography allows assessment of the cavernosal arteries and their spectral waveform evolution following intracavernosal injection of a pharmacostimulant in patients with erectile dysfunction (ED).[20–23] Depending on the institution, this may be performed in the office setting or by an ultrasound technician in a radiology suite, with subsequent interpretation of results by an urologist. In the authors' experience, the patient is brought to the radiology suite and a 1 mL injection of an alprostadil-papaverine-phentolamine mix using a 25-gauge needle is performed. The injection is made in either corpora cavernosa at the 3- or 9-o'clock position at the base of the penis. Following injection, a linear transducer set at 7 MHz or higher is used; scanning is typically performed on the ventral surface of the penis; however, the dorsal and lateral surfaces may be used if necessary.[23,24] Images and waveforms are obtained in both the longitudinal and the transverse planes from the base of the penis to the tip of the glans. Attention to the cavernosal arteries, integrity of the corpus cavernosa, and identification of plaques, tumors, and calcifications is important. Color Doppler ultrasonography is necessary for measuring the systolic velocity in the cavernosal arteries and for determining the preinjection (**Fig. 6**A) and postinjection diameters (see **Fig. 6**B) of the arteries. The thresholds for normal systolic and diastolic velocities of blood flow relating to the cavernosal arteries following injection of a pharmacostimulant are generally regarded as a peak systolic velocity (PSV) of greater than 25 to 35 cm/s and an end diastolic velocity (EDV) of less than 5 to 7 cm/s (see **Fig. 6**C).[20–23,25]

Arterial disease is one of the most common causes of ED with common predisposing factors including hypertension, diabetes mellitus, obesity, dyslipidema, smoking, and a sedentary lifestyle.[26,27] A PSV of less than 25 cm/s has been associated with a strong likelihood of severe arterial disease. A second cause of ED includes venous incompetence, or the finding of persistent diastolic flow and elevated EDV; an EDV greater than 5 to 7 cm/s is highly suggestive of a venous leak.[25] Third, penile Doppler ultrasonographic evaluation has been used in the diagnosis and treatment of Peyronie disease (PD), a benign, localized connective tissue disorder of unknown cause that causes fibrous thickening of the penile tunica albuginea. This fibrous thickening often leads to painful erections and erectile deformities. Evaluation in patients with PD provides an anatomic evaluation of the penile deformity and may identify concomitant ED, as ED has been associated with PD in as many as 80% of patients.[28] Chung and colleagues[29] evaluated 1500 men with ED over a 10-year period with penile Doppler ultrasonography, of which 891 men presented with PD and 609 men had ED. The authors found that men with ED had higher rates of diabetes and coronary artery disease; patients with impaired cavernosal arterial flow was observed in men with decreased penile rigidity and penile pain, and men with a higher EDV was associated with men having difficulty maintaining an erection and tunical thickening.

An underreported use of penile Doppler ultrasonography is for men with ED following a prostatectomy or cystectomy. Hekal and colleagues[30] evaluated 45 male patients with penile Doppler ultrasonography who had a cystectomy, including 21 patients with nerve-sparing technique and 24 patients with non-nerve-sparing technique over the course of 12 months postoperatively. PSVs were comparable between the 2 groups during

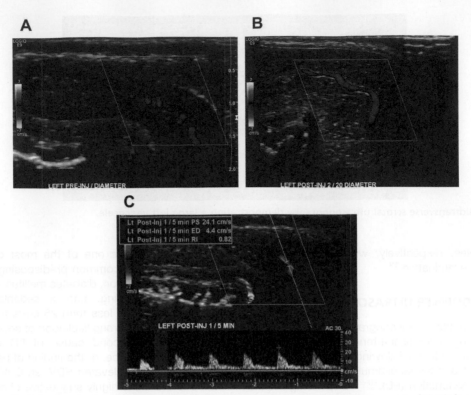

Fig. 6. Penile Doppler ultrasonography. (*A*) Prepharmacostimulant injection measurement of the left cavernosal artery diameter. (*B*) Postinjection measurement of the left cavernosal artery diameter. (*C*) Doppler ultrasonographic measurement of the PSV (*red*, 24.1 cm/s) and EDV (*blue*, 4.4 cm/s).

follow-up. EDV significantly deteriorated postoperatively compared to preoperative evaluation in both groups; however, gradual improvement in EDV was seen in the nerve-sparing group 12 months after surgery. Kawanishi and colleagues[31] evaluated 123 male patients with localized prostate cancer with penile Doppler ultrasonography before and after prostatectomy and found that 21 patients (17%) had normal erectile function before surgery and 9 (43%) of the 21 potent men had potency 4 to 6 weeks postoperatively. Finally, Ohebshalom and colleagues[32] analyzed 111 men with normal erectile function preoperatively within 6 months of prostatectomy with penile Doppler ultrasonography and found 32 patients (29%) had normal erectile hemodynamics after prostatectomy. In this cohort, 12 patients (11%) had a venous leak. When comparing patients with normal to those with abnormal hemodynamics, the mean International Index of Erectile Function scores were 25 and 17 ($P = .025$); the percentage of patients with functional erections for sexual activity without pharmacologic agents was 47% versus 22% ($P = .018$) and the percentage of patients responding to sildenafil citrate was 72% versus 43% ($P = .03$).[32]

PROSTATE ULTRASONOGRAPHY

Transrectal ultrasound (TRUS) of the prostate was first described in 1968 by Watanabe and colleagues,[33] and with expanded technology led to the first TRUS-guided sextant prostate biopsy by Hodge and colleagues[34] in 1989. TRUS is now used by most urologists to direct prostate biopsies accurately; although it cannot reliably detect prostate cancer, it is an inexpensive modality for imaging the prostate. In general, the patient is provided with either 3 days of a perioperative oral fluoroquinolone (eg, Ciprofloxacin) or a single-dose aminoglycoside (eg, Gentamicin) administered on the day of biopsy. A Fleets enema may be self-administered by the patient on the day of the biopsy. On the office procedure table, the patient is placed in the left lateral decubitus position with the buttock positioned slightly over the side of the table to allow adequate mobility of the transrectal ultrasound probe. With the patient appropriately positioned and draped, a digital rectal examination should be performed to assess for size, induration, nodules, and/or hypertrophy of the prostate gland. The rectal ultrasound probe, with adequate lubrication, is then slowly inserted into the rectum.

TRUS of the prostate is generally performed at very high frequencies of 5 to 10 MHz, much higher than imaging of other urologic structures (**Fig. 7**).[2] The echogenicity of structures within the prostate gland are compared relative to the medium-gray echogenicity of the peripheral zone—structures that are the same echogenicity are isoechoic: those that are brighter are hyperechoic and those that are darker are hypoechoic.[2] Peripheral zone palpable prostatic adenocarcinomas (PCa) typically are hypoechogenic[35,36]; however, most nonpalpable peripheral zone cancers do not demonstrate abnormal echo patterns. Transition zone tumors are even more isoechoic than peripheral zone cancers.[2] Following a general surveillance of the prostate assessing for these abnormalities, a measurement of the prostate in 3D is obtained to provide an accurate prostate volume. A local prostatic block is achieved using 1% lidocaine through a long spinal needle (eg, 7-inch, 22-gauge) using TRUS guidance along the biopsy channel of the transducer. Multiple techniques for injecting local anesthetic have been described and a common technique is to identify the level of the seminal vesicles near the bladder base at the junction of the seminal vesicles and prostate and to inject 5 mL lidocaine bilaterally.[37]

A biopsy gun or spring-driven, 18-gauge, needle core biopsy device is passed through the guide attached to the ultrasound probe and prostate biopsies are performed sequentially in this manner.[37] Inthe authors' experience, a 12-core, double sextant, biopsy is performed in either the transverse or the sagittal plane: 2 cores from each side of the prostate base, mid-gland and apex, are obtained. Numerous studies over the past 20 years have advocated for an extended core biopsy template over the traditional sextant biopsy. In 2000, Presti and colleagues[38] analyzed 483 patients in a prospective study and found that PCa detection rate increased from 80% to 96% when adding lateral cores from the base and mid gland.[39] Uno and colleagues[40] analyzed

313 patients who underwent TRUS-guided 14-core biopsy (standard 6 biopsy cores, 6 lateral cores, and 2 transition zone cores) and found 127 patients (40.6%) with PCa, 28 (22%) patients of which PCa would not have been detected by the sextant method alone. Depending on local guidelines, biopsy samples are placed in 10% formalin containers and sent to the pathology laboratory. After completing the biopsy, digital rectal pressure with gauze is sustained until adequate rectal hemostasis is achieved.

Office-based TRUS-guided prostate biopsy may be associated with considerable pain and anxiety for the patient. Although the procedure is most often only associated with minor complications, the patient's perception of the procedure may be traumatic and worrisome. Zisman and colleagues[41] prospectively enrolled 211 men undergoing TRUS-guided prostate biopsy in a study focusing on pain, anxiety, and ED associated with the procedure. They reported that 20% of patients reported pain during the procedure, which correlated with pain in the first 24 hours after biopsy. Inflammatory changes on biopsy and a younger patient correlated with persistent pain at 2 and 7 days after biopsy. Sixty-four percent of patients reported prebiopsy anxiety and this correlated with pain during the biopsy. ED was reported in 15% of previously potent men at 7 and 30 days postbiopsy.[41]

Given the level of anxiety and pain that may be associated with office-based TRUS-guided prostate biopsy, significant resources have been allocated to elucidating appropriate analgesia during the procedure. Ozden and colleagues[42] performed a prospective, randomized, placebo-controlled study analyzing the dose and injection location for periprostatic nerve block in 175 men. Seven groups of 25 men were allocated to receive 5 mL saline or 2.5, 5, or 10 mL 1% lidocaine injected at the prostate base or base and apical location. The authors reported that 10 mL local anesthetic injections provided better analgesia irrespective

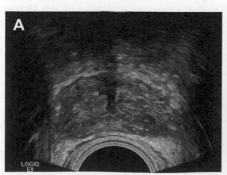
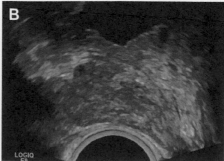

Fig. 7. Normal transrectal ultrasonography of the prostate in the (*A*) transverse and (*B*) sagittal planes.

of location.[42] Seckiner and colleagues[43] performed a prospective, randomized-controlled study comparing lidocaine and tramadol for periprostatic nerve blockage during TRUS-guided prostate biopsy in 90 patients. Group 1 (n = 30) received lidocaine; group 2 (n = 29) received tramadol, and group 3 (n = 31) received saline injection. Subsequently, visual pain scales were used to rate the patient's pain at 10 minutes postbiopsy; the mean pain scores of lidocaine, tramadol, and placebo groups were 1.73, 2.89, and 4.32 (P<.01), respectively, suggesting that tramadol may be as effective as lidocaine for providing biopsy analgesia. Meta-analyses advocate the use of adequate analgesia, primarily lidocaine, during TRUS-guided prostate biopsy.[44,45]

Modifications to the traditional gray-scale sonography have recently been developed, including color Doppler (**Fig. 8**A) and power Doppler

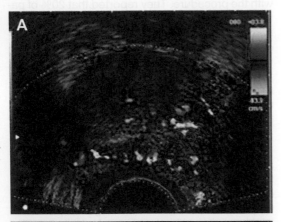

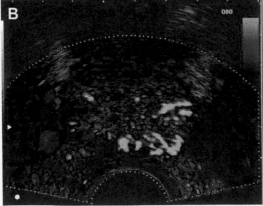

Fig. 8. Color Doppler (*A*) transrectal ultrasonography (TRUS) and power Doppler (*B*) TRUS identify a Gleason 4 + 4 = 8 adenocarcinoma in the left midgland (*arrow*). (*From* Trabulsi EJ, Halpern EJ, Gomella LG. Ultrasonography and biopsy of the prostate. In: Wein AJ, Kavoussi LR, Novick AC, editors. Campbell-Walsh urology. 10th edition. Philadelphia: Elsevier/Saunders; 2012. p. 2744; with permission.)

ultrasound (see **Fig. 8**B). Color Doppler ultrasonography depicts the velocity of blood flow in a directionally dependent manner and power Doppler imaging uses amplitude shift to detect both flow and velocity.[37] These advanced techniques to aid in ultrasound detection of PCa were developed because of radical prostatectomy specimens demonstrating increased microvessel density in PCa specimens.[46] Color and power Doppler ultrasound have unfortunately demonstrated mixed results as early studies' outcomes have not been replicated, demonstrating overall poor sensitivity (13%–86%) secondary to benign pathologic abnormality also showing ultrasound abnormalities.[39,47,48] Although outside the scope of the current article, contrast-enhanced agents and techniques have been applied to Doppler ultrasonography to attempt to increase the specificity and sensitivity of targeted ultrasound-guided prostate biopsy.[39,49,50]

Further advances in prostate ultrasonography include the use of 3D ultrasonography and elastography. 3D-TRUS requires a specialized endocavitary ultrasound probe; this technology allows simultaneous biplanar imaging of the prostate with computer reconstruction providing a coronal plane as well as a 3D image. Hamper and colleagues[51] compared 16 patients undergoing TRUS-guided prostate biopsy with 2-dimensional and 3D ultrasound subjectively reporting an improved ability to visualize hypoechoic lesions in 3D most notably in the coronal view. Furthermore, prostate volume calculations were believed to be more accurate, consistently 20% smaller than traditional dimensional volume calculations. More recent studies have suggested 84% sensitivity and 96% specificity for preoperative 3D ultrasonography detecting macroscopic extracapsular tumor extension of radical prostatectomy specimens.[52]

PCa is associated with increased cellular density and glandular architecture loss, which may result in a firmness or induration appreciated on digital rectal examination.[39] These findings result in a decreased elasticity of the tissue and may be detectable by elastography. This technique uses real-time ultrasonography of the prostate at baseline and under varying degrees of free-hand compression of the ultrasound probe against the prostate tissue. Through computerized calculations, an elastogram of the prostate is obtained, identifying regions with decreased tissue elasticity that may be suggestive of malignancy (**Fig. 9**). Two recent studies have reported the accuracy of elastography. In 2005, Konig and colleagues[53] analyzed 404 patients who underwent TRUS biopsy with subsequent generation of elastograms.

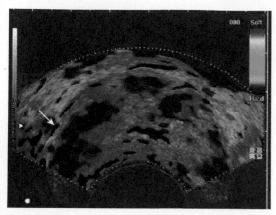

Fig. 9. Elastography demonstrates an area of decreased compliance in the right base consistent with an underlying malignancy (*blue near arrow*). The color scale in the upper right corner indicates relative tissue "firmness." Targeted biopsy of this region revealed a Gleason 4 + 4 = 8 adenocarcinoma. (*From* Trabulsi EJ, Halpern EJ, Gomella LG. Ultrasonography and biopsy of the prostate. In: Wein AJ, Kavoussi LR, Novick AC, editors. Campbell-Walsh urology. 10th edition. Philadelphia: Elsevier/Saunders; 2012. p. 2746; with permission.)

Of the 151 patients with PCa, 84% of patients had an abnormal elastogram. In 2008, Pallwein and colleagues[54] analyzed 492 patients who underwent elastography and TRUS biopsy and noted a sensitivity of 86% and specificity of 72% for detection of PCa on elastogram, corresponding to a negative predictive value of 91.4%.

SUMMARY

The use of office-based ultrasound continues to be an undisputable imaging modality for the clinical urologist when assessing the kidneys, bladder, scrotum, erectile function, and prostate. The lack of radiation exposure risk is advantageous to the operator and patient alike. With the advent of color Doppler and 3D ultrasonography, technology continues to evolve and broaden the indications for ultrasonography, ultimately improving patient care. Ultrasonography is increasingly being used in the office setting by urologists providing an imaging modality for initial diagnosis, interventional management, and longitudinal follow-up of urologic diseases.

REFERENCES

1. Kossoff G. Basic physics and imaging characteristics of ultrasound. World J Surg 2000;24:134–42.
2. Terris MK, Burnette J. Principles of prostate ultrasound. In: Jones JS, editor. Prostate cancer diagnosis—PSA, biopsy and beyond. New York: Human Press; 2013. p. 147–59.
3. Fulgham PF, Bishoff JT. Urinary tract imaging: basic principles. In: Wein AJ, Kavoussi LR, Novick AC, et al, editors. Campbell-Walsh urology. 10th edition. Philadelphia: Elsevier/Saunders; 2012. p. 99–139.
4. Resorlu B, Kara C, Resorlu EB, et al. Effectiveness of ultrasonography in the postoperative follow-up of pediatric patients undergoing ureteroscopic stone manipulation. Pediatr Surg Int 2011;27:1337–41.
5. Cost NG, Prieto JC, Wilcox DT. Screening ultrasound in follow-up after pediatric pyeloplasty. Urology 2010;76:175–9.
6. Riccabona M, Fritz G, Ring E. Potential applications of three-dimensional ultrasound in the pediatric urinary tract: pictorial demonstration based on preliminary results. Eur Radiol 2003;13:2680–7.
7. Parulkar BG, Hopkins TB, Wollin MR, et al. Renal colic during pregnancy: a case for conservative treatment. J Urol 1998;159:365–8.
8. Andreoiu M, MacMahon R. Renal colic in pregnancy: lithiasis or physiological hydronephrosis? Urology 2009;74:757–61.
9. White WM, Johnson EB, Zite NB, et al. Predictive value of current imaging modalities for the detection of urolithiasis during pregnancy: a multicenter, longitudinal study. J Urol 2013;189:931–4.
10. Mucksavage P, Ramchandani P, Malkowicz SB, et al. Is ultrasound imaging inferior to computed tomography or magnetic resonance imaging in evaluating renal mass size? Urology 2012;79:28–31.
11. O'Connor OJ, Fitzgerald E, Maher MM. Imaging of hematuria. AJR Am J Roentgenol 2010;195:W263–7.
12. McConnell JD, Barry MJ, Bruskewitz RC. Benign prostatic hyperplasia: diagnosis and treatment. Agency for Health Care Policy and Research. Clin Pract Guidel Quick Ref Guide Clin 1994;8:1–17.
13. Denis LJ. Future implications for the management of benign prostatic hyperplasia. Eur Urol 1994;25(Suppl 1):29–34.
14. Micallef M, Torreggiani WC, Hurley M, et al. The ultrasound investigation of scrotal swelling. Int J STD AIDS 2000;11:297–302.
15. Dudea SM, Ciurea A, Chiorean A, et al. Doppler applications in testicular and scrotal disease. Med Ultrason 2010;12:43–51.
16. Maizlin ZV, Belenky A, Kunichezky M, et al. Leydig cell tumors of the testis: gray scale and color Doppler sonographic appearance. J Ultrasound Med 2004;23:959–64.
17. Altinkilic B, Pilatz A, Weidner W. Detection of normal intratesticular perfusion using color coded duplex sonography obviates need for scrotal exploration in patients with suspected testicular torsion. J Urol 2013;189(5):1853–8.

18. Diamond DA, Zurakowski D, Bauer SB, et al. Relationship of varicocele grade and testicular hypotrophy to semen parameters in adolescents. J Urol 2007;178:1584–8.

19. Pierik FH, Dohle GR, van Muiswinkel JM, et al. Is routine scrotal ultrasound advantageous in infertile men? J Urol 1999;162:1618–20.

20. Halls J, Bydawell G, Patel U. Erectile dysfunction: the role of penile Doppler ultrasound in diagnosis. Abdom Imaging 2009;34:712–25.

21. Quam JP, King BF, James EM, et al. Duplex and color Doppler sonographic evaluation of vasculogenic impotence. AJR Am J Roentgenol 1989; 153:1141–7.

22. Bari V, Ahmed MN, Rafique MZ, et al. Evaluation of Erectile Dysfunction with Color Doppler Sonography. J Pak Med Assoc 2006;56:258–62.

23. Hattery RR, King BF, Lewis RW, et al. Vasculogenic impotence: duplex and colour Doppler imaging. Radiol Clin North Am 1991;29:629–45.

24. Pozniak MA, Lee FT Jr. Doppler imaging of the penis. In: Allan PL, editor. Clinical Doppler ultrasound. Philadelphia: Elsevier Health Sciences; 2006. p. 251–66.

25. Benson CB, Aruny JE, Vickers MA Jr. Correlation of duplex sonography with arteriography in patients with erectile dysfunction. Am J Roentgenol 1993; 160:71–3.

26. Roumeguere T, Wespes E, Carpentier Y, et al. Erectile dysfunction is associated with a high prevalence of hyperlipidemia and coronary heart disease risk. Eur Urol 2003;44:355–9.

27. El-Sakka AI. Association of risk factors and medical comorbidities with male sexual dysfunctions. J Sex Med 2007;4:1691–700.

28. Lopez JA, Jarow JP. Penile vascular evaluation of men with Peyronie's disease. J Urol 1993;149:53–5.

29. Chung E, Yan H, De Young L, et al. Penile Doppler sonographic and clinical characteristics in Peyronie's disease and/or erectile dysfunction: an analysis of 1500 men with male sexual dysfunction. BJU Int 2012;110:1201–5.

30. Hekal IA, El-Bahnasawy MS, Mosbah A, et al. Recoverability of erectile function in post-radical cystectomy patients: subjective and objective evaluations. Eur Urol 2009;55:275–83.

31. Kawanishi Y, Lee KS, Kimura K, et al. Effect of radical retropubic prostatectomy on erectile function, evaluated before and after surgery using colour Doppler ultrasonography and nocturnal penile tumescence monitoring. BJU Int 2001;88:244–7.

32. Ohebshalom M, Parker M, Waters B, et al. Erectile haemodynamic status after radical prostatectomy correlates with erectile functional outcome. BJU Int 2008;102:592–6.

33. Watanabe H, Kato H, Kato T, et al. Diagnostic application of transrectal ultrasonotomography for the prostate. Nihon Hinyokika Gakkai Zasshi 1968;59:273–9.

34. Hodge KK, McNeal JE, Terris MK, et al. Random systematic versus directed ultrasound guided transrectal core biopsies of the prostate. J Urol 1989;142:71–4.

35. Peterson AC, Terris MK. Urologic imaging without X-rays: ultrasonography, MRI, and nuclear medicine. 2008. Available at: eMedicine.com; http://www.emedicine.medscape.com/article/455553-overview. Accessed April 6, 2013.

36. Singer EA, Golijanin DJ, Davis RS, et al. What's new in urologic ultrasound? Urol Clin North Am 2006;33: 279–86.

37. Trabulsi EJ, Halpern EJ, Gomella LG. Ultrasonography and biopsy of the prostate. In: Wein AJ, Kavoussi LR, Novick AC, et al, editors. Campbell-walsh urology. 10th edition. Philadelphia: Elsevier/Saunders; 2012. p. 2735–47.

38. Presti JC Jr, Chang JJ, Bhargava V, et al. The optimal systematic prostate biopsy scheme should include 8 rather than 6 biopsies: results of a prospective trial. J Urol 2000;163:163–6.

39. Trabulsi EJ, Sackett D, Gomella LG, et al. Enhance transrectal ultrasound modalities in the diagnosis of prostate cancer. Urology 2010;76:1025–33.

40. Uno H, Nakano M, Ehara H, et al. Indications for extended 14-core transrectal ultrasound-guided prostate biopsy. Urology 2008;71:23–7.

41. Zisman A, Leibovici D, Kleinmann J, et al. The impact of prostate biopsy on patient well-being: a prospective study of pain, anxiety and erectile dysfunction. J Urol 2001;165:445–54.

42. Ozden E, Yaman O, Gogus C, et al. The optimum doses of and injection locations for periprostatic nerve blockade for transrectal ultrasound guided biopsy of the prostate: a prospective, randomized, placebo controlled study. J Urol 2003;170:2319–22.

43. Seckiner I, Sen H, Erturhan S, et al. A prospective, randomized controlled study comparing lidocaine and tramadol in periprostatic nerve blockage for transrectal ultrasound-guided prostate biopsy. Urology 2011;78:257–60.

44. Autorino R, De Sio M, Di Lorenzo G, et al. How to decrease pain during transrectal ultrasound guided prostate biopsy: a look at the literature. J Urol 2005;174:2091–7.

45. Hergan L, Kashefi C, Parsons JK. Local anesthetic reduces pain associated with transrectal ultrasound-guided prostate biopsy: a meta-analysis. Urology 2007;69:520–5.

46. Bigler SA, Deering RE, Brawer MK. Comparison of microscopic vascularity in benign and malignant prostate tissue. Hum Pathol 1993;24:220–6.

47. Halpern EJ, Strup SE. Using gray-scale and color and power Doppler sonography to detect prostate cancer. AJR Am J Roentgenol 2000;174:623–7.

48. Nelson ED, Slotoroff CB, Gomella LG, et al. Targeted biopsy of the prostate: the impact of color Doppler imaging and elastography on prostate cancer detection and Gleason score. Urology 2007;70:1136–40.

49. Mitterberger M, Pinggera GM, Horninger W, et al. Comparison of contrast enhanced color Doppler targeted biopsy to conventional systematic biopsy: impact on Gleason score. J Urol 2007;178:464–8.

50. Aigner F, Pallwein L, Mitterberger M, et al. Contrast-enhanced ultrasonography using cadence-contrast pulse sequencing technology for targeted biopsy of the prostate. BJU Int 2009;103:458–63.

51. Hamper UM, Trapanotto V, DeJong MR, et al. Three-dimensional US of the prostate: early experience. Radiology 1999;212:719–23.

52. Mitterberger M, Pinggera GM, Pallwein L, et al. The value of three-dimensional transrectal ultrasonography in staging prostate cancer. BJU Int 2007;100:47–50.

53. Konig K, Scheipers U, Pesavento A, et al. Initial experiences with real-time elastography guided biopsies of the prostate. J Urol 2005;174:115–7.

54. Pallwein L, Mitterberger M, Pinggera G, et al. Sonoelastography of the prostate: comparison with systematic biopsy findings in 492 patients. Eur J Radiol 2008;65:304–10.

Index

Note: Page numbers of article titles are in **boldface** type.

A

Alcohol abusers
  OBA in
    preoperative evaluation for, 507
Allergy(ies)
  OBA in patients with
    preoperative evaluation for, 507
Anesthesia/anesthetics
  office-based, **497–519**. *See also* Office-based
    anesthesia (OBA)
  for office-based sperm retrieval for infertility,
    570–571
  prior history of
    OBA in patients with
      preoperative evaluation for, 507
  in TRUS–guided PB, 460–461
  in ureteroscopy in office-based management of
    kidney stones, 491
  for vasectomy, 560
Antibiotics
  in office-based management of kidney
    stones, 482
  in office-based management of nonmuscle
    invasive bladder cancer, 476
Asthma
  OBA in patients with
    preoperative evaluation for, 504–505

B

Behavioral therapy
  office-based, **613–635**
    for LUTS, **613–635**
      assessment before, 614–617
      BT, 623
      drug therapy with, 632
      introduction, 613–614
      lifestyle modifications, 618–623
      PFMT, 613–614, 623–627
        pre- and postprostatectomy, 627–632
      stimulation, 632
      urgency reduction strategies, 623
Benign prostatic hyperplasia
  office-based therapy for, 594–595
Biofeedback
  coding for, 610
Biomarker(s)
  voided

in nonmuscle invasive bladder cancer
  surveillance, 475–476
Bladder
  overactive. *See* Overactive bladder (OAB)
Bladder cancer
  low-grade
    management of
      costs in, 474
  noninvasive
    incidence of, 473–474
    natural history of, 473–474
  nonmuscle invasive
    office-based management of,
      473–479
      antibiotics in, 476
      drug resistance in, 476
      effectiveness of, 474–475
      follow-up care in, 475
      imaging for surveillance in, 476
      lifestyle modification in, 476
      narrow-band imaging in, 476–477
      patient selection for, 474
      tolerability of, 474–475
      tumor surveillance in, 475
      voided biomarkers for surveillance in,
        475–476
      watchful waiting of identified bladder
        tumors in, 475
  prevalence of, 473
Bladder catheterization, irrigation, and instillation
  procedures
  coding for, 606–607
Bladder emptying function
  invasive assessment of
    in urodynamic testing, 550–551
Bladder storage function
  assessment of
    in urodynamic testing, 547–549
Bladder training (BT)
  for LUTS, 623
Bladder ultrasonography
  office-based, 639
Blood glucose
  in OBA preoperative laboratory testing, 508
Bone-targeting therapy
  office-based, 596–597
Botulinum toxin
  intradetrusor injection of
    for incontinence, 595

Urol Clin N Am 40 (2013) 649–656
http://dx.doi.org/10.1016/S0094-0143(13)00106-7
0094-0143/13/$ – see front matter © 2013 Elsevier Inc. All rights reserved.

United States Postal Service

Statement of Ownership, Management, and Circulation
(All Periodicals Publications Except Requestor Publications)

1. Publication Title: Urologic Clinics of North America

2. Publication Number: 0 0 0 - 7 1 1

3. Filing Date: 9/14/13

4. Issue Frequency: Feb, May, Aug, Nov

5. Number of Issues Published Annually: 4

6. Annual Subscription Price: $339.00

7. Complete Mailing Address of Known Office of Publication (Not printer) (Street, city, county, state, and ZIP+4®):
Elsevier Inc.
360 Park Avenue South
New York, NY 10010-1710

Contact Person: Stephen R. Bushing
Telephone (Include area code): 215-239-3688

8. Complete Mailing Address of Headquarters or General Business Office of Publisher (Not printer):
Elsevier Inc., 360 Park Avenue South, New York, NY 10010-1710

9. Full Names and Complete Mailing Addresses of Publisher, Editor, and Managing Editor (Do not leave blank)

Publisher (Name and complete mailing address):
Linda Belfus, Elsevier, Inc., 1600 John F. Kennedy Blvd. Suite 1800, Philadelphia, PA 19103-2899

Editor (Name and complete mailing address):
Stephanie Donley, Elsevier, Inc., 1600 John F. Kennedy Blvd. Suite 1800, Philadelphia, PA 19103-2899

Managing Editor (Name and complete mailing address):
Adrianne Brigido, Elsevier, Inc., 1600 John F. Kennedy Blvd. Suite 1800, Philadelphia, PA 19103-2899

10. Owner (Do not leave blank. If the publication is owned by a corporation, give the name and address of the corporation immediately followed by the names and addresses of all stockholders owning or holding 1 percent or more of the total amount of stock. If not owned by a corporation, give the names and addresses of the individual owners. If owned by a partnership or other unincorporated firm, give its name and address as well as those of each individual owner. If the publication is published by a nonprofit organization, give its name and address.)

Full Name	Complete Mailing Address
Wholly owned subsidiary of	1600 John F. Kennedy Blvd., Ste. 1800
Reed/Elsevier, US holdings	Philadelphia, PA 19103-2899

11. Known Bondholders, Mortgagees, and Other Security Holders Owning or Holding 1 Percent or More of Total Amount of Bonds, Mortgages, or Other Securities. If none, check box ☐ None

Full Name	Complete Mailing Address
N/A	

12. Tax Status (For completion by nonprofit organizations authorized to mail at nonprofit rates) (Check one)
The purpose, function, and nonprofit status of this organization and the exempt status for federal income tax purposes:
☐ Has Not Changed During Preceding 12 Months
☐ Has Changed During Preceding 12 Months (Publisher must submit explanation of change with this statement)

PS Form 3526, September 2007 (Page 1 of 3 (Instructions Page 3)) PSN 7530-01-000-9931 PRIVACY NOTICE: See our Privacy policy in www.usps.com

---

13. Publication Title: Urologic Clinics of North America

14. Issue Date for Circulation Data Below: August 2013

15. Extent and Nature of Circulation

			Average No. Copies Each Issue During Preceding 12 Months	No. Copies of Single Issue Published Nearest to Filing Date
a. Total Number of Copies (Net press run)			1,394	1,198
b. Paid Circulation (By Mail and Outside the Mail)	(1)	Mailed Outside-County Paid Subscriptions Stated on PS Form 3541. (Include paid distribution above nominal rate, advertiser's proof copies, and exchange copies)	585	523
	(2)	Mailed In-County Paid Subscriptions Stated on PS Form 3541 (Include paid distribution above nominal rate, advertiser's proof copies, and exchange copies)		
	(3)	Paid Distribution Outside the Mails Including Sales Through Dealers and Carriers, Street Vendors, Counter Sales, and Other Paid Distribution Outside USPS®	408	380
	(4)	Paid Distribution by Other Classes Mailed Through the USPS (e.g. First-Class Mail®)		
c. Total Paid Distribution (Sum of 15b (1), (2), (3), and (4))		▶	993	903
d. Free or Nominal Rate Distribution (By Mail and Outside the Mail)	(1)	Free or Nominal Rate Outside-County Copies Included on PS Form 3541	83	85
	(2)	Free or Nominal Rate In-County Copies Included on PS Form 3541		
	(3)	Free or Nominal Rate Copies Mailed at Other Classes Through the USPS (e.g. First-Class Mail)		
	(4)	Free or Nominal Rate Distribution Outside the Mail (Carriers or other means)		
e. Total Free or Nominal Rate Distribution (Sum of 15d (1), (2), (3) and (4))		▶	83	85
f. Total Distribution (Sum of 15c and 15e)		▶	1,076	988
g. Copies not Distributed (See instructions to publishers #4 (page #3))		▶	318	210
h. Total (Sum of 15f and g)		▶	1,394	1,198
i. Percent Paid (15c divided by 15f times 100)			92.29%	91.40%

16. Publication of Statement of Ownership
☐ If the publication is a general publication, publication of this statement is required. Will be printed in the November 2013 issue of this publication.
☐ Publication not required

17. Signature and Title of Editor, Publisher, Business Manager, or Owner
Stephen R. Bushing
Stephen R. Bushing – Fulfillment/Inventory Specialist
Date: September 14, 2013

I certify that all information furnished on this form is true and complete. I understand that anyone who furnishes false or misleading information on this form or who omits material or information requested on the form may be subject to criminal sanctions (including fines and imprisonment) and/or civil sanctions (including civil penalties).

PS Form 3526, September 2007 (Page 2 of 3)

Moving?

Make sure your subscription moves with you!

To notify us of your new address, find your **Clinics Account Number** (located on your mailing label above your name), and contact customer service at:

Email: journalscustomerservice-usa@elsevier.com

800-654-2452 (subscribers in the U.S. & Canada)
314-447-8871 (subscribers outside of the U.S. & Canada)

Fax number: 314-447-8029

Elsevier Health Sciences Division
Subscription Customer Service
3251 Riverport Lane
Maryland Heights, MO 63043

*To ensure uninterrupted delivery of your subscription, please notify us at least 4 weeks in advance of move.

ELSEVIER

Printed and bound by CPI Group (UK) Ltd, Croydon, CR0 4YY

03/10/2024

01040309-0004